WIC Nutrition Risk Criteria: A Scientific Assessment

Committee on Scientific Evaluation of
WIC Nutrition Risk Criteria

Food and Nutrition Board

INSTITUTE OF MEDICINE

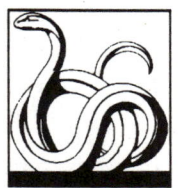

NATIONAL ACADEMY PRESS
Washington, D.C. 1996

NATIONAL ACADEMY PRESS • 2101 Constitution Avenue, N.W. • Washington, DC 20418

NOTICE: The project that is the subject of this report was approved by the Governing Board of the National Research Council, whose members are drawn from the councils of the National Academy of Sciences, the National Academy of Engineering, and the Institute of Medicine. The members of the committee responsible for the report were chosen for their special competences and with regard for appropriate balance.

This report has been reviewed by a group other than the authors according to procedures approved by a Report Review Committee consisting of members of the National Academy of Sciences, the National Academy of Engineering, and the Institute of Medicine.

The Institute of Medicine was chartered in 1970 by the National Academy of Sciences to enlist distinguished members of the appropriate professions in the examination of policy matters pertaining to the health of the public. In this, the Institute acts under both the Academy's 1863 congressional charter responsibility to be an adviser to the federal government and its own initiative in identifying issues of medical care, research, and education. Dr. Kenneth I. Shine is president of the Institute of Medicine.

This study was supported under contract no. 59-3198-3-044 from the Food and Nutrition Service, U.S. Department of Agriculture.

Library of Congress Catalog Card No. 95-72317
International Standard Book Number 0-309-05385-4

Additional copies of this report are available from:

National Academy Press
2101 Constitution Avenue, N.W.
Box 285
Washington, DC 20055

Call 800-624-6242 or 202-334-3313 (in the Washington, D.C. metropolitan area) or visit the online bookstore at *http://www.nas.edu/nap/online/*.

Copyright 1996 by the National Academy of Sciences. All rights reserved.

Printed in the United States of America

The serpent has been a symbol of long life, healing, and knowledge among almost all cultures and religions since the beginning of recorded history. The image adopted as a logotype by the Institute of Medicine is based on a relief carving from ancient Greece, now held by the Staatlichemuseen in Berlin.

COMMITTEE ON SCIENTIFIC EVALUATION OF WIC NUTRITION RISK CRITERIA

RICHARD E. BEHRMAN (*Chair*),* Center for the Future of Children, David and Lucile Packard Foundation, Los Altos, California
BARBARA ABRAMS, School of Public Health, University of California, Berkeley
A. SUE BROWN (through February 1995), Commission on Health Care Finance, Government of the District of Columbia, Washington, D.C.
MARY ELLEN COLLINS, Brigham and Women's Hospital, Boston, Massachusetts
CATHERINE COWELL, School of Public Health, Columbia University, New York, New York
BARBARA DEVANEY, Mathematica Policy Research, Inc., Plainsboro, New Jersey
LEON GORDIS,* School of Hygiene and Public Health, The Johns Hopkins University, Baltimore, Maryland
JEAN-PIERRE HABICHT, Division of Nutritional Sciences, Cornell University, Ithaca, New York
K. MICHAEL HAMBIDGE, Center for Human Nutrition, University of Colorado Health Sciences Center, Denver
GAIL G. HARRISON, School of Public Health, University of California, Los Angeles
JEAN YAVIS JONES, Congressional Research Service, Library of Congress, Washington, D.C.
ROY M. PITKIN,* School of Medicine, University of California, Los Angeles
ERNESTO POLLITT, Department of Pediatrics, University of California, Davis
KATHLEEN M. RASMUSSEN, Division of Nutritional Sciences, Cornell University, Ithaca, New York
EARNESTINE WILLIS, MACC Fund Research Center and Department of Pediatrics, Medical College of Wisconsin, Milwaukee

Staff
ROBERT EARL, Study Director (through November 1995)
CAROL WEST SUITOR, Study Director (beginning November 1995)
SANDRA A. SCHLICKER, Senior Program Officer (beginning November 1995)
SHEILA A. MOATS, Research Associate
KIMBERLY M. BREWER, Research Assistant (beginning September 1995)
GERALDINE KENNEDO, Project Assistant

---

* Member, Institute of Medicine

FOOD AND NUTRITION BOARD

CUTBERTO GARZA (*Chair*), Division of Nutritional Sciences, Cornell University, Ithaca, New York
JOHN W. ERDMAN, JR. (*Vice Chair*), Division of Nutritional Sciences, College of Agriculture, University of Illinois, Urbana
PERRY L. ADKISSON,[†] Department of Entomology, Texas A&M University, College Station
LINDSAY H. ALLEN, Department of Nutrition, University of California, Davis
DENNIS M. BIER, USDA Children's Nutrition Research Center, Baylor College of Medicine, Houston, Texas
FERGUS M. CLYDESDALE, Department of Food Science and Nutrition, University of Massachusetts, Amherst
MICHAEL P. DOYLE, Center for Food Safety and Quality Enhancement, University of Georgia, Griffin
JOHANNA T. DWYER, Frances Stern Nutrition Center, New England Medical Center, Boston, Massachusetts
SCOTT M. GRUNDY, Center for Human Nutrition, University of Texas Southwestern Medical Center, Dallas
K. MICHAEL HAMBIDGE, Center for Human Nutrition, University of Colorado Health Sciences Center, Denver
JANET C. KING,[*] USDA Western Human Nutrition Research Center, Presidio of San Francisco, California
SANFORD A. MILLER, Graduate Studies and Biological Sciences, University of Texas Health Science Center, San Antonio
ALFRED SOMMER,[*] School of Hygiene and Public Health, Johns Hopkins University, Baltimore, Maryland
STEVE L. TAYLOR (*Ex officio*), Food Processing Center, University of Nebraska, Lincoln
VERNON R. YOUNG,[†] Laboratory of Human Nutrition, School of Science, Massachusetts Institute of Technology, Cambridge

---

[*] Member, Institute of Medicine
[†] Member, National Academy of Sciences

Staff
ALLISON A. YATES, Director (beginning July 1994)
CATHERINE E. WOTEKI, Director (through December 1993)
BERNADETTE M. MARRIOTT, Associate Director and Interim Director (through June 30, 1994)
GAIL SPEARS, Administrative Assistant (beginning September 1994)
MARCIA S. LEWIS, Administrative Assistant (through August 1994)
JAMAINE L. TINKER, Financial Associate

Acknowledgments

This report represents the collaborative efforts of many individuals, particularly the study committee and staff whose names appear at the beginning of this document. Completion of this study was a complex task and it required substantial dedication and effort by all those who participated in its completion.

The committee wishes to acknowledge the assistance of the National Association of WIC Directors (NAWD) for furnishing volumes of information about nutrition risk criteria in use in state WIC programs. NAWD's president during the majority of the study, Alice Lenihan, was particularly helpful and supportive. The committee wants to express their appreciation of the input received from the entire WIC community, too numerous to mention by name, through public meetings, site visits, additional information about nutrition risk criteria, and informal communications.

Drs. Robert Kuczmarski and Anne Looker of the National Center for Health Statistics (NCHS), Centers for Disease Control and Prevention, U.S. Department of Health and Human Services, made presentations to the committee on upcoming data from the third National Health and Nutrition Examination Survey and revision of NCHS infant and child growth charts. Dr. Tiefu Shen of the Division of Nutritional Sciences, Cornell University, and Cyn O'Malley and Suzan Carmichael of the School of Public Health, University of California, Berkeley, provided substantial assistance with the development of the chapter on anthropometric risk criteria.

This report was sponsored by the Food and Consumer Service, U.S. Department of Agriculture (USDA). Without their vision for the need to undertake this scientific assessment, this report would not have become a reality. The committee acknowledges their commitment to the WIC program and their support of this project, particularly the support of project officers Jay Hirschman and Dr. Janet Tognetti Schiller. In addition, the committee recognizes other major informational contributions of several USDA staff: Donna Hines, Julie Kresge, Michele Lawler, Elaine Lynn, and Debra Whitford.

The committee also wishes to express its appreciation to the staff of the Food and Nutrition Board of the Institute of Medicine, whose tireless efforts on our behalf were so critical to the committee's deliberations and the production of this report. Our appreciation goes to Robert Earl, who provided administrative support to the committee. The committee is especially grateful for the substantial efforts of Dr. Carol Suitor, who, with the assistance of Dr. Sandra Schlicker and Kim Brewer, worked closely with committee members to complete the analysis and finalize the report. The efforts of Sheila Moats, Geraldine Kennedo, Susan Knasiak, and Dr. Allison Yates on behalf of the committee are also deserving of our heartfelt thanks.

RICHARD E. BEHRMAN, *Chair*
Committee on Scientific Evaluation of
WIC Nutrition Risk Criteria

Contents

SUMMARY 1
  Committee Process and Structure of the Report, 3
  Principles of Nutrition Risk Assessment, 5
  General Conclusions, 7
  Recommendations for Specific Nutrition Risk Criteria, 9
  Recommendations for Future Research and Action, 20

1 OVERVIEW 23
  Charge to the Committee, 24
  The WIC Program, 25
  Overview of the Report and the Committee Process, 34
  References, 38

2 POVERTY AND NUTRITION RISK 41
  Definition of Poverty, 41
  Prevalence of Poverty, 43
  Poverty and Nutrition Risk for Women, 43
  Poverty and Nutrition Risk for Infants and Children, 45
  Effects of WIC Program Participation, 47
  References, 49

3 PRINCIPLES UNDERLYING THE NUTRITION RISK CRITERIA FOR WIC ELIGIBILITY 53
  Principles of Nutrition Risk Assessment, 53

WIC Nutrition Risk Criteria, 60
Priority System of the WIC Program, 60
Summary and Implications, 63
References, 65

4 ANTHROPOMETRIC RISK CRITERIA 67
Use of Anthropometric Measures in the WIC Program, 67
Maternal Anthropometric Risk Criteria, 70
- Prepregnancy Underweight, 70
- Low Maternal Weight Gain, 73
- Maternal Weight Loss During Pregnancy, 79
- Prepregnancy Overweight, 80
- High Gestational Weight Gain, 84
- Maternal Short Stature, 87
- Postpartum Underweight, 89
- Postpartum Overweight, 92
- Abnormal Postpartum Weight Change, 96

Anthropometric Risk Criteria for Infants and Children, 97
- Low Birth Weight, 97
- Small for Gestational Age, 100
- Short Stature, 104
- Underweight, 110
- Low Head Circumference, 114
- Large for Gestational Age, 117
- Overweight, 118
- Slow Growth, 123

Summary and Conclusions, 125
References, 128

5 BIOCHEMICAL AND OTHER MEDICAL RISK CRITERIA 149
Criteria Related to Nutrient Deficiencies, 154
- Anemia, 154
- Failure to Thrive and Other Nutrient Deficiency Diseases, 159

Medical Conditions Applicable to the Entire WIC Population, 166
- Gastrointestinal Disorders, 166
- Diabetes Mellitus, 169
- Thyroid Disorders, 170
- Chronic Hypertension, 172
- Renal Disease, 174
- Cancer, 175
- Central Nervous System Disorders, 177
- Genetic and Congenital Disorders, 179

Inborn Errors of Metabolism, 181
Chronic or Recurrent Infections, 183
HIV Infection and AIDS, 185
Recent Major Surgery, Trauma, Burns, or Severe Acute Infections, 188
Other Medical Conditions, 190
Conditions Related to the Intake of Specific Foods, 192
Food Allergies, 192
Food Intolerances, 194
Conditions Specific to Pregnancy, 195
Pregnancy at a Young Age, 195
Pregnancy Age Older Than 35 Years, 197
Closely Spaced Pregnancies, 197
High Parity, 200
History of Preterm Delivery, 204
History of Postterm Delivery, 206
History of Low Birth Weight, 206
History of Neonatal Loss, 207
History of Previous Birth of an Infant with a Congenital or Birth Defect, 207
Lack of Prenatal Care, 208
Multifetal Gestation, 210
Fetal Growth Restriction, 211
Preeclampsia and Eclampsia, 213
Placental Abnormalities, 214
Conditions Specific to Infants and/or Children, 215
Prematurity, 215
Hypoglycemia, 217
Potentially Toxic Substances, 218
Long-Term Drug-Nutrient Interactions or Misuse of Medications, 218
Maternal Smoking, 220
Alcohol and Illegal Drug Use, 226
Lead Poisoning, 229
Summary, 232
References, 233

6 DIETARY RISK CRITERIA 251

Inappropriate Dietary Patterns, 253
Dietary Patterns That Fail to Meet Dietary Guidelines for Americans, 253
Vegetarian Diets, 259
Highly Restrictive Diets, 260

Inappropriate Infant Feeding, 261
Inappropriate Use of Nursing Bottle, 265
Inappropriate Diets in Children, 268
Excessive Caffeine Intake, 269
Pica, 270
Inadequate Diet, 272
Food Insecurity, 279
Definition of Food Insecurity, 279
Summary, 283
References, 283

7 **PREDISPOSING NUTRITION RISK CRITERIA**   295
Homelessness, 297
Migrancy, 304
Passive Smoking, 309
Low Level of Maternal Education and Illiteracy, 311
Maternal Depression, 314
Battering, 317
Child Abuse or Neglect, 319
Child of a Young Caregiver, 321
Child of a Mentally Retarded Parent, 323
Summary, 325
References, 325

8 **CONCLUSIONS AND RECOMMENDATIONS**   335
General Conclusions, 336
Recommendations for Specific Nutrition Risk Criteria, 337
Recommendations for Future Research and Action, 350

APPENDIXES

A	Participants at the First Public Meeting, May 19, 1994	353
B	Participants at the Second Public Meeting, September 19–20, 1994	355
C	WIC Program: Common Nutritional Risk Criteria	357
D	Definitions of Yield and Sensitivity of Cutoff Points for Nutrition Risk	359
E	Biographical Sketches	361

ACRONYMS   371

INDEX OF RISK CRITERIA   373

List of Tables and Figures

TABLES

S-1 Nutrition Risk Criteria and Committee Recommendations for the Specific WIC Population, by Category of Nutrition Risk, 10
1-1 WIC Program Participation by Subgroup and Federal Costs, 1974–1993, 35
3-1 Nutrition Risk Criteria Defined by WIC Program Regulations, 61
3-2 The WIC Priority System, 62
4-1 Summary of Anthropometric Risk Criteria in the WIC Program and Use by States, 68
4-2 Summary of Anthropometric Risk Criteria as Predictive of Risk or Benefit Among Pregnant and Postpartum Women, 70
4-3 Summary of Anthropometric Risk Criteria as Predictive of Risk or Benefit Among Infants and Children, 98
4-4 Summary of Anthropometric Risk Criteria and Committee Recommendations for the Specific WIC Population, 126
5-1 Summary of Biochemical and Other Medical Risk Criteria in the WIC Program and Use by States, 150
5-2 Summary of Broad Categories of Biochemical and Other Medical Risk Criteria as Predictive of Risk or Benefit Among Women, Infants, and Children, 153
5-3 Cutoff Points for Anemia Used in the WIC Program and Recommended Cutoff Points from the Centers for Disease Control and Prevention and the Institute of Medicine for Women, Infants, and Children, 158
5-4 Summary of Medical Risk Criteria and Committee Recommendations for the Specific WIC Population, 160

6-1 Summary of Broad Dietary Risk Criteria in the WIC Program and Use by States, 252
6-2 Summary of Broad Dietary Risk Criteria as Predictive of Risk or Benefit Among Women, Infants, and Children, 253
6-3 Summary of Broad Dietary Risk Criteria and Committee Recommendations for the Specific WIC Population, 266
7-1 Summary of Predisposing Risk Criteria in the WIC Program and Use by States, 296
7-2 Summary of Predisposing Risk Criteria as Predictive of Risk or Benefit Among Women, Infants, and Children, 297
7-3 Summary of Dietary Risk Criteria and Committee Recommendations for the Specific WIC Population, 298
8-1 Nutrition of Risk Criteria and Committee Recommendations for the Specific WIC Population, by Category of Nutrition Risk, 338
8-2 Committee Recommendations for Changes in Risk Criteria, 347

FIGURES

S-1 WIC program components, services, benefits, and projected outcomes, 2
1-1 WIC program components, services, benefits, and projected outcomes, 26

Summary

The Special Supplemental Nutrition Program for Women, Infants, and Children (WIC) provides specific supplemental foods, nutrition education, and social service and health care referrals to low-income pregnant, breastfeeding, and postpartum women, infants, and children up to age 5 years who are at nutrition risk. The WIC program is based on the premise that many low-income individuals are at risk of poor nutrition and health outcomes because of insufficient nutrition during the critical growth and development periods of pregnancy, infancy, and early childhood. The WIC program is a *supplemental* food and nutrition program to help meet the special needs of low-income women, infants, and children during these periods. Income below 185 percent of the poverty level is one of the standards of eligibility for the WIC program. A summary of WIC program components, services, and anticipated outcomes is provided in Figure S-1.

All WIC program participants must be determined to be at nutrition risk on the basis of a medical or nutrition assessment by a physician, nutritionist, dietitian, nurse, or some other competent professional authority. Using nutrition risk as a requirement for certification is a unique feature of the WIC program. Public Law 94-105 broadly defines nutrition risk as "(a) detrimental or abnormal nutritional conditions detectable by biochemical or anthropometric measures, (b) other documented nutritionally related medical conditions, (c) dietary deficiencies that impair or endanger health, or (d) conditions that predispose persons to inadequate nutritional patterns or nutritionally related medical conditions."

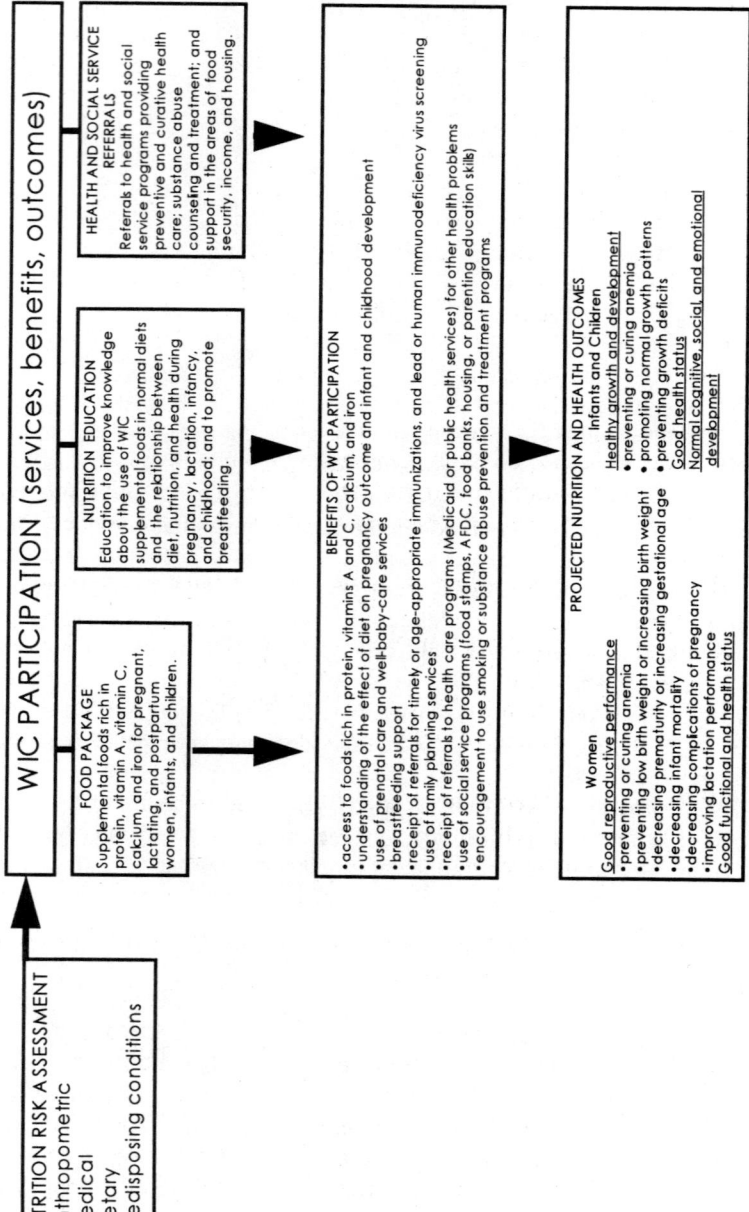

FIGURE S-1 WIC program components, services, benefits, and projected outcomes.

Nutrition risk criteria also provide the basis for a seven-level priority system for eligible women, infants, and children. If a local WIC agency reaches its maximum caseload given its level of funding, the WIC priority system is used to maintain a waiting list of eligible applicants. As program openings become available, they can be filled from the waiting list. In general, priority is given to anthropometric, hematologic, and clinical evidence of medically based nutrition risks over dietary-based nutrition risks; to pregnant and breastfeeding women and infants over children; and to children over postpartum women.

In the summer of 1993, the Food and Nutrition Service of the U.S. Department of Agriculture (now the Food and Consumer Service [FCS]) requested that the Food and Nutrition Board (FNB) of the Institute of Medicine conduct a comprehensive review of the scientific basis for the nutrition risk criteria used in the WIC program. In October 1993, the FNB established the Committee on the Scientific Evaluation of WIC Nutrition Risk Criteria. The committee was charged with conducting a study that included the following tasks:

- Performing a critical review of the literature surrounding the various nutrition risk criteria used by the WIC program.
- Developing scientific consensus (where possible) regarding the nutrition risk criteria used by the WIC program, taking into account the preventive nature of the program.
- Identifying specific segments of the WIC population at risk for each criterion.
- Identifying gaps in the scientific knowledge base for the current nutrition risk criteria used by the WIC program.
- Formulating recommendations regarding appropriate criteria and, if applicable, recommendations of numerical values for determining who is at risk for each criterion.
- Identifying critical areas for future research.
- Identifying the practicality of consensus recommendations for nutrition risk criteria for the variety of WIC program delivery settings.

COMMITTEE PROCESS AND STRUCTURE OF THE REPORT

Over the course of the study, the committee met five times, conducted two public meetings, participated in many conference calls, and made site visits to local WIC program clinics. The committee began its deliberations by reviewing the WIC program. Since the federal WIC program does not have a uniform set of nutrition risk criteria (where a risk criterion is defined as a risk indicator and its cutoff point), the committee obtained a list of nutrition risk criteria used by WIC state agencies in 1992. It categorized these into (1) anthropometric, (2) biochemical and other medical, (3) dietary, and (4) predisposing risks to reflect the definition of nutrition risk in federal WIC program regulations. Using terms based on this list, the committee conducted bibliographic searches of the scientific literature and compiled and critically reviewed research findings. In reviewing each risk criterion, the committee examined three issues: (1) Is there scientific evidence that the criterion serves as an indicator of nutrition and health risk? (2) Does the criterion serve as an indicator of nutrition and health benefit from participation in the WIC program? (3) What cutoff value, if any, is scientifically justified? The relationship between poverty and nutrition risk is also discussed in the report because it is a separate standard for WIC program eligibility. Poverty is not a WIC nutrition risk criterion and was not reviewed as one.

The two public meetings gathered information from WIC program administrators, staff, and participants as well as from researchers in the fields related to the risk criteria under study. The public meetings and the visits to WIC clinics provided valuable information about the use of nutrition risk criteria in the WIC setting.

Chapter 1 of the committee's report on its study describes the structure and function of the WIC program and provides an overview of the committee's task. Chapter 2 reviews linkages between low income and risk of inadequate nutrition. Chapter 3 discusses the principles of nutrition risk assessment that guided the committee in conducting its review and provides the framework used to develop the committee's recommendations. Chapters 4 through 7 cover the nutrition risk criteria used by the WIC program: anthropometric, biochemical and medical, dietary, and predisposing risks. Chapter 8 provides conclusions and recommendations regarding nutrition risk criteria and recommendations for research and action.

The concept of nutrition risk assessment is integral to the design and operation of the WIC program. Nutrition risk is a criterion for program eligibility, and nutrition risk criteria are used to assign a priority level to women, infants, and children. By serving those at the highest priority levels first, the WIC priority system is used to allocate limited program resources among eligible individuals. In addition, the nutrition risk assessments are used to tailor the WIC intervention and, in some cases, to monitor the health and nutrition status of program participants.

This report is a scientific assessment of the WIC nutrition risk criteria as they are currently used to establish WIC eligibility and the priority of the WIC eligible individuals. This scientific assessment is the basis for the final chapter's general conclusions, recommendations for specific nutrition risk criteria, and recommendations for future research and action.

The framework that was used in the scientific assessment conducted for this report has two key features. The first is the exposition and utilization of the concept of potential to benefit from the delivery of interventions and services provided by the WIC program. The second is the explicit consideration of the concepts of yield of risk, yield of benefit, and sensitivity of the nutrition risk criteria used by the WIC program, which are described below.

PRINCIPLES OF NUTRITION RISK ASSESSMENT

A nutrition risk assessment is used to determine eligibility for participation in the WIC program. Nutrition risk assessment uses a risk criterion; a risk criterion is defined by a risk indicator and a cutoff point. A risk indicator is any measurable characteristic or circumstance that is associated with an increased likelihood of poor outcomes, such as poor nutrition status, poor health, or death. In some cases (e.g., low hemoglobin level), a risk indicator could also be considered to be an outcome. The cutoff point may be the presence or absence of the condition (e.g., a diagnosis of diabetes mellitus) or a value chosen from many possibilities for a specified population (e.g., a hemoglobin value of 11.0 gm/dl for women in their first trimester of pregnancy).

The committee agreed that nutrition risk criteria used in the WIC program should serve both as indicators of nutrition and health risk and as indicators of nutrition and health benefit. *Indicators of nutrition and health risk* should select those who have the greatest need for the services provided by the WIC program because they are either more unhealthy or poorly nourished at the time of assessment or are at future risk of ill health, overnutrition, or undernutrition. *Indicators of nutrition and health benefit* are those that improve the efficacy of participation in the WIC program by selecting those potential participants most likely to benefit from participation over those less likely to benefit from participation.

Once a risk indicator is chosen as a predictor of benefit, a cutoff point for the indicator is set as the level below or above which individuals are eligible for participation in the WIC program. Four important concepts in selecting cutoffs for the nutrition risk indicators used by the WIC program are yield of benefit, yield of risk, sensitivity, and efficacy of WIC interventions:

1. *Yield of benefit*: the percentage of those truly at risk who will actually experience nutrition and health benefit among all those, with or without the risk, who are selected by a nutrition risk indicator and its cutoff point. Individuals are considered truly at risk if they would have a bad outcome without an intervention.

2. *Yield of risk*: the percentage of those truly at risk who are identified at risk.

3. *Sensitivity*: the percentage identified of all those who could benefit from the WIC program.

4. *Efficacy of WIC interventions*: the percentage of individuals selected for the WIC program whose bad outcomes will be prevented or reduced.

Yield of benefit can be high only if the yield of risk is high and the WIC program can prevent or reduce bad outcomes for those at risk. A perfect yield of risk occurs at the cutoff point at which all those selected for participation in the WIC program are truly at risk. A perfect yield of risk, however, implies that many who could benefit are not selected. Identification of all who could benefit is called perfect sensitivity. In general, there is a trade-off between yield of risk and sensitivity, and it is usually impossible to achieve both maximum yield of risk (serving only those truly at risk) and perfect sensitivity (identification of all those at true risk). Overall yield of benefit is affected both by the yield of risk and the efficacy of the interventions, since it is the product of the yield of risk and the efficacy.

These concepts of yield of risk, yield of benefit, and sensitivity, in conjunction with the concepts of indicators of risk and indicators of benefit, have implications that underlie both the assessments of the nutrition risk criteria used by the WIC program and the development of the report's conclusions and recommendations. Ideally, risk indicators and cutoff points should be chosen such that the highest proportion of those who are truly at risk can be identified and the highest proportion of those identified can benefit from WIC program participation. With limited program resources, cutoff points should be set with less than perfect sensitivity to increase yield, recognizing that as cutoff points become more restrictive, some individuals who could benefit from WIC services will not be served.

The following decision process underlies the committee's recommendations. This process could be used to review other risk criteria that the WIC program may be asked to approve in the future.

• For nutrition risk criteria for which there is good evidence of both nutrition and health risk and benefit from the WIC program, the committee recommends use of these criteria by all state WIC programs.

• For nutrition risk criteria for which the risk indicator is a predictor of both nutrition and health risk and benefit from the WIC program but for which cutoffs have been set so that many individuals selected are not truly at risk, the committee recommends using the risk indicator with more stringent cutoff values.

• For risk criteria for which there is strong evidence of nutrition and health risk but uncertain evidence of benefit, the committee recommends using the nutrition risk criteria and conducting further research on the benefit from the WIC program.

• For risk criteria for which there is good evidence of nutrition and health risk and benefit from the WIC program, but poor ability to identify those at risk with current methods, the committee recommends that action be taken to develop better assessment tools. Pending this result, the committee recommends

using the best available methods to identify the risk, using scientifically justifiable cutoff values.
- For risk criteria for which there is strong evidence of nutrition and health risk but no direct or indirect evidence of benefit, either theoretical or empirical, the committee recommends discontinuing use of these risk criteria.
- For risk criteria with weak evidence of risk or benefit, the committee recommends discontinuing use of these criteria.

The WIC program is a broad-based and comprehensive food and nutrition program with three main components: (1) supplemental foods, (2) nutrition education, and (3) referrals to health care and social service providers. Thus, evidence of benefit from the WIC program, either theoretical or empirical, could be from any of the three program components. In making its recommendations for each nutrition risk criterion, however, the committee decided that evidence of benefit from the WIC program should reflect the ability of an individual with that risk to benefit (avert bad outcomes) from the WIC food package or, in some cases, from nutrition education.

Benefit from only the referral services of the WIC program was not considered sufficient to justify the use of a nutrition risk criterion. Three main reasons for this decision follow: (1) the provision of supplemental foods and nutrition education account for nearly all the WIC program costs; (2) it is difficult to justify the provision of a monthly food package worth approximately $30 per WIC participant unless there is evidence that the individual can benefit from the food package or the nutrition education that accompanies the provision of food; and (3) the WIC program is designed to be only an adjunct to good health care and is not itself a comprehensive health program. Nonetheless, the committee respects the comprehensive nature of the program.

GENERAL CONCLUSIONS

The committee reached seven general conclusions about the WIC nutrition risk criteria and priority system:

- *A body of scientific evidence supports a majority of the nutrition risk criteria used by the WIC program.* For some of the risk criteria, however, there are serious gaps in the evidence.
- *Nutrition risk criteria used by many states have a high sensitivity and low yield of benefit.* This is because the prevalence of many of the risk conditions is low and the cutoffs used are generous, resulting in both the selection of many of those who have the risk condition (high sensitivity) and the selection of many individuals who do not have the risk condition (low yield of risk, which results in low yield of benefit).

- *Use of generous cutoff points or loosely defined conditions in categories designated by federal regulation to receive high priority for eligibility may result in denial of services to individuals who are actually at higher nutrition risk.* When resources are limited, individuals in lower priority categories may not be served even if their true risk is very high, while those in high priority categories must be served. Very generous cutoff points produce a low yield of benefit without any increase in sensitivity (serving more of those truly at risk). Loosely defined risk conditions are those that encompass a broad range of medical problems with varying degrees of nutrition risk or potential to benefit from WIC participation. Such loosely defined nutrition risk criteria include endocrine disorders, renal disease, chronic and recurrent infections, food allergies, and genetic and congenital disorders.
- *There is some inconsistency between the WIC program's goals, design, and implementation.* The goal of the WIC program is one of primary prevention—to prevent the occurrence of health problems. Through the use of nutrition risk criteria, the WIC priority system is designed in principle to be a secondary/tertiary prevention program to reduce or cure identified risk. However, through the use of generous cutoff points, loosely defined risk conditions, and a priority system that places pregnant women and infants at the highest priorities, in general, the WIC program operates as a primary prevention program for pregnant women and infants and a secondary and tertiary prevention program for children and postpartum women.
- *The WIC priority system should be reexamined.* Many individuals now classified in low priority categories have more potential to benefit from WIC services than some individuals placed in higher priority categories. For example, a child of a mentally retarded parent (currently priority VII) or an anemic child age 3 years with a very low hemoglobin (currently priority III) may have a greater potential to benefit than an infant classified as anemic (currently priority I) by a criterion with a too generous cutoff point.
- *It is important that the WIC program reevaluate the criteria in use every 5 to 10 years and change cutoffs and incorporate new criteria as necessary.* This is because the yield of risk of a criterion increases as the prevalence of the risk in the population increases, and it decreases as the prevalence of the risk in the population decreases. For example, the yield of risk of the nutrition risk criterion for poor growth has decreased over time as the prevalences of wasting and stunting have declined. The addition of homelessness as a nutrition risk criterion by the WIC program reflects, in part, increases in the prevalence of homelessness.
- *There is a need to identify or develop additional nutrition risk criteria that select those individuals who are at risk of developing specific health and nutrition problems if they do not receive WIC benefits.* Since the WIC program is believed to be a major contributor to the decline in the prevalence of health and nutrition problems (for example, iron deficiency anemia), it is important to

identify practical indicators of the risk of developing the problem so that the WIC program can maintain its preventive function. Dietary risk criteria or predisposing risk criteria may do this, but data are limited. Setting high cutoff points for anemia or poor growth does not effectively identify those at risk of developing the problem.

In addition, the committee emphasizes the importance of the systematic collection of data about the prevalence of individuals meeting specific WIC nutrition risk criteria.

RECOMMENDATIONS FOR SPECIFIC NUTRITION RISK CRITERIA

Table S-1 summarizes the committee's recommendations for use of nutrition risk criteria, cutoff values, and the segments of the population to which they apply. For greater specificity, the name of the criterion used occasionally differs from that used by the WIC program. The recommendations are intended to apply to all states. Exceptions may be made if the meaning of the criterion in a particular context is different or the condition (e.g., pica) is common in one state and uncommon in another. Brief supplementary information about these recommendations follows for each of the categories of nutrition risk criteria. The full report provides the basis for each recommendation.

Anthropometric Risk Criteria

Anthropometric risk criteria are used in the WIC program to assess individuals for nutrition risk and to monitor their nutrition status or their response to WIC program interventions over time. The committee's review indicated that most of the WIC anthropometric risk indicators are predictors both of nutrition and health risks and of benefit from participation in the WIC program. The cutoff points used for anthropometric risk indicators among WIC programs vary substantially, however, with resulting effects on yield. Therefore, the committee recommends that cutoff points for anthropometric measures be limited to those that are scientifically justified. It further points out that there is no obvious justification for the use of symmetric cutoff points (for example, at the 5th and 95th percentiles).

Risk criteria for which there was very little evidence of nutrition risk or benefit from WIC participation include maternal short stature, abnormal postpartum weight change, and infants large for gestational age. Therefore, the committee recommends discontinuing use of these nutrition risk criteria.

TABLE S-1 Nutrition Risk Criteria and Committee Recommendations for the Specific WIC Population, by Category of Nutrition Risk

Risk Criterion	Committee Recommendation	Pregnant Women	Postpartum Women Lactating	Postpartum Women Nonlactating	Infants	Children
Anthropometric Risk Criteria						
Women						
Prepregnancy underweight	Use with cutoff value of IBW <90% or BMI <19.8	✓				
Low maternal weight gain	Use with cutoff value of <0.9 kg/mo for nonobese and <0.45 kg/mo for obese	✓				
Maternal weight loss during pregnancy	Use with cutoff value of >2 kg first trimester, >1 kg 2nd or 3rd trimesters	✓				
Prepregnancy overweight	Use with cutoff value of IBW >120% or BMI >26	✓	✓	✓		
High gestational weight gain	Use with cutoff value of >3 kg/mo	✓	✓	✓		
Maternal short stature	Do not use					
Postpartum underweight	Use with cutoff value of IBW <90% or BMI <19		✓	✓		
Postpartum overweight	Use with cutoff value of IBW >120% or BMI >26 after 6 weeks postpartum		✓	✓		
Abnormal postpartum weight change	Do not use					

Infants and Children

Criterion	Specification		
Low birth weight	Use with cutoff value of <2,500 g	✓	✓
Small for gestational age	Use with cutoff value of <10th percentile	✓	✓
Short stature	Use with cutoff value of <5th percentile	✓	✓
Underweight	Use with cutoff of 5th percentile	✓	✓
Low head circumference	Use with cutoff value of <5th percentile	✓	✓
Large for gestational age	Do not use		
Overweight	Use with cutoff value of >95th percentile	✓	✓
Slow growth	Use with cutoff value of <3rd percentile	✓	✓

Biochemical and Other Medical Risk Criteria

Criteria Related to Nutrient Deficiencies

Criterion	Specification			
Anemia	Use with CDC or IOM cutoffs	✓	✓	✓
Failure to thrive	Use[a]		✓	✓
Nutrient deficiency diseases	Use[a]		✓	✓

Medical Conditions Applicable to the Entire WIC Population[b]

Criterion	Specification			
Gastrointestinal disorders	Use	✓	✓	✓
Nausea and vomiting during pregnancy	Use only if serious and prolonged	✓	✓	✓
Diabetes mellitus	Use	✓	✓	✓
Gestational diabetes	Use	✓		

Continued

TABLE S-1 Continued

Risk Criterion	Committee Recommendation	Pregnant Women	Postpartum Women Lactating	Postpartum Women Nonlactating	Infants	Children
Biochemical and Other Medical Risk Criteria (Continued)						
Medical Conditions Applicable to the Entire WIC Population[b] (Continued)						
Thyroid disorders	Use	✓	✓	✓	✓	✓
Chronic hypertension	Use	✓	✓	✓	✓	✓
Renal disease	Use, but not for chronic urinary tract infections	✓	✓	✓	✓	✓
Cancer	Use	✓	✓	✓	✓	✓
Central nervous system disorders	Use	✓	✓	✓	✓	✓
Genetic and congenital disorders	Use	✓	✓	✓	✓	✓
Pyloric stenosis	Do not use					
Inborn errors of metabolism	Use[a]	✓	✓	✓	✓	✓
Chronic or recurrent infections	Use, with exceptions	✓	✓	✓	✓	✓
Upper respiratory infections	Do not use					
Bronchitis	Do not use					
Otitis media	Do not use					
Urinary tract infections	Do not use					
HIV infections and AIDS	Use	✓	✓	✓	✓	✓
Recent major surgery, trauma, burns, or severe acute infections	Use	✓	✓	✓	✓	✓

Other medical conditions (juvenile rheumatoid arthritis, lupus erythematosus, and cardiorespiratory disorders)	Use		✓	✓	✓	

Conditions Related to the Intake of Specific Foods

Food allergies	Use	✓	✓	✓	✓	
Celiac disease	Use	✓	✓	✓	✓	
Lactose intolerance	Use	✓	✓			
Other food intolerance	Do not use					
Asthma	Do not use					

Conditions Specific to Pregnancy

Pregnancy at a young age	Use with cutoff value of 2 years postmenarche	✓	✓			
Pregnancy age older than 35 years	Do not use					
Closely spaced pregnancies	Use with an interconceptional interval of 6 months (9 months if concurrently lactating)	✓				
High parity	Do not use					
History of preterm delivery	Use	✓				
History of postterm delivery	Do not use					
History of low birth weight	Use	✓				
History of neonatal loss	Do not use					
History of birth with congenital or birth defect	Use	✓				

Continued

13

TABLE S-1 Continued

Risk Criterion	Committee Recommendation	Pregnant Women	Postpartum Women Lactating	Postpartum Women Nonlactating	Infants	Children
Biochemical and Other Medical Risk Criteria (Continued)						
Conditions Specific to Pregnancy (Continued)						
Lack of prenatal care	Use with cutoff value of care beginning after 1st trimester or long intervals between visits[c]	✓				
Multifetal gestation	Use	✓				
Fetal growth restriction	Use	✓		✓		
Preeclampsia and eclampsia	Do not use					
Placental abnormalities	Do not use					
Conditions Specific to Infants and/or Children						
Prematurity	Use with cutoff value of ≤37 weeks' gestation; do not use for children				✓	✓
Hypoglycemia	Use				✓	✓
Potentially Toxic Substances						
Long-term drug-nutrient interactions	Use for selected drugs	✓	✓			
Maternal smoking	Use, with cutoff of any smoking[c,d]	✓	✓			
Alcohol and illegal drug use	Use with cutoff of any use[c,e]	✓	✓			
Lead poisoning	Use with cutoff value of >10 μg/dl	✓	✓	✓	✓	✓

Dietary Risk Criteria

Failure to meet Dietary Guidelines	Use; develop valid assessment tools		✓		✓
Vegan diets	Use		✓		✓
Other vegetarian diets	Do not use		✓		✓
Highly restrictive diets	Use		✓		
Inappropriate infant feeding	Use		✓✓		
Early introduction of solid foods	Use		✓		
Feeding cow milk during 1st 12 months	Use		✓		
No dependable source of iron after 4–6 months	Use		✓✓		
Improper dilution of formula	Use		✓		
Feeding other foods low in essential nutrients	Use		✓		
Lack of sanitation in preparation of nursing bottles	Use		✓		
Infrequent breastfeeding as sole source of nutrients	Use		✓		
Inappropriate use of nursing bottle	Use				
Excessive caffeine intake	Do not use	✓			
Pica	Use			✓	

Continued

TABLE S-1 Continued

Risk Criterion	Committee Recommendation	Pregnant Women	Postpartum Women Lactating	Postpartum Women Nonlactating	Infants	Children
Dietary Risk Criteria *(Continued)*						
Inadequate diet	Do not use; use diet recall or FFQ to tailor nutrition education; develop valid assessment tools					
Food insecurity	Use; develop valid assessment tools	✓	✓	✓	✓	✓
Predisposing Risk Criteria						
Homelessness	Use	✓	✓	✓	✓	✓
Migrancy	Use	✓	✓	✓	✓	✓
Passive smoking	Do not use					
Low level of maternal education or illiteracy	Use	✓	✓	✓	✓	✓
Maternal depression	Add	✓	✓	✓		
Battering	Use	✓	✓	✓		
Child abuse or neglect	Use				✓	✓
Child of a young caregiver	Use				✓	✓
Child of a mentally retarded parent	Use				✓	✓

NOTE: ✓ = subgroup to which the recommendation applies; IBW = ideal body weight; BMI = body mass index; CDC = Centers for Disease Control; IOM = Institute of Medicine; FFQ = food frequency questionnaire.

[a] This criterion merits higher priority among children. [b] Diagnosis of the condition is the cutoff point used.
[c] This criterion merits lower priority.
[d] Two committee members (Barbara Abrams and Barbara Devaney) preferred to (1) set a higher cutoff point that would more clearly identify women whose cigarette use places them at higher risk of poor outcomes and (2) maintain this criterion at high priority.
[e] Three committee members (Barbara Abrams, Barbara Devaney, and Roy Pitkin) preferred to (1) set a higher cutoff point that would more clearly identify women whose alcohol use places them at higher risk of poor outcomes and (2) maintain these criteria at high priority.

Biochemical and Other Medical Risk Criteria

In general, the biochemical and other medical risk criteria predict nutrition and health risk, with varying degrees of benefit. The most common concern of the committee was the lack of scientific justification for the generous cutoff points for biochemical and certain other medical risk criteria currently used by many state WIC agencies.

Of the biochemical and other medical risk criteria, anemia is used most frequently in the WIC program to establish the eligibility of women, infants, and children to participate in the program. Cutoff values for anemia vary substantially among state WIC agencies, with little or no scientific justification for variation from standard definitions. The committee recommends that anemia continue to be used as a risk criterion in the WIC program but discourages the use of high cutoff points because of the resulting low yield from increased iron intake. That is, the high cutoff values for anemia used by many state WIC programs result in the inclusion of many who do not have and are not at risk of anemia and, thus, are unlikely to benefit from provision of WIC supplemental food.

Many biochemical and other medical nutrition risks are documented as the result of diagnosis by a medical care provider of an existing condition that affects nutritional needs or may be improved by dietary management. These diagnosed conditions are reported to WIC program staff. The committee recommends that most of these nutrition risk criteria continue to be used in the WIC program, using cutoff points that generally are documentation or diagnosis of the disease or disorder.

Maternal cigarette, alcohol, and illegal drug use among pregnant and lactating women pose significant health risks but uncertain benefit from participation in the WIC program. On an interim basis, the committee recommends that these criteria be used in the WIC program, with a cutoff of "any use."[1]

Risk criteria for which there was risk and benefit only under specific conditions included long-term drug-nutrient interactions and chronic and recurrent infections. The committee feels that these criteria were too vague to be useful in their current form. It recommends that a listing of drugs for which there are clear drug-nutrient interactions or potential for misuse be developed. The use of other medications would not be associated with nutrition risk or benefit, and thus their use would not provide a basis for eligibility. For chronic and recurrent infections, evidence of risk and benefit was available only for

---

[1] Three committee members preferred to set higher cutoff points that would more clearly delineate women whose substance use places them at higher risk for poor outcomes. Barbara Abrams and Barbara Devaney preferred to set higher cutoff points for cigarette and alcohol use; Roy Pitkin preferred a higher cutoff point only for alcohol use.

certain chronic infections for which there were documented nutrition deficits, and the committee recommends that states should clearly define "chronic" or "recurrent" in determining cutoff points for these indicators.

Risk criteria for which there was very limited evidence of nutrition risk or benefit from participation in the WIC program included food intolerance other than lactose intolerance, high age at conception, previous placental abnormalities, history of postterm delivery, high parity, preeclampsia and eclampsia, and prematurity as a risk criterion for children ages 1 to 5 years. The committee recommends that these nutrition risk criteria no longer be used in the WIC program.

Dietary Risk Criteria

Three major categories of dietary risk criteria are reviewed: inappropriate dietary patterns, inadequate diets, and food insecurity. Risk criteria classified as inappropriate dietary patterns are listed in Table S-1. The committee found that there are clear health and nutrition risks associated with selected inappropriate dietary patterns and that the potential to benefit from participation in the WIC program is high. For women and for children at least 2 years of age, failure to meet Dietary Guidelines for Americans is a dietary risk criterion that receives increased attention in this report.

As long as the food provided by the supplemental food package is eaten, the WIC program is likely to improve the diets of those WIC participants with inadequate diets. In the WIC setting, however, diet recalls and food frequency questionnaires that compare estimated nutrient intake with Recommended Dietary Allowances have poor ability to ascertain who actually has inadequate diets. Thus, even though the WIC program is likely to improve dietary intake, the committee recommends discontinuing use of *inadequate diets* as a nutrition risk criterion because it has a very low yield. Nonetheless, diet recalls or food frequency questionnaires are useful in the WIC program for identifying foods commonly consumed and providing a starting point for nutrition education.

Food insecurity is defined as the lack of predictable, sustainable access in socially acceptable ways to enough food of adequate quality to sustain health. Although this risk criterion is just beginning to be used by state WIC agencies, and there is limited evidence to evaluate causal links to nutrition and health risk, the committee believes that there is a fundamental value to addressing the risk to health and nutrition related to a lack of access to food. The benefit of participation in the WIC program for those at risk of food insecurity is high. Therefore, the committee recommends use of food insecurity as a nutrition risk criterion in the WIC program. At present, however, there is insufficient scientific evidence on which to select a cutoff point that would identify those most likely to benefit from the WIC program.

Predisposing Nutrition Risk Criteria

Currently, predisposing nutrition risk criteria receive a low priority within the WIC program. The use of predisposing nutrition risk criteria warrants additional attention. If an individual has a predisposing risk but no other risk, he or she will be placed in a priority category that is usually unserved by the WIC program. This may limit the WIC program's ability to serve as a preventive program. Additional attention to the predisposing nutrition risk criteria is warranted because (1) they have a high yield for risk and a high, but as yet unknown, potential for benefit from WIC services and (2) the prevalence of some of these factors (e.g., homelessness) is increasing, thus increasing the overall yield of these criteria.

The committee supports the use of most of the predisposing risk criteria that have been used in the WIC program (see Table S-1).

The committee recommends that a diagnosis of depression be added as a predisposing risk criterion for women, and that diagnosed maternal depression be added as a predisposing risk criterion for infants and children. Because of the lack of evidence that nutrition will benefit those exposed to passive smoking, the committee recommends that this risk criterion no longer be used in the WIC program.

RECOMMENDATIONS FOR FUTURE RESEARCH AND ACTION

Research Recommendations

Regarding the nutrition risk criteria reviewed in the report, the committee recommends the following areas for future research:

- Develop anthropometric standards (including weight change velocity) for pregnant and lactating women, including adolescents. These standards should be suitable to assess the likelihood that these women would benefit from nutrition intervention and to achieve improved reproductive outcomes.
- Evaluate whether the use of a combination of criteria (e.g., an anthropometric risk criterion plus a dietary risk criterion) may be more effective than the use of a single risk criterion in predicting a benefit from participation in the WIC program.
- Evaluate whether overweight or obese mothers and their infants and children benefit from current WIC program interventions. The prevalence of overweight and obesity among low-income women, infants, and children is increasing over time, and the health and nutrition risks of obesity are well-documented.
- Evaluate the yields of benefit for the various cutoff points used for anthropometric risk criteria—recognizing that there is no obvious justification

for symmetric high and low cutoff points. It is possible that current cutoff points are so generous that the yield of benefit from WIC program interventions is low.

• Examine how the WIC program affects nutrition outcomes for individuals with selected medical risk factors.

• Determine the extent to which women who use cigarettes, alcohol, and/or illegal drugs benefit from the WIC program and the level of use of these substances that should be set as the cutoff point, if applicable.

• Invest in the development and validation of practical dietary assessment instruments that can be used across WIC programs for the identification of inappropriate dietary patterns, inadequate dietary intake, and food insecurity, recognizing that adaptations may be needed for culturally diverse populations.

• Examine the utility of predisposing factors (such as homelessness, migrancy, low level of maternal education, child abuse and neglect, and maternal depression) as predictors of benefit from WIC program services.

Action Recommendations

In addition to these research recommendations, the committee recommends the following actions be taken by the Food and Consumer Service, U.S. Department of Agriculture, to provide guidance to state WIC agencies in the development of nutrition risk criteria:

• Adopt scientifically justified cutoff values for anemia and for anthropometric criteria among women, infants, and children, realizing that they may be different across populations as prevalences change.

• Define *preterm* consistently as delivery before the end of the 37th postmenstrual week for both mothers and their infants.

• Adopt scientifically justified cutoff points for *young maternal age* (chronological or gynecological, or both), because increased risks associated with births to these women cannot be entirely explained by poverty.

• Distinguish among some of the broadly defined medical and dietary conditions used by the WIC program in order to identify eligible WIC participants truly at high nutrition risk. These broad nutrition risk categories include *endocrine disorders, renal disease, chronic and recurrent infections, food allergies,* and *genetic and congenital disorders.* They include a broad range of medical problems with varying degrees of nutrition risk or potential to benefit from participation in the WIC program. Similarly, the category *inappropriate diet* includes some behaviors for which little nutrition risk is evident. The list in Table S-1 distinguishes among criteria in the broad nutrition risk categories.

• Appoint an expert committee to provide guidance on cutoff points for cigarette, alcohol, and illegal drug use that will identify pregnant and lactating women who are most likely to benefit from the WIC program. Members of the expert committee should have expertise in substance abuse during pregnancy and lactation, assessment and treatment of substance abuse, public policy, nutrition, and epidemiology.

• Identify the specific drugs that place individuals at nutrition risk with prolonged use and for which WIC program interventions could provide some benefit. The current nutrition risk criteria *drug-nutrient interactions and inappropriate use of medications* are too broadly defined and likely to produce very low yield of benefit.

• Disseminate information about risk criteria widely.

• Consider changing the current WIC priority system to give higher priority to those nutrition risk criteria identified in this report as having strong relationships to risk and potential to benefit and lower priority to nutrition risk criteria with weaker relationships to risk and potential to benefit.

1. *Risk criteria that merit higher priority*: vegan diets, highly restrictive diets, selected aspects of inappropriate infant feeding, food insecurity, homelessness, child of a mentally retarded parent.

2. *Risk criteria that merit higher priority among children*: nutrient deficiency diseases, failure to thrive, inborn errors of metabolism, gastrointestinal disorders.

3. *Risk criteria that merit lower priority*: mild nausea and vomiting during pregnancy; lack of prenatal care; cigarette, alcohol, and illegal drug use.[2]

Such a change in the priority system would require disaggregating the current categories (anthropometric, medical, dietary, and predisposing) that are used for ranking each risk criterion into one of seven priorities. It would also mean that in some cases children could be given priority over pregnant women. Such a change should improve the targeting of the program in terms of both risk and benefit.

---

[2] Three committee members (Barbara Abrams, Barbara Devaney, and Roy Pitkin) prefer retaining high priority for the criteria *alcohol use* and *illegal drug use*. Barbara Abrams and Barbara Devaney prefer retaining the high-priority level for the criterion *cigarette use* as well. See footnote 1 concerning cutoff points for these criteria.

1

Overview

The Special Supplemental Nutrition Program for Women, Infants, and Children (the WIC program; originally the Special Supplemental Food Program for Women, Infants, and Children) provides supplemental foods, nutrition education, and social service and health care referrals to five categories of low-income individuals (categorical criteria): pregnant, breastfeeding, and postpartum women, infants (0 through 12 months of age), and children (13 months up to 5 years of age) if they are identified at nutrition risk. The WIC program is based on the premise that many low-income people are at risk of poor nutrition and health outcomes because of insufficient nutrition during the critical growth and developmental periods of pregnancy, infancy, and early childhood. The WIC program is a *supplemental* food and nutrition program to help meet the special needs of low-income women, infants, and children during these periods.

In addition to categorical criteria and income standards, eligibility for participation in the WIC program requires evidence of nutrition risk. To become a participant, each applicant must be determined to be at nutrition risk on the basis of a medical or nutrition assessment conducted by a competent professional authority such as a physician, physician assistant, nutritionist, dietitian, nurse, or state or locally medically trained health official (7 CFR Subpart A, Section 246.2). Public Law 94-105 broadly defines nutrition risk as "(a) detrimental or abnormal nutritional conditions detectable by biochemical or anthropometric measures, (b) other documented nutritionally related medical conditions, (c) dietary deficiencies that impair or endanger health, or (d) conditions that predispose persons to inadequate nutritional patterns or nutritionally related medical conditions." Each state, territorial, or tribal WIC agency uses specific criteria for nutrition risk assessment within these guidelines.[1]

The criteria (nutrition risk indicators and their cutoff points) used for nutrition risk assessments vary widely across states. Over the years, concerns have been expressed about this variation and the resulting potential for unequal access to the program on the basis of geographic residence (GAO, 1979, 1980; USDA, 1986). As a result, the U.S. Congress in 1989 mandated that the U.S. Department of Agriculture (USDA), in consultation with state WIC agency directors and other nutrition experts, conduct a review of the nutrition risk criteria used by the WIC program (Public Law 101-147). USDA then reviewed a selected group of 14 existing nutrition risk criteria and published a compilation of these reviews in 1991 to fulfill this legislative mandate (USDA, 1991). In its 1992 report, the National Advisory Council on Maternal, Infant, and Fetal Nutrition commented on the 1991 reviews and made recommendations regarding existing nutrition risk criteria. In particular, it recommended that homelessness, migrancy, and alcohol and drug abuse be included as independent nutrition risk criteria (USDA, 1992).

CHARGE TO THE COMMITTEE

With continued concern over the variation among nutrition risk criteria across state WIC programs, the Food and Nutrition Service (FNS; now the Food and Consumer Service [FCS], USDA) requested that the Institute of Medicine (IOM) review the scientific basis for the nutrition risk criteria used in the WIC program. In October 1993, the Food and Nutrition Board of the IOM established the Committee on the Scientific Evaluation of WIC Nutrition Risk Criteria. The committee was charged with conducting a study to include the following:

- Performing a critical review of the literature surrounding the various nutrition risk criteria used by the WIC program.
- Developing scientific consensus (where possible) regarding the nutrition risk criteria used by the WIC program, taking into account the preventive nature of the program.
- Identifying specific segments of the WIC population at risk for each criterion.
- Identifying gaps in the scientific knowledge base for current nutrition risk criteria used by the WIC program.

---

[1] Throughout this report, the generic terms *state WIC agency* and *state agency* are used to denote programs or program requirements that apply uniformly to state, territorial, or tribal WIC programs.

- Formulating recommendations regarding appropriate criteria and, if applicable, recommendations of numerical values for determining who is at risk for each criterion.
- Identifying critical areas for future research.
- Identifying the practicality of consensus recommendations for nutrition risk criteria for the variety of WIC program delivery settings.

This report responds to these tasks.

THE WIC PROGRAM

Program Benefits

The WIC program is a broad-based and comprehensive food and nutrition program providing three main benefits to participants: (1) supplemental foods, (2) nutrition education, and (3) referrals to health care and social service providers. The WIC program serves as an adjunct to available health care to prevent the occurrence of nutrition-related health problems and to improve the health status of participants. Thus, in standard public health terms, the WIC program serves as both a secondary prevention and tertiary prevention program by providing risk appraisal and risk reduction (secondary prevention) and by providing treatment or rehabilitation to individuals with a diagnosed health condition (tertiary prevention) (Kaufman, 1990).

The structure of the program's components is shown in Figure 1-1 and includes the following anticipated benefits:

- For pregnant women, the WIC food supplements are expected to improve their nutrition status during pregnancy, which, in turn, is expected to improve pregnancy outcomes and enhance the nutrition status of both mother and infant.
- For breastfeeding women, the WIC food supplements (basic or enhanced breastfeeding food packages) are expected to provide nutrients to meet the special dietary needs of mothers who are breastfeeding, improve lactation performance, and enhance the nutrition status of both mother and infant.
- For nonbreastfeeding, postpartum women, the WIC food supplements are expected to improve their nutrition status, thus reducing the incidence of health problems associated with the physical demands of the postpartum period and improving health and nutrition status during the interconceptional period.
- For infants and children, the WIC food supplements are expected to reduce the prevalence of iron deficiency anemia, improve diets, and improve physical and mental growth and development.

WIC PARTICIPATION (services, benefits, outcomes)

NUTRITION RISK ASSESSMENT
- anthropometric
- medical
- dietary
- predisposing conditions

FOOD PACKAGE
Supplemental foods rich in protein, vitamin A, vitamin C, calcium, and iron for pregnant, lactating, and postpartum women, infants, and children.

NUTRITION EDUCATION
Education to improve knowledge about the use of WIC supplemental foods in normal diets and the relationship between diet, nutrition, and health during pregnancy, lactation, infancy, and childhood; and to promote breastfeeding.

HEALTH AND SOCIAL SERVICE REFERRALS
Referrals to health and social service programs providing preventive and curative health care; substance abuse counseling and treatment; and support in the areas of food security, income, and housing.

BENEFITS OF WIC PARTICIPATION
- access to foods rich in protein, vitamins A and C, calcium, and iron
- understanding of the effect of diet on pregnancy outcome and infant and childhood development
- use of prenatal care and well-baby-care services
- breastfeeding support
- receipt of referrals for timely or age-appropriate immunizations, and lead or human immunodeficiency virus screening
- use of family planning services
- receipt of referrals to health care programs (Medicaid or public health services) for other health problems
- use of social service programs (food stamps, AFDC, food banks, housing, or parenting education skills)
- encouragement to use smoking or substance abuse prevention and treatment programs

PROJECTED NUTRITION AND HEALTH OUTCOMES

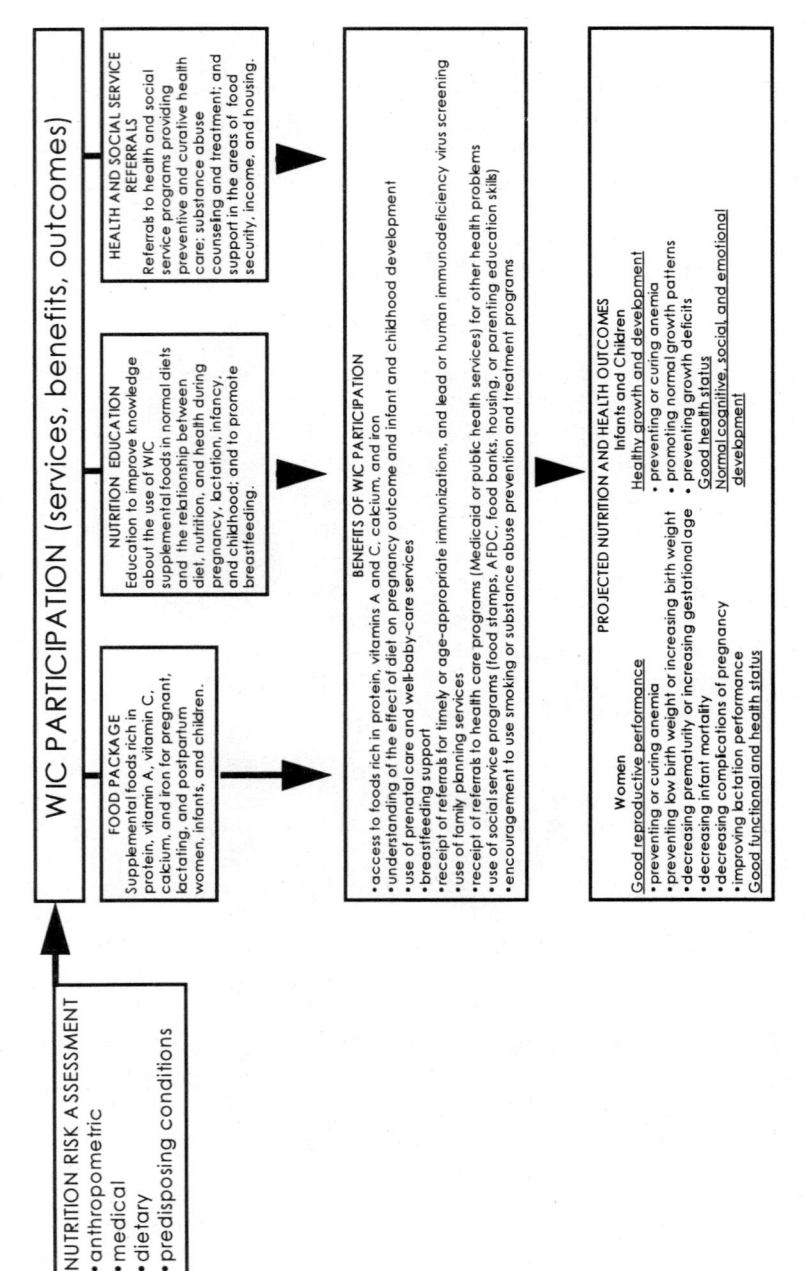

Women
<u>Good reproductive performance</u>
- preventing or curing anemia
- preventing low birth weight or increasing birth weight
- decreasing prematurity or increasing gestational age
- decreasing infant mortality
- decreasing complications of pregnancy
- improving lactation performance
<u>Good functional and health status</u>

Infants and Children
<u>Healthy growth and development</u>
- preventing or curing anemia
- promoting normal growth patterns
- preventing growth deficits
<u>Good health status</u>
<u>Normal cognitive, social, and emotional development</u>

FIGURE 1-1 WIC program components, services, benefits, and projected outcomes.

- The nutrition education component of the WIC program is expected to stress the relationship between nutrition and good health, with special emphasis on the needs of pregnant, postpartum, and breastfeeding women, infants, and children under 5 years of age; to assist individuals at nutrition risk in achieving positive changes in food habits; and to take into account ethnic, cultural, and geographic food preferences.
- Referrals to health care providers are expected to promote good health care among participants. For pregnant women, the health care referral system is expected to increase their use of prenatal and postpartum care; for breastfeeding and postpartum women, infants, and children, the WIC program is expected to facilitate their access to routine preventive as well as other health care services, such as immunization, family planning, smoking cessation, and drug treatment and counseling programs.
- Social service referrals to substance abuse treatment and counseling, housing assistance, Medicaid, Aid to Families with Dependent Children (AFDC), and food stamps are expected to aid in addressing the full range of the health and nutrition needs of low-income women and their children.

Supplemental food is provided in the form of food or, more commonly, a food instrument (either a voucher or a check) that can be used to purchase food in a store. The food instrument identifies the quantities of specific foods, including brand names, that can be redeemed with that instrument. WIC food packages include various combinations of iron-fortified infant formula or milk and cheese, eggs, iron-fortified adult or infant cereals, fruit or vegetable juices rich in vitamin C, and dried peas or beans and peanut butter.

The food packages contain food sources of specific nutrients that are assumed to be lacking in the diets of the population potentially eligible to participate in the WIC program: protein, vitamin A, vitamin C, calcium, and iron. WIC program regulations require tailored food packages that provide specified types and amounts of food appropriate for seven categories of participants: (1) infants from birth to 3 months of age, (2) infants from 4 to 12 months of age, (3) women, infants, and children with special dietary needs, (4) children from 1 year of age to the 5th birthday, (5) pregnant women, (6) postpartum nonbreastfeeding mothers, and (7) breastfeeding mothers (basic or enhanced food package). The amounts and types of food in each package vary by type of recipient (e.g., breastfeeding versus nonbreastfeeding mothers) and their individual nutrition need. USDA regulations specify the maximum amounts for each food package. Competent professional authorities at the local level tailor WIC food packages to meet specific individual needs, based on guidance from state WIC agencies. Special formulas or medical foods may be provided if medically indicated for infants, children, and women with special dietary needs.

Monthly food packages for infants who are not being breastfed may contain up to 403 fluid ounces of concentrated, liquid, iron-fortified infant formula (or powdered or ready-to-feed formula in equivalent amounts), 24 ounces of dry iron-fortified infant cereal, and 63 fluid ounces of vitamin C-rich infant juice (or equivalent amounts of adult-strength fluid or concentrated juice). Monthly food packages for pregnant and breastfeeding women may contain up to 28 quarts of fluid milk (with substitutions allowed for cheese and evaporated, skim, or dry milk), 2.5 dozen eggs (or egg powder), 36 ounces of dry, iron-fortified cereal, 276 ounces of fluid vitamin C-rich juice, and either 1 pound of dried beans or peas or 18 ounces of peanut butter.

Children 1 to 5 years of age receive the same foods (and allowable substitutions as stated above) in the same quantities except for fluid milk (up to 24 quarts). The enhanced food package for breastfeeding women adds cheese (1 pound) in addition to fluid milk, provides more juice (a total of 322–336 fluid ounces), includes both dried beans or peas and peanut butter, adds 26 ounces of canned tuna fish, and adds fresh, frozen, or canned carrots (2 pounds fresh or frozen or two 16- to 20-ounce cans).

The WIC program also provides nutrition education to improve the nutrition status of participants. Local agencies must spend at least one-sixth of WIC program administrative funds on nutrition education and counseling. WIC agencies must offer at least two nutrition education sessions to a participating woman in each 6-month certification period. However, participants cannot be denied food supplements if they do not attend the specified nutrition education sessions. Programs to promote breastfeeding and to foster successful lactation performance are an important part of the WIC program's nutrition education efforts, and program resources are specifically earmarked for this purpose. Federal funds designated for WIC nutrition services and program administration may be used to purchase breastfeeding aids such as breast pumps for use by breastfeeding women.

To qualify as a provider of WIC program services, the local agency must arrange for health care services to be available and accessible to low-income women, infants, and children. The WIC program advises clients about the types of health care available, the locations of health care facilities, how they can receive health care, and why it is beneficial. Many WIC program service sites are located at or adjacent to public health clinics.

In summary, the overarching goal of the WIC program is to improve the nutrition and health status of women, infants, and children, which in turn should improve pregnancy outcomes and promote optimal child growth and development. Although supplemental food assistance is the cornerstone of the WIC program, nutrition education and health care and social service referrals are also integral components of benefit to WIC participants.

WIC Program Eligibility Criteria

Eligibility for participation in the WIC program is based on categorical criteria, income criteria, and evidence of nutrition risk. To be eligible on the basis of the categorical criteria, an individual must be either (1) a pregnant woman, (2) a breastfeeding woman less than 1 year postpartum, (3) a nonbreastfeeding, postpartum woman up to 6 months after delivery, (4) an infant up to 1 year of age, or (5) a child 1 year of age to the 5th birthday.

States have the option of setting eligibility on the basis of income at the income level required to obtain free or reduced-price health services, provided that the income levels used range from between 100 and 185 percent of the federal poverty level. Nearly all states currently use income at 185 percent of the poverty level as the eligibility threshold on the basis of income. Some states have given their local agencies authority to set their own income eligibility thresholds, within the 100 to 185 percent range (if they use lower income eligibility thresholds for free or reduced-price health care in their local areas), and to use weekly, monthly, or annual income as the basis for eligibility. In addition, categorically eligible individuals can become income eligible for participation in the WIC program through participation in the Medicaid, Food Stamps, or Aid to Families with Dependent Children programs (known as *adjunct* or *automatic eligibility*).

The participant must be determined to be at nutrition risk on the basis of a medical or nutrition assessment by a competent professional, such as a physician, a nutritionist, a nurse, or some other health professional. Each state WIC agency establishes and uses specific assessment criteria for nutrition risk within federal guidelines. The minimum information that must be collected on each WIC program participant includes: height (length for infants), weight, and results from a blood test for iron deficiency anemia (infants younger than 6 months are exempt from the blood test). Eligibility can be determined on the basis of data collected at the local agency or with referral data from a competent professional not on staff at the local agency. The cutoff values used to determine nutrition risk vary widely across states.

Legislative and Programmatic History of the WIC Program

By the late 1960s, the federal focus on feeding low-income Americans had expanded dramatically to reflect the decade's War on Poverty programs, and policymakers were becoming more interested in the relationship between nutrition and health. School food programs, commonly referred to as school "feeding" programs, began to be called child "nutrition" programs following enactment of the Child Nutrition Act of 1966.

More emphasis on diet, nutrition, and health followed the publication of the final report of the White House Conference on Food, Nutrition, and Health (WHC, 1970). In 1969, largely in response to growing concerns about malnutrition and related health problems among low-income pregnant women and children, and because of the political pressures generated by the 1968 Poor People's Campaign, USDA began what was later to be called the Commodity Supplemental Food Program. This program provided free, government-purchased commodities to low-income, nutritionally at-risk pregnant women, new mothers, and children under 6 years of age.

At approximately the same time, physicians began to notice an increase in the number of young, pregnant women or mothers and infants arriving at public health clinics who, after clinical examination, were determined to have a variety of symptoms but no overt evidence of disease (Leonard, 1994). These patients' primary complaint was a lack of food for their families. In 1968, a group including community-based public health physicians; staff of the Bureau of Women and Children of the then U.S. Department of Health, Education, and Welfare; and staff of the then Consumer and Marketing Service, USDA, met to discuss the problem. The suggestion was made to build food commissaries attached to neighborhood health clinics and to stock them with commodity foods and infant formula. Food prescribed via vouchers by clinic physicians or staff would provide low-income women, infants, and children with a supplemental food package at the same time that they received health care services. USDA opened a demonstration commissary-clinic in Atlanta, Georgia, in the fall of 1968. Later, another health clinic-food distribution program began in Baltimore, Maryland, through the Johns Hopkins University School of Medicine.

Expansion of these demonstration projects was given statutory authority by the U.S. Congress in 1972 (Public Law 92-433). Thus, the WIC program officially began as a 2-year pilot program linking health care to food assistance for low-income pregnant women, nursing mothers, infants, and preschool-age children considered to be at health risk because of poor nutrition. It was authorized under Section 17 of the Child Nutrition Act and was to supplement the Food Stamp Program and two other smaller programs that served similar target groups.

The WIC program made cash grants to state health departments or comparable health agencies for distribution to the local agencies operating the programs. During the initial years, eligible recipients were low-income pregnant and postpartum women, infants (to age 1 year), and children (ages 1 to 4 years) who were determined by competent professionals to be at nutrition risk because of inadequate nutrition and inadequate income. Participants received specified food items either directly by picking them up at WIC centers or through home delivery, or by using coupons or vouchers to redeem specific food items at local grocery stores. Recipients had to live in areas that were served by clinics or other health facilities that had been determined to have significant numbers of infants and pregnant and postpartum women at nutrition risk. The 1972 law also required that the benefits of the program be evaluated and reported to Congress.

A special task force was established to design the program, and on July 11, 1973, this task force published initial regulations. These regulations required local clinics to apply for WIC program grants through their state departments of health. The USDA's Food and Nutrition Service designed the eligibility criteria used by state agencies for participants and the contents of the monthly supplemental food package (i.e., the kinds and amounts of food). Between August and December 1973, a total of 216 WIC programs were approved.

National Expansion

The WIC program's legislative history shows an increasing focus on the preventive nature of the WIC program. The 1975 Amendments to the National School Lunch Act of 1946 and the Child Nutrition Act of 1966 restated the WIC program's purpose: "to provide supplemental nutritious food as an adjunct to good health care during such critical times of growth and development in order to prevent the occurrence of health problems" (Public Law 94-105). These amendments also liberalized eligibility, extending the period for breastfeeding mothers to 1 year postpartum and that for nonbreastfeeding mothers to 6 months postpartum, and raising the age limit for children from the fourth birthday to the fifth birthday. In addition, the law provided for a National Advisory Council on Maternal, Infant, and Fetal Nutrition, with members to be appointed by the Secretary of Agriculture.

The 1978 amendments further reinforced the preventive focus of the WIC program by amending the purpose to add "to prevent the occurrence of health problems and improve the health status of these persons" (Public Law 95-627). The 1978 law reiterated the earlier provision requiring nutrition risk determination by specifying that individuals would not be eligible solely on the basis of low income but also had to exhibit evidence of nutrition risk, as determined by a competent professional authority. State agencies were given the responsibility to include in their state plans a description of the methods used to determine nutrition risk.

Maximum income levels for eligibility in the WIC program were set by the 1978 amendments. Previously, the law was silent on this issue, but by regulation USDA had set the income limit for eligibility at the same level as that locally determined for eligibility to receive free or reduced-price health care. (In most cases, states set this level at between 100 and 200 percent of the poverty level.) The 1978 law set the income ceiling for eligibility for participation in the WIC program at the ceiling used for eligibility for reduced-price school meals under the National School Lunch Act (Public Law 79-396); the ceiling was then

195 percent of the Secretary of Agriculture's income poverty guidelines, adjusted annually to reflect changes in the Consumer Price Index.

Subsequent to the 1978 law, USDA changed its regulations, permitting states to set income criteria for eligibility in local WIC agencies at the same levels as those set for free or reduced-price health care, provided these were no higher than the income level set for reduced-price school lunches and no lower than 100 percent of the poverty guidelines published by the U.S. Department of Health and Human Services (*Federal Register,* February 10, 1994, 59(28): 6277–6278).

Other Programmatic and Administrative Changes During the 1970s

In an effort to increase the nutrition education component of the WIC program, the 1978 amendments required the Secretary of Agriculture to ensure that nutrition education be provided to all adult participants in the WIC program. It required the state agency to provide training to the individuals who provided such nutrition education and to use not less than one-sixth of federal administrative funds for nutrition education activities. State agencies were also required to evaluate annually their nutrition education programs and to provide nutrition education materials in relevant non-English languages in areas with substantial non-English-speaking, low-income populations.

A competent professional (e.g., physician, nutritionist, dietitian, or registered nurse) was made responsible for both certifying nutrition need and prescribing the appropriate foods to be provided to participants. The Secretary of Agriculture was required to issue regulations on the types of supplemental food that could be made available through the WIC program. To the degree possible, the Secretary was directed to ensure that the fat, sugar, and salt contents of foods be appropriate.

Programmatic and Administrative Changes During the 1980s

The Omnibus Budget Reconciliation Act (OBRA) of 1980 included a provision extending funding authority for the WIC program through fiscal year (FY) 1984 and changing the authorization from a specified ceiling to the amount approved through the annual appropriations process (Public Law 96-499). The OBRA of 1981 (Public Law 97-35) reduced the maximum income levels that states could use to define eligibility for WIC program participation by lowering the income level for eligibility for reduced-price school lunches from 195 to 185 percent of the poverty guidelines. This law also reduced the number of required items that states had to include in their annual program plan in order to receive WIC program funds.

The Hunger Prevention Act of 1988 added new provisions for the WIC program dealing with service to homeless people. These provisions require coordination among local agencies to provide outreach to eligible homeless mothers, infants, and children as part of each state's WIC program plan. They also permit states to adopt methods for the delivery of benefits to homeless people and to adapt WIC food packages to meet the special needs of homeless participants. This law also added a demonstration project that provided for 3-year grant awards to 10 states to assist them to implement and operate a program that gave coupons, with a value of up to $20 annually, to WIC program participants to redeem for fresh fruits and vegetables at local farmers' markets.

Programmatic and Administrative Changes During the 1990s

The Healthy Meals for Healthy Americans Act of 1994 (Public Law 103-488) reauthorized the WIC program through FY 1998 and established several provisions to improve program management and accessibility. The legislation officially changed the name of the WIC program to the Special Supplemental Nutrition Program for Women, Infants, and Children. It also provided state WIC agencies the option of allowing pregnant women who meet the income standards for eligibility to be temporarily eligible to participate in the program and to receive immediate certification for participation in the program. Full determination of nutrition risk for such women would follow within 60 days and benefits would be discontinued if it was shown that the pregnant woman did not meet the eligibility criteria for nutrition risk.

In April 1995, USDA published final rules incorporating homelessness and migrancy as nutrition risk conditions. The regulation also codified the name change included in the Healthy Meals for Healthy Americans Act and modified the definition of nutrition risk to include more medical and health conditions previously categorized as predisposing nutrition risks as direct nutrition risks (*Federal Register*, April 19, 1995, 60(75):19,487–19,491).

Program Size

The WIC program operates in each of the 50 states, the District of Columbia, Puerto Rico, Guam, the American Virgin Islands, and 33 American Indian tribal organizations. In total, the WIC program is operated through more than 2,000 local agencies and more than 10,000 service sites nationwide. During 1995, the program was expected to serve an average of 6.8 million women, infants, and children.

USDA estimated that 7.5 million people were eligible for participation in the WIC program in 1984 (USDA, 1987). Actually participating in the WIC program in 1984 were 3.05 million women, infants, and children, or 40 percent of those estimated to be eligible. Although the WIC program served only about 40 percent of eligible participants in 1984, it served considerably larger proportions of the high-risk and very-low-income populations eligible to participate in the program. Among those being served, the WIC program was found to target its services best among the groups designated for higher priority service. The Congressional Budget Office estimated that it would have cost a total of $3.75 billion in FY 1992 to serve all of those eligible and likely to apply for the program. This would have required $1.15 billion (44 percent) more than the $2.6 billion actually appropriated for the program in FY 1992.

The WIC program has been one of the fastest growing of the federal nutrition programs. Federal WIC program funding nearly quadrupled between 1980 and 1993, rising from about $725 million in FY 1980 to more than $2.8 billion in FY 1993. During that same period, total participation rose from 1.9 million to 5.9 million individuals (see Table 1-1). The average monthly food benefit doubled between 1974 and 1984. In 1989, following legislative mandates that required states to implement competitive bids for infant formula, average food package costs declined somewhat from a high of $33 per month and stabilized at approximately $30 per month.

OVERVIEW OF THE REPORT AND THE COMMITTEE PROCESS

The first three chapters of this report cover an overview of the committee's task, the relationship of low income to nutrition risk, and principles for defining nutrition risk, respectively. Chapters 4 through 7 examine the scientific basis for WIC nutrition risk criteria: a description of each risk criterion, the prevalence of the condition in the U.S. population and WIC participants (if available), factors associated with the condition, the criterion as an indicator of nutrition and health risk, the criterion as an indicator of nutrition and health benefit, the use of the risk criterion in the WIC program setting, and the committee's recommendation for each risk criterion. Chapter 8 provides the committee's conclusions and recommendations.

The committee met five times, held many conference calls, conducted two public meetings (see Appendixes A and B for detailed information), made site visits to local WIC program clinics, and exchanged much written information. The USDA's FCS provided a wealth of programmatic information to the committee through formal presentations and written materials.

The committee began by reviewing the WIC program. It obtained a list of nutrition risk criteria used by WIC state agencies in 1992. This list is considerably more detailed than both the risks specified by federal regulation and the prioritized list of risk criteria provided by FCS (see Appendix C). The committee examined more than 74 nutrition risk criteria, categorized into anthro-

TABLE 1-1 WIC Program Participation by Subgroup and Federal Costs, 1974–1993

Fiscal Year	Number of Participants (thousands)					Average Monthly Food Benefit/Person	Federal Cost (millions)	
	Women	Infants	Children	Total[a]		Current Dollars[b]	Constant 1992 Dollars[c]
1974	17	26	44	88	15.68	9.90	—
1975	55	103	186	344	18.58	82.80	—
1976	81	148	291	520	19.60	142.50	—
1977	165	213	471	848	20.80	255.90	597.10
1978	240	308	633	1,181	21.99	379.60	827.50
1979	312	389	782	1,483	24.09	525.40	1,039.60
1980	411	507	995	1,913	25.43	724.70	1,261.90
1981	446	585	1,088	2,119	27.84	874.40	1,370.10
1982	478	623	1,088	2,189	28.83	948.20	1,384.50
1983	542	730	1,265	2,537	29.62	1,123.10	1,583.50
1984	657	825	1,563	3,045	30.58	1,386.30	1,876.70
1985	655	874	1,600	3,138	31.69	1,488.90	1,945.60
1986	712	945	1,665	3,312	31.82	1,580.50	2,014.30
1987	751	1,019	1,660	3,429	32.68	1,663.60	2,016.70
1988	815	1,095	1,683	3,593	33.28	1,802.40	2,145.90
1989	952	1,260	1,907	4,118	30.14	1,929.40	2,192.20
1990	1,035	1,413	2,069	4,517	30.20	2,125.90	2,301.00
1991	1,120	1,559	2,214	4,893	29.84	2,301.10	2,370.90
1992	1,221	1,684	2,505	5,411	30.20	2,566.50	2,566.50
1993	1,365	1,742	2,813	5,920	29.77	2,819.50	2,737.00

[a] Total participation may not equal sum of categories because of rounding.
[b] Includes funding for WIC studies, surveys, and pilot projects.
[c] Constant dollars were calculated using the FY 1992 CPI-U (Consumer Price Index-Universal).

SOURCE: USDA (1994).

pometric, biochemical and medical, dietary, and predisposing risks. The committee conducted bibliographic searches of the scientific literature and critically reviewed research findings surrounding risk criteria.

In reviewing each nutrition risk criterion, the committee examined two issues: the risk criterion as an indicator of nutrition and health risk and the risk criterion as an indicator of health and nutrition benefit from participation in the WIC program, as explained in detail in Chapter 3. The potential to benefit from the services provided by the WIC program is a key feature of the committee's approach. This approach differs from the approach that has guided the development of risk criteria used by WIC programs: assessing poor outcomes only. The application of the concept of potential to benefit moves the program focus from curative (tertiary prevention) to risk reduction (secondary prevention). Utilizing such an approach can provide for more efficient targeting of the scarce resources available to the WIC program and also improve outcomes.

The committee did not specifically examine two nutrition risk criteria used to certify infants for the WIC program: (1) breastfeeding mother and infant dyad and (2) infant of a mother eligible for the WIC program or of a mother at nutrition risk during pregnancy. Together, these two risk criteria account for 78 percent of all infants certified for the WIC program (Randall and Boast, 1994). Because of their nature, however, these two nutrition risk criteria do not fit with either the charge to the committee or the framework used to assess the WIC nutrition risk criteria. Specifically, these two risk criteria do not have a scientific literature that examines the nutrition and health risks associated with these conditions. In practice, these two criteria implicitly serve to certify nearly all income-eligible infants. Thus, Chapter 2 of this report, which examines the relationship between poverty and nutrition risk, may be viewed, in part, as presenting the nutrition and health risks for infants certified on the basis of either a breastfeeding mother or a mother eligible or participating in the WIC program during pregnancy. Moreover, the evidence presented in Chapter 2 on the effectiveness of the WIC program for infants can be used to infer the degree to which these two risk criteria for infants serve as indicators of health and nutrition benefit from the WIC program.

Throughout its work, the committee faced a number of limitations regarding the use of currently available data on nutrition risks in the WIC program setting. The scientific literature addressing the anthropometric, biomedical and medical, dietary, and predisposing risks for poor nutrition and health status among women, infants, and children is imperfect and incomplete. Interpretation of studies is a challenge because of the difficulty of obtaining accurate and reliable estimates of nutrition status. Furthermore, during reproduction, growth, and development, the effect of a nutritional insult may be based on its timing or severity, but the critical time frame may not be understood. Health outcomes related to pregnancy, lactation, and growth are difficult to measure accurately and reliably. Even if measurements of excellent quality could be obtained, the complex interrelationships between genetic, social, cultural, economic, and nutrition factors make it difficult to isolate the independent effect of nutrition on human health and development. Non-nutrition-related variables need to be controlled or otherwise considered when studies are conducted or analyzed, but often they are not. These limitations made it especially important for the com-mittee to develop a clear framework for its decision-making process. This framework is presented at the end of Chapter 3.

Many of the studies assessing an indicator of nutrition and health risk were observational and could identify associations but not causal relationships. However, carefully designed observational studies that control for confounding variables and that have adequate sample sizes can serve as excellent sources of understanding about how medical, anthropometric, dietary, and predisposing factors are associated with nutrition and health status.

Well-controlled, randomized experiments that intervene to improve nutrition status in pregnant or lactating mothers, infants, or children provide the best opportunity to test causal relationships and assess indicators of nutrition and health benefit. However, that type of study is usually extremely expensive, complex to design, and difficult to carry out in the field. A variety of problems can influence their results and the interpretation of those results. For example, the food supplement may replace part of the diet rather than supplement it, the length of treatment may be too short, the timing of supplementation may be inappropriate, or the composition or quantity of the supplementation may not be correctly related to the degree of poor nutrition. In addition, problems with compliance, loss to follow-up, unanticipated interventions in the control group, and other sources of inconsistency and bias can limit the ability to interpret study results. Finally, it may not be feasible to conduct controlled studies in the populations with the highest likelihood of responding. Nevertheless, the available studies attempting to control for nondiet factors form the backbone of researchers' understanding of nutrition intervention and, when available, were emphasized in the reviews.

Names, definitions, and cutoff points used with nutrition risk criteria vary substantially across research studies, and these made comparison of results a difficult task. Additionally, the committee identified few studies that attempted to quantify the efficacy of a particular indicator of nutrition risk or benefit, for example, by examining its yield or sensitivity as an assessment variable (see Chapter 3). Estimates of the prevalence of many of the conditions that pose nutrition or health risks among the WIC program population or the population eligible for participation in the WIC program were not easy to obtain.

Little of the available literature specifically addressed the WIC program population. For many nutrition risk indicators, the only data available were from populations outside of the United States with substantially higher prevalences of undernutrition, and the relevance of these studies to the WIC program population had to be considered.

When WIC program evaluations or other studies of WIC program populations were available, they focused almost entirely on perinatal outcomes; on the whole, data on lactating or postpartum women, infants, or children were lacking. Studies of the WIC program addressing perinatal outcomes almost exclusively addressed birth outcomes, such as birth weight. Thus, those studies did not contribute information about the impact of the WIC program on indicators such as hematocrit concentration or maternal weight gain, nor were data available to address how subgroups of women with such problems as homelessness or substance abuse respond to WIC program interventions.

The public meetings were designed to solicit information from WIC program administrators, staff, and participants as well as from researchers in the fields related to the nutrition risk criteria under study (see Appendixes A and B). Through the public meetings and visits to WIC program clinics, the committee obtained valuable information about the use of nutrition risk criteria in WIC clinics, the methods of conducting nutrition assessments and determining appropriate nutrition and health interventions, and practical considerations. The presentations made at the public meetings also provided the committee with information about the nutrition risk criteria being developed by some states or criteria that had been disallowed by the FCS.

REFERENCES

GAO (U.S. General Accounting Office). 1979. Special Supplemental Food Program for Women, Infants, and Children (WIC). Pub. No. CED-79-55. Washington, D.C.: U.S. Government Printing Office.

GAO (U.S. General Accounting Office). 1980. Better Management and More Resources Needed to Improve Federal Efforts to Improve Pregnancy Outcome. Pub. No. HRD-80-24. Washington, D.C.: U.S. Government Printing Office.

Kaufman, M., ed. 1990. Nutrition in Public Health: A Handbook for Developing Programs and Services. Rockville, Md.: Aspen Publishers, Inc.

Leonard, R. 1994. Recalling WIC program's 1960s humble beginnings. CNI Weekly Report 24(15):4–7.

Randall, B., and L. Boast. 1994. Study of WIC Participant and Program Characteristics, 1992. Office of Analysis and Evaluation, food and Nutrition Service, U.S. Department of Agriculture. Washington, D.C.: U.S. Department of Agriculture.

USDA (U.S. Department of Agriculture). 1986. 1986 Biennial Report on the Special Supplemental Food Program for Women, Infants and Children and on the Commodity Supplemental Food Program. National Advisory Council on Maternal, Infant, and Fetal Nutrition. Food and Nutrition Service. Washington, D.C.: USDA.

USDA (U.S. Department of Agriculture). 1987. Estimation of Eligibility for the WIC Program: Report of the WIC Eligibility Study. Summary of Data, Methods, and Findings. Office of Analysis and Evaluation, Food and Nutrition Service. Contract No. 53-3198-3-138. Washington, D.C.: USDA.

USDA (U.S. Department of Agriculture). 1991. Technical Papers: Review of WIC Nutritional Risk Criteria. Prepared for the Food and Nutrition Service by the Department of Family and Community Medicine, College of Medicine, University of Arizona, Tucson. Washington, D.C.: USDA.

USDA (U.S. Department of Agriculture). 1992. 1992 Biennial Report on the Special Supplemental Food Program for Women, Infants and Children and on the Commodity Supplemental Food Program. National Advisory Council on Maternal, Infant, and Fetal Nutrition. Food and Nutrition Service. Washington, D.C.: USDA.

USDA (U.S. Department of Agriculture). 1994. Annual Historical Review. Washington, D.C: USDA.

WHC (White House Conference on Food, Nutrition, and Health). 1970. Final Report: White House Conference on Food, Nutrition, and Health. Washington, D.C.: U.S. Government Printing Office.

2

Poverty and Nutrition Risk

An underlying premise of the WIC program (Special Supplemental Nutrition Program for Women, Infants, and Children) is that low income predisposes women, infants, and children to poor nutrition status and health outcomes. By using both an income standard of up to 185 percent of the federal poverty level and nutrition risk criteria in determining eligibility for participation in the WIC program, the WIC program attempts to target scarce program resources to those individuals with limited economic resources who are at the highest risk of poor outcomes. Before reviewing (in subsequent chapters) the scientific evidence relating to the nutrition risk criteria used to establish eligibility for participation in the WIC program, this chapter presents evidence of low income, or poverty, as a predisposing nutrition risk factor for women, infants, and children.

DEFINITION OF POVERTY

Considerable controversy exists over how to define and measure poverty. A recent expert panel defined poverty as "economic deprivation," reflecting inadequate economic resources for the consumption of basic goods and services (NRC, 1995). Poverty standards are generally called *absolute* measures and are based on the assumption that there is some objective minimum level of either income or consumption such that if economic resources are less than this minimum standard, individuals and families do not have adequate resources to satisfy their basic needs (Ruggles, 1990). Families and individuals are classified as being in poverty if their incomes are less than official poverty thresholds. The poverty measure was initially constructed by determining the cost of a nutritionally adequate low-cost food plan (then the Economy Food Plan, now the

Thrifty Food Plan) designed by the U.S. Department of Agriculture (USDA) for families of different sizes and compositions and then multiplying the cost by a factor of three. This approach was based on analysis of the 1955 Household Food Consumption Survey, which showed that food consumption represents one-third of family income (Orshansky, 1963, 1965). Official poverty thresholds are derived by using the Consumer Price Index (CPI) to update this measure annually.

Over time, several criticisms of official poverty statistics have emerged, each with different implications for estimating the prevalence of poverty. The first type of criticism is conceptual and questions whether absolute measures of poverty truly reflect what is meant by being poor in U.S. society. Alternative poverty measures include both relative and subjective measures and may better reflect current living and consumption standards (Ruggles, 1990). However, such measures rarely have been considered official measures of poverty.

A second and more common criticism of official poverty statistics focuses on the specific components used to construct the poverty thresholds (Lewit, 1993; NRC, 1995; Ruggles, 1990). Three specific issues are important. First, current poverty thresholds are based on 1955 food consumption and expenditure patterns and do not reflect the resources required for a minimally adequate standard of living today. Second, measures of family income do not account for in-kind benefits such as food stamps, free or reduced-price school meals under the child nutrition programs, donated USDA commodity food, Medicaid, and public housing subsidies, nor do they consider fixed expenses, such as child care and child support, taxes, housing, and medical expenses. Since the 1960s, when the poverty concept was introduced, there has been tremendous growth both in the value of benefits from in-kind programs and in fixed expenses.

Finally, the CPI, as opposed to an index based on the price of food, is used to update poverty thresholds. If poverty is theoretically linked only with having a minimally adequate amount of food, then official poverty statistics will overstate the prevalence of poverty during periods of rapid inflation in the price of nonfood items. In addition, use of the CPI alone to update poverty thresholds ignores the substantial geographic variation in the cost of housing.

Despite considerable controversy over official poverty thresholds and statistics, the measures in use form the basis for determining the size of the population in need, designing and evaluating antipoverty programs, and assessing economic well-being over time. Poverty guidelines used as the basis for determining income eligibility in the WIC program are those published annually by the U.S. Department of Health and Human Services (*Federal Register*, February 19, 1994, 59(28):6277–6278).

PREVALENCE OF POVERTY

Compared with other industrialized nations, poverty in the United States is widespread and disproportionately affects children. In 1993, the poverty rate—the percentage of individuals with a family income less than the federal poverty line—was 15.1 percent for the U.S. population and 22.7 percent for children under 18 years of age (U.S. Bureau of the Census, 1995). The poverty rate for children in the United States is generally considered to exceed the rate for children in almost all other industrialized countries: during the 1980s, the poverty rate of U.S. children was more than three times the poverty rates of children in Sweden and Switzerland and more than twice the poverty rates of children in Germany and Norway (Duncan, 1991).

Trends in poverty among children show that the rate increased through the 1970s, 1980s, and early 1990s, despite uninterrupted economic growth from 1982 through 1989 and the recent recovery from the 1990–1991 economic recession (Children's Defense Fund, 1991, 1994; Duncan, 1991; Li and Bennett, 1994). In 1993, poverty among children was more prevalent than in any year since 1965. Increases in poverty are particularly dramatic among very young children. More than 1 in 4 children under 6 years of age is poor, and among very young poor children, nearly half live in families with an income less than 50 percent of the poverty level (Center on Budget and Policy Priorities, 1994).

The implications for the WIC program of the high prevalence of measured poverty among women, infants, and children are dramatic. In 1993, 9.5 million infants and children 1 to 4 years of age—almost one-half of all infants and children in this age group—lived in families within the WIC program's guidelines for eligibility on the basis of income and as defined by WIC state agencies (Trippe and Schirm, 1994). The WIC program served only 4.6 million, or half, of these income eligible infants and young children. The largest discrepancy between the number of people eligible for participation on the basis of income and the number served occurs for children 1 to 4 years of age. The discrepancy results from the fact that the WIC program is not fully funded.

POVERTY AND NUTRITION RISK FOR WOMEN

Evidence linking poverty and nutrition risk for women served by the WIC program is obtained almost exclusively from the relationship between poverty and (1) poor perinatal outcomes and (2) risk factors for poor perinatal outcomes. The relationship between low income and poor perinatal outcomes is well established in the literature. Using median family income within census tracts identified from birth certificates, Gould and LeRoy (1988) analyzed rates of low birth weight for large cohorts of births in Los Angeles County from 1982 to 1983 and found that median family income was a strong predictor of the relative risk of low birth weight. For both black and white infants, increases in median family income were associated with decreases in the percentage of low-birth-weight infants. These differences persisted after controlling for maternal age and education and the adequacy of the prenatal care that was received. Other studies also confirm the relationship between geographic variation in perinatal outcomes and socioeconomic status (Brooks, 1980; Gortmaker, 1979; Knox et al., 1980).

In addition, cross-sectional data collected over the past decade, such as the National Longitudinal Survey of Youth (NLSY) and the National Maternal and Infant Health Survey, include data on family income and such birth outcomes as birth weight, adequacy of prenatal care, and infant mortality. Starfield and colleagues (1991) used data from the NLSY to examine the effects of income and race on the risk of low birth weight. The risk of low birth weight among poor women was higher than that among nonpoor women, especially for white mothers. In addition, the study findings show the importance of factors antecedent to pregnancy, such as long-term poverty or poverty before pregnancy, in understanding variations in the risk of low birth weight.

Although the relationship between poverty and poor perinatal outcomes is well established, the mechanisms by which poverty or low socioeconomic status exerts an influence on perinatal outcome are less clear. Poverty is likely to affect perinatal outcomes in one or more of the following ways: restricting access to health care; affecting nutrition before, during, and after pregnancy; and producing stress, which can result in other risk factors such as smoking, teen pregnancy, drug use or abuse, poor mental health, and inadequate shelter and living conditions.

As confirmation of these potential mechanisms, Gould and LeRoy (1988) found that median family income is strongly associated with risk factors for low birth weight, including the percentage of teen pregnancies and increases in the percentage of women with late or no prenatal care. The Institute of Medicine (IOM) also concluded that risk factors for low birth weight are greatest for women of low socioeconomic status (IOM, 1985, 1988). Data from the Pregnancy Nutrition Surveillance System indicate that low-income women receive less prenatal care and receive care later in pregnancy than higher-income women (Kim et al., 1992).

With regard to dietary status, findings from analyses of the Continuing Survey of Food Intakes of Individuals (CSFII) conducted in 1985 and 1986 and from the second National Health and Nutrition Examination Survey (NHANES II) suggest that diet quality differs between low-income and higher-income women. Block and Abrams (1993) analyzed CSFII dietary data from 4 nonconsecutive days for women ages 19 to 50 years and found that for every nutrient analyzed (protein, vitamin A, vitamin E, vitamin C, vitamin B_6, folate, calcium, iron, and zinc), the proportion of women with intakes less than 70 percent of the Recommended Dietary Allowance (RDA) and the proportion of women with intakes less than 100 percent of the RDA were greater in the lowest-income group.[1] The women showed marked differences in fruit and vegetable consumption: 82 percent of the women in the higher-income group reported eating a vegetable at least once in the 4 nonconsecutive days, compared with only 54 percent of the women in the lowest-income group. Women in the lowest-income group were half as likely to report consuming a dark green vegetable (7 versus 14 percent) and were significantly less likely to report consuming any fruit or juice in the 4 days (67 versus 87 percent). In addition, an analysis of NHANES II dietary data for white non-Hispanic women found that the risk of a poor diet was increased by poverty (Guendelman and Abrams, 1995).

POVERTY AND NUTRITION RISK FOR INFANTS AND CHILDREN

Poverty among children is associated with impaired growth and cognitive development. Empirical evidence shows that poverty is related to almost all indicators of child growth and development and to almost all intervening risk factors for delayed growth and development.

Cross-sectional data from early national surveys of U.S. children document the deficits in nutrition status as determined by height and weight for children living in poverty (Jones et al., 1985). Cycle II of the Health Examination Survey, 1963–1965, examined children 6 to 11 years of age and found that the mean height and weight for low-income children was lower than the mean height and weight for higher-income children (Hamill et al., 1972). The Ten-State Nutrition Survey, 1968–1970, further confirmed this finding; these data showed that children from families with an income less than 150 percent of the poverty level were more often of low weight and short stature than children from families with incomes above this cutoff (CDC, 1972). Likewise, the Preschool Nutrition Survey, 1968–1970, found decreased growth in children living in low-income families (Owen et al., 1974). Finally, data from the first and second National Health and Nutrition Examination Surveys (NHANES I, 1971–1975, and NHANES II, 1976–1980) also show lower mean values for all of the growth measures examined—height, weight, triceps skinfold thickness, and subscapular skinfold thickness—for children living in homes below the poverty threshold compared with the mean values for children living in homes above the poverty threshold (Jones et al., 1985). Between the NHANES I and NHANES II

---

[1] It is important to note the limitations of using the proportion meeting the RDA in assessing dietary status. The RDAs for most dietary components are set so that the recommended amount will meet the needs of most healthy individuals. However, the nutrition requirements of individuals vary considerably, and many people remain healthy even if the amount of a nutrient consumed is less than the RDA. With the exception of food energy, a usual intake below the RDA does not necessarily signal a nutrient deficiency (NRC, 1989).

surveys, however, the differences in children's growth measures by poverty status declined in magnitude.

More recently, data from the NLSY suggest that the income-related deficits in growth and development are more severe for children living in chronic or persistent poverty than for children experiencing short-term poverty (Miller and Korenman, 1994). NLSY data include measures of family income for each year from 1978 to 1990 and measures of height, weight, and cognitive development of children in 1986, 1988, and 1990. Miller and Korenman (1994) reported both a higher prevalence of wasting (low weight-for-height) and stunting (low height-for-age) among poor children than among nonpoor children and greater differentials according to long-term rather than short-term measures of poverty. These detrimental effects of chronic poverty persist after controlling for other mediating factors such as maternal age and education, family structure, race, height and weight of the mother, and newborn birth weight.

Data from the Pediatric Nutrition Surveillance System (PedNSS) of the U.S. Centers for Disease Control and Prevention also show a higher-than-expected prevalence of stunting among low-income children under 5 years of age (Yip et al., 1992). Although the PedNSS data do not show a higher-than-expected prevalence of wasting among low-income children, these data are collected only for children who participate in public health and nutrition programs and may underestimate the prevalence among all low-income children.

Among the nutrition deficiencies of infants and children, iron deficiency anemia is one of the most prevalent and important U.S. public health problems (IOM, 1993). The prevalence of anemia among low-income infants and young children (through 2 years of age) participating in public health programs in 1991 ranged between 20 and 30 percent, compared to 5 percent for the nation as a whole (Yip et al., 1992). Although anemia can be caused by many factors, most cases (80 to 90 percent) can be attributed to iron deficiency.

Studies also find a relationship between measures of cognitive development of children and socioeconomic status or income. Research on iron deficiency anemia, which is more prevalent among low-income children than among higher-income children, consistently shows that infants and young children with iron deficiency anemia score lower than iron-replete controls on a wide range of psychological tests (Lozoff, 1990; Oski and Honig, 1978; Pollitt, 1994). The literature on nutrition status and cognitive development also suggests that stunting is associated with cognitive deficits among children (Wachs, 1995; Wilson, 1981).

Two recent studies examined the effects of poverty on cognitive development and found that children who experience long-term or persistent poverty score lower on IQ tests and other cognitive measures than children who experience transitory poverty, who in turn score lower than children who were never poor (Duncan et al., 1994; Miller and Korenman, 1993).

In summary, the available literature provides strong evidence that children born into poverty are at greater risk of impaired growth and delays in cognitive development. As is the case for women, the actual mechanism by which poverty exerts a biologic influence on child health outcomes is through one or more of the following: nutrition and dietary quality, limited access to health care, and exposure to such other risk factors as passive smoking, inadequate housing, and poor food preparation facilities.

Interestingly, despite the overwhelming evidence documenting the deficits in growth among children in low-income families, income is not strongly related to variations in energy or nutrient intake. The many studies that examine the relationship between family income and children's nutrient intake report either no effect of household income or small positive effects (Adrian and Daniel, 1976; Basiotis et al., 1983; DHHS/USDA, 1986). Data from NHANES I and NHANES II found lower mean values of all growth measures for children in families with incomes below the poverty level but no differences in intakes of food energy between poor and nonpoor children (Jones et al., 1985). Recent analyses based on the 1987–1988 Nationwide Food Consumption Survey show similar results. For example, in a study of nutrient intakes over 3 days among children 1 to 10 years of age, household income had no significant effect on either micronutrient intakes or any measures of dietary quality after controlling for social and demographic characteristics (Johnson et al., 1994).

Certain dietary differences by poverty status, however, are found for children. Using 4 days of dietary intake data from the 1985–1986 CSFII, Cook and Martin (1995) found that the proportions of low-income children with intakes less than 70 percent of the RDA are significantly higher than the proportions of nonpoor children for 10 of 16 nutrients examined. In addition, CSFII data also suggest that low-income children have diets that are very high in fat and cholesterol. Thompson and Dennison (1994) found that children in families with incomes less than 130 percent of the poverty level were more likely to have fat intakes exceeding 40 percent of their total food energy intakes, consume higher amounts of saturated fat, and have higher cholesterol intakes than children in higher-income households.

EFFECTS OF WIC PROGRAM PARTICIPATION

Through the provision of supplemental nutritious foods, nutrition education, and health and social service referrals, the WIC program is expected to improve the nutrition status of low-income women, infants, and children by addressing the risk factors for poor outcomes. Evidence on poverty and nutrition risk for pregnant women and infants, in conjunction with fairly convincing evidence of the positive effects of the WIC program on perinatal outcomes and the prevalence of iron deficiency anemia, suggests that eligibility for participation in the WIC program could rely solely on income for pregnant women and infants.

Numerous studies have found positive effects of prenatal WIC program participation on perinatal outcomes, although the magnitude of these effects varies owing to differences in methodologic approaches. In particular, controlling for the confounding effects of self-selection in WIC program evaluations has proved to be extremely difficult (Devaney et al., 1992), and virtually no studies have been able to disentangle the impacts of prenatal WIC program participation from those of underlying differences between participants and nonparticipants. By far the most common perinatal outcome examined is birth weight, and most studies find a significant effect of prenatal WIC program participation on birth weight (Devaney et al., 1992; Edozien et al., 1979; Kennedy et al., 1982; Metcoff et al., 1985). Several studies also examined the effects of prenatal participation in the WIC program on health care costs after birth and found substantial savings in Medicaid costs during the first 60 days after birth resulting from participation in the WIC program during pregnancy (Devaney et al., 1990, 1992).

In the National WIC Evaluation, Rush (1988) compared longitudinal data for 5,205 prenatal WIC program participants with those for 1,358 non-WIC program participants at prenatal clinics across the country. The findings for prenatal WIC program participants were as follows: no statistically significant effect on newborn birth weight; increased infant head circumference; increased birth weight and head circumference with better WIC program quality; no statistically significant effect on gestational age; appreciable but not statistically significant reduction in the incidence of fetal death; and increased maternal intakes of protein, iron, calcium, and vitamin C (four of the five nutrients targeted by the WIC program).

In contrast to the large body of literature examining the effects of prenatal participation in the WIC program, fewer studies focus on the effects of WIC program participation on infants and children, and these usually were conducted with small samples of infants and children from local areas. Nevertheless, some of the studies reported positive effects of participation in the WIC program, especially among infants. Data from PedNSS indicate that the prevalence of anemia among low-income children decreased during the 1980s, a finding largely attributed to improvements in iron nutrition status and to the positive effects of the WIC program (Yip et al., 1987, 1992). In the National WIC Evaluation, Rush (1988) found significant effects of participation in the WIC program on children's height and weight-for-height (kg/m^2 among children who had entered the WIC program in utero or by age 3 months). Children's intakes of iron, vitamin C, thiamin, niacin, and vitamin B$_6$ were improved if they participated in the WIC program (Rush, 1988).

The WIC program's priority system is currently designed to serve pregnant women and infants first, then children. As a result, coverage rates among infants and pregnant women whose incomes make them eligible for participation in the WIC program are very high (e.g., an estimated 96 percent of eligible infants participate) (Trippe and Schirm, 1994). In a recent report to the U.S. Congress, the U.S. General Accounting Office (GAO) recommended that pregnancy itself be used as a nutrition risk criterion for low-income women and, on the basis of estimates of program costs and expected benefits, estimated that the federal government would save $24 million if all pregnant women whose incomes made them eligible for the WIC program were served by the program (GAO, 1992).

Subsequently, the additional provision in the legislation reauthorizing the WIC program in 1994 gives the states the option of certifying pregnant women whose incomes make them eligible for participation as presumptively eligible for WIC program services, even if the results from health and nutrition screenings are not known. Screening results, however, must be available within 60 days and must establish nutrition risk.

REFERENCES

Adrian, J., and R. Daniel. 1976. Impact of socioeconomic factors on consumption of selected food nutrients in the United States. Am. J. Agric. Econ. 58:31–38.

Basiotis, P., M. Brown, S.R. Johnson, and K.J. Morgan. 1983. Nutrient availability, food costs, and food stamps. Am. J. Agric. Econ. 65:684–693.

Block, G., and B. Abrams. 1993. Vitamin and mineral status of women of childbearing potential. Ann. N.Y. Acad. Sci. 678:244–254.

Brooks, C.H. 1980. Social, economic, and biologic correlates of infant mortality in city neighborhoods. J. Health Soc. Behav. 21:2–11.

CDC (Center for Disease Control). 1972. Ten-State Nutrition Survey, 1968–1970. III. Clinical, Anthropometry, Dental. DHEW Pub. No. (HSM) 72-8131. Atlanta: CDC.

Center on Budget and Policy Priorities. 1994. Despite Economic Recovery, Poverty and Income Trends are Disappointing in 1993. Washington, D.C.: Center on Budget and Policy Priorities.

Children's Defense Fund. 1991. Child Poverty in America. Washington, D.C.: Children's Defense Fund.

Children's Defense Fund. 1994. The State of America's Children, 1994. Washington, D.C.: Children's Defense Fund.

Cook, J.T., and K.S. Martin. 1995. Difference in Nutrient Adequacy Among Poor and Nonpoor Children. Center on Hunger, Poverty and Nutrition Policy. Medford, Mass.: Tufts University School of Nutrition.

Devaney, B., L. Bilheimer, and J. Schore. 1990. The Savings in Medicaid Costs for Newborns and Their Mothers from Prenatal Participation in the WIC Program, Vol. I. Office of Analysis and Evaluation, Food and Nutrition Service, U.S. Department of Agriculture. Washington, D.C.: U.S. Government Printing Office.

Devaney, B., L. Bilheimer, and J. Schore. 1992. Medicaid costs and birth outcomes: The effects of prenatal WIC participation and the use of prenatal care. J. Policy Anal. Manage. 11:573–592.

DHHS/USDA (U.S. Department of Health and Human Services and U.S. Department of Agriculture). 1986. Nutrition Monitoring in the United States. A progress report from the Joint Nutrition Monitoring Evaluation Committee. DHHS Pub. No. (PHS) 86-1255. Hyattsville, MD: National Center for Health Statistics.

Duncan, G. 1991. The Economic Environment of Childhood. Pp. 23–50 in Children in Poverty: Child Development and Public Policy, A.C. Huston, ed. Cambridge: Cambridge University Press.

Duncan, G.J., J. Brooks-Gunn, and P.K. Klebanov. 1994. Economic deprivation and early childhood development. Child Dev. 65:296–318.

Edozien, J.C., B.R. Switzer, and R.B. Bryan. 1979. Medical evaluation of the Special Supplemental Food Program for Women, Infants, and Children. Am. J. Clin. Nutr. 32:677–692.

GAO (U.S. General Accounting Office). 1992. Early Intervention: Federal Investments Like WIC Can Produce Savings. GAO Pub. No. HRD 92-18. Washington, D.C.: U.S. Government Printing Office.

Gortmaker, S.L. 1979. Poverty and infant mortality in the United States. Am. Sociol. Rev. 44:280–297.

Gould, J.B., and S. LeRoy. 1988. Socioeconomic status and low birthweight: A racial comparison. Pediatrics 82:896–904.

Guendelman, S., and B. Abrams. 1995. Dietary intake among Mexican-American women: Generational differences and a comparison with white non-Hispanic women. Am. J. Public Health 85:20–25.

Hamill, P.V.V., F.E. Johnston, and S. Lemeshow. 1972. Height and Weight of Children: Socioeconomic Status, United States. National Center for Health Statistics. HSM 75-1601. Vital Health Stat. 11(119).

IOM (Institute of Medicine). 1985. Preventing Low Birthweight. Report of the Committee to Study the Prevention of Low Birthweight, Division of Health Promotion and Disease Prevention. Washington, D.C.: National Academy Press.

IOM (Institute of Medicine). 1988. Prenatal Care: Reaching Mothers, Reaching Infants. Report of the Committee to Study Outreach for Prenatal Care, Division of Health Promotion and Disease Prevention. Washington, D.C.: National Academy Press.

IOM (Institute of Medicine). 1993. Iron Deficiency Anemia: Recommendations for the Prevention, Detection, and Management Among U.S. Children and Women of Childbearing Age. Report of the Committee on the Prevention, Detection, and Management Among U.S. Children and Women of Childbearing Age, Food and Nutrition Board. Washington, D.C.: National Academy Press.

Johnson, R.K., H. Guthrie, H. Smiciklas-Wright, and M.Q. Wang. 1994. Characterizing nutrient intakes of children by sociodemographic factors. Public Health Rep. 109:414–420.

Jones, D.Y., M.C. Nesheim, and J-P. Habicht. 1985. Influences in child growth associated with poverty in the 1970s: An examination of HANES I and HANES II, cross-sectional U.S. national surveys. Am. J. Clin. Nutr. 42:714–724.

Kennedy, E.T., S. Gershoff, R. Reed, and J.E. Austin. 1982. Evaluation of the effect of WIC supplemental feeding on birth weight. J. Am. Diet. Assoc. 80: 220–227.

Kim, I., D.W. Hungerford, R. Yip, S.A. Kuester, C. Zyrkowski, and F.L. Trowbridge. 1992. Pregnancy nutrition surveillance system—United States, 1979–1990. Morbid. Mortal. Weekly Rep. 41(SS-7):25–41.

Knox, E.G., T. Marshall, S. Kane, A. Green, and R. Mallett. 1980. Social and health care determinants of area variations in perinatal mortality. Community Med. 2:282–290.

Lewit, E.M. 1993. Child indicators: Children in poverty. Future Child. 3(1):176–182.

Li, J., and N. Bennett. 1994. Young Children in Poverty: A Statistical Update. New York: Columbia University National Center for Children in Poverty.

Lozoff, B. 1990. Has iron deficiency been shown to cause altered behavior in infants? Pp. 107–131 in Brain Behavior and Iron in the Infant Diet, J. Dobbing, ed. London: Springer-Verlag.

Metcoff, J., P. Costiloe, W.M. Crosby, S. Dutta, H.H. Sandstead, D. Milne, C.E. Bodwell, and S.H. Majors. 1985. Effect of food supplementation (WIC) during pregnancy on birth weight. Am. J. Clin. Nutr. 41:933–947.

Miller, J.E., and S. Korenman. 1993. Poverty, Nutrition Status, Growth and Cognitive Development of Children in the United States. Princeton, N.J.: Office of Population Research, Princeton University.

Miller, J.E., and S. Korenman. 1994. Poverty and children's nutrition status in the United States. Am. J. Epidemiol. 140:233–243.

NRC (National Research Council). 1989. Recommended Dietary Allowances, 10th ed. Report of the Subcommittee on the Tenth Edition of the Recommended Dietary Allowances, Food and Nutrition Board, Commission on Life Sciences. Washington, D.C.: National Academy Press.

NRC (National Research Council). 1995. Measuring Poverty: A New Approach. Report of the Panel on Poverty and Family Assistance: Concepts, Information Needs, and Measurement Methods, Committee on National Statistics, Commission on Behavioral and Social Sciences and Education. Washington, D.C.: National Academy Press.

Orshansky, M. 1963. Children of the poor. Social Security Bull. 26:3–13.

Orshansky, M. 1965. Counting the poor: Another look at the poverty profile. Social Security Bull. 28:3–29.

Oski, F.A., and A.S. Honig. 1978. The effects of therapy on developmental scores of iron-deficient infants. J. Pediatr. 92:21–25.

Owen, G.M., K.M. Kram, P.J. Garry, J.E. Lowe, and A.H. Lubin. 1974. A study of nutritional status of preschool children in the United States, 1968–1970. Pediatrics 53:597–646.

Pollitt, E. 1994. Poverty and child development: Relevance of research in developing countries to the United States. Child Dev. 65:283–295.

Ruggles, P. 1990. Drawing the Line: Alternative Poverty Measures and Their Implications for Public Policy. Washington, D.C.: The Urban Institute Press.

Rush, D. 1988. The National WIC Evaluation: An Evaluation of the Special Supplemental Food Program for Women, Infants, and Children. Research Triangle Park, N.C.: Research Triangle Institute.

Starfield, B., S. Shapiro, J. Weiss, K.Y. Liang, K. Ra, D. Paige, and X.B. Wang. 1991. Race, family income, and low birth weight. Am. J. Epidemiol. 134:1167–1174.

Thompson, F.E., and B.A. Dennison. 1994. Dietary sources of fats and cholesterol in U.S. children ages 2 through 5 years. Am. J. Public Health 84:799–806.

Trippe, C., and A. Schirm. 1994. Number of Infants and Children in WIC Income-Eligible Families in 1993 and 1992 Based on March 1994 CPS and Revised March 1993 CPS. Memorandum to Office of Analysis and Evaluation, Food and Nutrition Service, U.S. Department of Agriculture (USDA). Contract No. 53-3198-3-038-243. Washington, D.C.: USDA.

U.S. Bureau of the Census. 1995. Income, Poverty, and Valuation of Non-Cash Benefits: 1993. Current Population Reports, Consumer Income, Series P-60, No. 188. Washington, D.C.: U.S. Government Printing Office.

Wachs, T.D. 1995. Relation of mild-to-moderate malnutrition to human development: Correlational studies. J. Nutr. 125(suppl.):2245S–2254S.

Wilson, A.B. 1981. Longitudinal Analysis of Diet, Physical Growth, Verbal Development and School Performance. Malnourished Children of the Rural Poor. Boston: Auburn House.

Yip, R., N.J. Binkin, L. Fleshood, and F.L. Trowbridge. 1987. Declining prevalence of anemia among low-income children in the United States. J. Am. Med. Assoc. 258:1619–1623.

Yip, R., I. Parvanta, K. Scanlon, E.W. Borland, C.M. Russell, and F.L. Trowbridge. 1992. Pediatric nutrition surveillance system—United States, 1980–1991. Morbid. Mortal. Weekly Rep. 41(SS-7):1–24.

3

Principles Underlying the Nutrition Risk Criteria for WIC Eligibility

The WIC program (Special Supplemental Nutrition Program for Women, Infants, and Children) uses three criteria for program eligibility: (1) categorical status as pregnant, breastfeeding, or postpartum women; infants; or children under age 5 years; (2) income less than or equal to 185 percent of the poverty level (or adjunct eligibility, see Chapter 1); and (3) evidence of nutrition risk. Eligibility on the basis of categorical status is based on the special importance of nutrition during the critical growth and development periods of pregnancy, infancy, and childhood. Eligibility on the basis of income is based on the evidence presented in Chapter 2, which shows that low income predisposes women, infants, and children to both poor nutrition status and poor health outcomes. The WIC program's nutrition risk criteria are intended to target its limited resources to low-income individuals who either already have poor outcomes or are at the greatest risk of poor outcomes.

This chapter presents the committee's underlying principles concerning the use of nutrition risk criteria for eligibility for participation in the WIC program, a description of current WIC nutrition risk criteria, a discussion of the current WIC priority system, and the framework adopted by the committee as the basis for its recommendations for the use of specific nutrition risk criteria.

PRINCIPLES OF NUTRITION RISK ASSESSMENT

Nutrition risk assessment uses a risk criterion. A risk criterion is defined by a risk indicator and a cutoff point. A risk indicator is any measurable characteristic or circumstance that is associated with a poor outcome or an increased likelihood of such outcomes such as poor nutrition status, poor health, or death. Risk indicators may have causal relationships or may merely be associated with poor outcomes. For example, maternal undernutrition, short interpregnancy interval, and poverty are all risk indicators for low birth weight (a poor outcome). Maternal undernutrition (a risk indicator) has a causal linkage with low birth weight. Short interpregnancy interval (a risk indicator) does not itself cause low birth weight but may contribute to maternal nutrition depletion and may therefore contribute to the risk of low birth weight. Similarly, poverty (a risk indicator) is strongly associated with low birth weight, but the linkage is indirect.

Some risk indicators (e.g., homelessness) use categorical or dichotomous cutoff points. Others, such as maternal undernutrition, have no clearly defined threshold, so several factors need to be considered in setting cutoff points, as discussed below.

Purpose of Nutrition Risk Criteria in the WIC Program

To target the limited resources of the WIC program, competent professional authorities assess women, infants, and children who are eligible for participation on the basis of income by using a set of nutrition risk criteria. The committee agreed that the WIC program's nutrition risk criteria should serve two major purposes: (1) *to identify those at nutrition and health risk,* and (2) *to identify those most likely to derive specific health benefits from food, nutrition education, and/or referrals provided through the WIC program.* To identify those at nutrition risk, criteria should select those who have greater need for the services of the WIC program either because they are currently more unhealthy or poorly nourished or because they are at greater risk of future ill health or malnutrition than those excluded by the screening. Moreover, nutrition risk criteria should select those most likely to benefit from the WIC program from among potential participants who are at risk of poor outcomes. In other words, the nutrition risk criteria used in the WIC program should serve both as *indicators of nutrition and health risk* and as *indicators of nutrition and health benefit*. The committee did not consider other uses of these indicators (Habicht and Pelletier, 1990), but it is important to recognize that information obtained from WIC nutrition risk assessments assists in the determination of the content of WIC interventions (food package, nutrition education, and health and social service referrals).

Identifying Nutrition Risk Indicators

The selection of risk indicators requires an examination of the pathways from the determinants to the undesirable outcomes, the intervention points for

WIC program activities, evidence for efficacy of the interventions, and various interactions among determinants and interventions.

For example, suppose a child is not growing properly and it is found that the mother is underweight. If the cause of both the maternal thinness and the child's poor growth is hunger because of destitution, providing food or resources to acquire food will address the problem. If the cause of the mother's thinness is a lack of appetite resulting from drug abuse and the child's poor growth is due to neglect, then focusing on the mother's drug abuse may improve the child's growth. If the cause of the mother's thinness is tuberculosis that infected her child and resulted in poor child growth, then curing the child's tuberculosis is the solution to curing the poor growth. Curing the mother's tuberculosis in the first place, however, would have prevented the child's infection. Finally, if the cause of the mother's thinness is chronic malnutrition that led to an undersized newborn with poor growth potential but the mother is feeding her child adequately now, none of the WIC program's interventions will improve the child's growth. However, the low birth weight likely would have been prevented if the mother had consumed a better diet during pregnancy.

Examination of causal pathways and possible interventions is a key step in identifying risk indicators that predict nutrition and health risk. In the example given above, one such indicator is maternal thinness. However, this indicator alone does not provide sufficient information to determine whether a child will benefit from a given intervention to prevent or cure poor child growth. Information from other indicators can help determine which children might experience improved growth from WIC program participation. Thus, use of more than one indicator may help to identify those with potential to benefit.

Requiring that an indicator be in the pathway between a cause and a biologic impact is compatible with a preventive program, but that requirement may be too narrow. An indicator may be distantly related to the causal pathway and still be an excellent targeting indicator. In the previous example, with maternal underweight as an indicator of risk of poor child growth, one of the pathways was not causal. Maternal underweight was only a proxy for a mother at risk of neglecting her child because of drug abuse.

In another example, short stature of immigrant women whose growth was stunted in their own childhood may be an excellent indicator of mothers who may benefit during pregnancy and whose children may benefit thereafter from participation in the WIC program. These immigrants are likely to be poor, often have other family members who are ill, and need to be informed to make the most of their resources in an unfamiliar country. The WIC program can be an effective intervention to prevent poor nutrition and ill health among these women and their children. Both short stature and potential to benefit from WIC program participation are independently related to recent immigration, but there is no causal link between them. Furthermore, no interventions will affect maternal stature.

A priori theoretical considerations for identifying predictors of health benefit sometimes fail. Criteria may not predict benefit because those who could most benefit from a program do not participate. Such was the case for a recently completed smoking cessation trial, in which the heavy smokers benefited less from the intervention than less heavy smokers (COMMIT Research Group, 1995). The best risk indicator for the ill effects of smoking was heavy smoking, whereas the best predictor of benefit from a smoking cessation intervention was light to moderate smoking.

At other times, the biological basis may differ from the intuitive explanation. For example, Winkvist (1992) found that malnourished, thin pregnant women who weighed the least showed no weight gain from an improved diet, in contrast to a considerable weight gain in less malnourished, thin women. This is because the beneficial effects of improved diets are deflected to the fetus in the more malnourished women. Moreover, this finding implies that low prepregnancy weight may be a poor predictor of maternal weight response to food supplementation during pregnancy, but it may be a good predictor of improved birth weight. Thus, the actual responsiveness of an indicator to interventions should not always be viewed as a proxy for the indicator's ability to predict nutrition or health benefit. This example shows that it is important to consider all outcomes in selecting an indicator of benefit. In this case, improvements in the diets of severely malnourished pregnant women result in clear benefits to the fetus.

Setting Cutoff Points for Nutrition Risk Indicators

Once a risk indicator is chosen as a predictor of nutrition and health benefit, a cutoff point for the indicator is set at the level below (or above, depending upon the indicator) which individuals are eligible for participation in the WIC program.

In general, more stringent cutoff points can be chosen to increase the potential of risk indicators to select those individuals who will benefit. This increase occurs for two reasons. The first relates to the degree of risk. In general, the greater the risk predicted by an indicator, the greater the expected nutrition and health benefit for the individual chosen (see above for some exceptions). As an extreme example, moderate thinness, reflecting moderate malnutrition, may predict that the woman will become more physically active if she becomes better nourished, whereas severe thinness, reflecting severe malnutrition, may predict that she will avoid death if she becomes better nourished. Preventing death is a greater benefit than increasing physical activity. Thus, the more stringent a cutoff point—that is, the further a cutoff point is from the average for a healthy person—the greater the likely benefit to the individual.

The second reason for increased potential to benefit with more stringent cutoffs points relates to yield. The term *yield* is used to identify the percentage who will actually experience nutrition and health benefit of those individuals selected by a risk indicator and its cutoff point.[1] By moving the cutoff point toward levels that predict worse conditions, the *percentage* of those chosen who will benefit will be greater. As the cutoff point is made progressively more stringent, it will reach a point such that all those chosen will benefit—a perfect yield of 100 percent.

Increasing the yield of nutrition risk criteria helps target scarce resources. A perfect yield occurs at any cutoff point at which all of those selected for participation in the WIC program can benefit and nobody who cannot benefit is selected. A perfect yield, however, means that there is a high likelihood that many who could benefit are not selected. Identification of all who could benefit is called perfect *sensitivity* of the risk assessment. Ideally, the value of the cutoff point would be set so that as many as possible who could benefit would be served (high sensitivity) and most of those served would experience nutrition and health benefit (high yield).

In general, there is a trade-off between yield and sensitivity. For example, consider the risk criterion for a child's poor growth, as defined by height-for-age less than the 5th percentile according to standard growth references.[2] Low height-for-age, also called stunting, is generally considered to reflect long-term nutrition status. Setting the cutoff point at the 5th percentile has implications for both sensitivity and yield. Only children with height-for-age at or less than the 5th percentile would be selected. Sensitivity is imperfect (< 100 percent) if some children who are taller than the cutoff point are still smaller than their genetic potential. These stunted children would not be selected by the 5th percentile cutoff point, yet they could benefit from better nutrition and, consequently, participation in the WIC program.

The yield using this cutoff point may also be quite low. Estimates of the prevalence of height-for-age less than the 5th percentile among low-income children in the United States range from 6 to 7 percent (Yip et al., 1992). As-

---

[1] A similar concept is called the *positive predictive value* (Last, 1988) when it is applied to an indicator predicting the risk of death or the presence of disease. However, because of the confusion that arises when the term *positive predictive value* is applied to predict a benefit instead of a risk, the committee concluded that the concept of *yield* is easier to grasp in the sense that moving the cutoff point toward a higher level of prediction of benefits yields a greater percentage of those who can benefit. For simplicity, in this report, the committee calls the positive predictive value of risk the yield of risk and differentiates between the yield of risk and the yield of benefit.

[2] All reference standards are imprecise, and those used in this example have been well enough studied so that the imprecisions are recognized (e.g., Gorstein et al., 1994).

suming that 5 percent of healthy, well-nourished children have height-for-age less than the 5th percentile, then only 1 to 2 percent of the low-income children are actually stunted, resulting in a yield of risk of only 17 percent (1/6) to 29 percent (2/7). If the cutoff point is increased to the 10th percentile, the sensitivity of the higher cutoff point is higher: additional children who are stunted will be selected by the more generous cutoff point. However, the yield of the risk criterion will decline, since fewer of the additional children selected are stunted and therefore will not experience improved growth from participation in the WIC program. In contrast, if the cutoff point is lowered to the 2nd percentile, the yield will improve (more of those selected could benefit from improved nutrition), but the sensitivity will decline (a larger number of children who could benefit are above the cutoff point and will not be selected).

Thus, the yield of a risk criterion increases with the prevalence of the risk in the population. For instance, using the above example of the cutoff point at the 5th percentile of height-for-age, if 30 of 100 children were below the cutoff point, the number of children with stunted growth would be 25 (30 − 5), and the yield will be 83 percent (25/30). It is therefore important to monitor the prevalence of changing risk conditions, including medical conditions and social conditions such as homelessness, and to make changes in the WIC program nutrition risk criteria as appropriate. Possible changes in response to the changing prevalence of risks include adding new risk indicators, for example, homelessness, or changing cutoff points, for example, moving the cutoff point for height-for-age below the 5th percentile as the prevalence of poor growth declines.

The WIC program typically uses several risk criteria in addition to the income screen to determine eligibility for participation in the program. For instance, adding hemoglobin assessments to anthropometric assessments will identify anemic children who are not identified by slow growth. If this process identifies more individuals who can benefit without increasing the percentage who cannot, the yield will not decrease, and such a combination of risk criteria also improves sensitivity.

It is usually impossible to achieve both perfect sensitivity (identification of all who could benefit) and maximum yield (of those selected, all could benefit). The question, then, is how to choose the best cutoff point. When resources are sufficient to serve everybody selected, the cutoff point with perfect sensitivity is the logical cutoff point. A less stringent cutoff point would not be scientifically justified because it would decrease the yield without increasing the sensitivity. However, any cutoff point with perfect sensitivity includes a high percentage of individuals who will not benefit.

If resources are limited, however, cutoff points should be set with less than perfect sensitivity to increase yield—recognizing that as the cutoff points become more restrictive, some individuals who could derive nutrition and health benefits from participation in the WIC program will not be served. In general, cutoff points should be chosen so that the highest percentage of those selected are at risk and can benefit from WIC program services. This most efficient cutoff point will nevertheless include a number of participants who will not benefit (false positives) and will exclude some who can benefit (false negatives). The numbers of false positives and false negatives can be reduced by using improved criteria or combinations of criteria, but they can never be reduced to zero. Excessive lowering of cutoff points to reduce false positives would be counterproductive, since it would prevent access to services by many who truly need them. It must be recognized that unmet needs of prevention or cure that result from imperfect sensitivity may have costs that would outweigh the costs of providing services to the false positives if sensitivity were improved. This would be a strong argument for increasing resources to the WIC program to increase overall coverage. However, such considerations are beyond the purview of this report.

In evaluating the use of nutrition risk criteria in the WIC program, it is important to note that the *yield of a risk criterion* refers to the yield of benefit and is actually the product of the *yield of risk* and the *efficacy* of the WIC program for individuals with that risk:

Yield of benefit =
[Yield of risk] × [The proportion of individuals truly at risk who will benefit from the WIC program]

That is, the yield of risk is the percentage of those truly at-risk who are identified at risk by the risk criterion. These truly at risk people are individuals who would be sure to have a bad outcome without intervention. The proportion of those at risk who will benefit from the WIC program is the *efficacy* of the WIC program for individuals with that risk. (See Appendix D for more detailed information.)

Nutrition risk criteria can vary considerably in these two components. In the United States, some anthropometric criteria (e.g., low height-for-age) have poor yields in terms of identifying those at risk but good yields in terms of benefiting those truly at risk. Other nutrition risk criteria (e.g., homelessness and overweight) have good yields in terms of identifying those with the risk but poor or unknown yields in terms of benefiting those at risk. Overall yield of benefit will be very low if the yield of risk and the efficacy are both low.

It might appear from the above discussion that the criteria with the highest risk yield will also have the highest benefit yield for the same outcome, intervention, and sensitivity. This is not necessarily the case. Recent research involving length and weight at age 3 months shows that length is the better predictor of deficits in adult stature that are due to childhood malnutrition. However, weight is the better predictor of response of stature to an improved diet (Ruel et al., in press). This finding means that the two different indicators have different yields for deficits in stature that are preventable by better diet. The intervention had better efficacy for those deficits in stature that were predicted by weight than for those predicted by length.

WIC NUTRITION RISK CRITERIA

According to federal regulation, each participant in the WIC program must be determined to be at nutrition risk on the basis of a medical and/or nutrition assessment by a competent professional authority. At a minimum, federal regulations require that the following nutrition and health data be collected on each potential participant: height or length, weight, and a hematologic test for anemia (hematocrit, hemoglobin, or free erythrocyte protoporphyrin concentration). Hematologic tests are not required for infants under 6 months of age. For pregnant women, this minimum set of nutrition and health information must be collected during pregnancy and, if the woman was given presumptive eligibility, within 60 days from prior certification. Collection of data on women certified as postpartum or breastfeeding must be collected after they give birth (7 CFR, Subpart C, Section 246.7(d)(1)). At the state or local agency's discretion, the blood test is not required for children who were determined to be within the normal range at their last program certification, but it must be performed every 12 months.

WIC program regulations define nutrition risk as shown in Table 3-1.

PRIORITY SYSTEM OF THE WIC PROGRAM

Because the WIC program is not an entitlement program, participation is limited by funding levels, which have never been adequate to serve all eligible applicants. Once a local agency is serving its maximum caseload, federal regulations require that a waiting list of eligible applicants be maintained. As program openings become available, they are to be filled from the waiting list according to a seven-point priority system.

Federal regulations specify a seven-point priority system, in which all priorities are related to nutrition risk (Table 3-2). Priorities I through VI are used by all states. State WIC agencies may, at their discretion, expand the priority system to include Priority VII. Individuals who qualify for participation in the WIC program under Priority I are served first, then those in Priority II, and then in each subsequent priority, until program resources are exhausted. A state WIC agency may also assign subpriorities within each of the seven priority levels. In general, priority is given to anthropometric, hematologic, and clinical evidence

TABLE 3-1 Nutrition Risk Criteria Defined by WIC Program Regulations

Conditions Detectable by Biochemical or Anthropometric Measurements:
- anemia
- underweight
- overweight
- abnormal patterns of weight gain in a pregnant woman
- low birth weight in an infant
- stunting in an infant or child

Other Documented Medical Conditions:
- clinical signs of nutrition deficiencies
- metabolic disorders
- preeclampsia in a pregnant woman
- failure to thrive in an infant
- chronic infections in any person
- alcohol or drug abuse or mental retardation in women
- lead poisoning
- history of high-risk pregnancies or factors associated with high risk-pregnancies (such as smoking; conception before 16 months postpartum; history of low birth weight; premature births, or neonatal loss; adolescent pregnancy; or current multiple pregnancy)
- congenital malformations in infants or children
- infants born to women with alcohol or drug abuse histories or mental retardation

Dietary Nutrition Risk Criteria:
- inadequate dietary patterns assessed by a 24-hour dietary recall, dietary history, or food frequency checklist

Predisposing Nutrition Risk Criteria:
- homelessness or migrancy

SOURCE: 7 CRF Subpart C, Section 246.7 (e)(2).

of medically based nutrition risks over dietary-based nutrition risks; to pregnant and breastfeeding women and all infants over children; and to children over postpartum women[3] (7 CFR Subpart C, Section 246.7 (d)(4)).

The use of a priority system of risk criteria can help to achieve the highest yield in the face of limited program resources. For the system to be most effective, nutrition risk criteria that have high yield would be given priority in assigning eligibility. The WIC priority system reflects a preference for

---

[3] Furthermore, local agencies whose caseloads force them to serve only individuals given the top priorities frequently serve children according to age. Some clinics serve children who are 1 to 2 years of age but not children 3 years of age and older, or some agencies serve participants up to 12 months of age and then serve them only one certification period beyond their first birthday, up to 18 months of age.

TABLE 3-2 The WIC Priority System

Priority	
I	Pregnant and breastfeeding women and infants at nutrition risk as demonstrated by anthropometric or hematologic measurements or by other documented nutrition-related medical condition.[a]
II	Infants up to 6 months of age whose mothers participated in the WIC program during pregnancy or who would have been eligible to participate under Priority I.[a]
III	Children at nutrition risk, as demonstrated by anthropometric or hematologic measurements or other documented medical condition. At the state's option, this priority can also include high-risk postpartum women.
IV	Pregnant and breastfeeding women and infants at nutrition risk as demonstrated by inadequate dietary pattern. At the state's option, this priority can also include high-risk postpartum women or pregnant or breastfeeding women and infants who are at nutrition risk solely because of homelessness or migrancy.
V	Children at nutrition risk because of inadequate dietary pattern. At the state's option, this priority can also include high-risk postpartum women or children who are at nutrition risk solely because of homelessness or migrancy.
VI	Postpartum women, not breastfeeding, at nutrition risk on the basis of either medical or dietary criteria, unless they are assigned to higher priorities at the state's discretion. This priority, at the state's option, may also include postpartum women who are at nutrition risk solely because of homelessness or migrancy.
VII	Individuals certified for WIC program participation solely because of homelessness or migrancy and, at the state agency option, previously certified participants whose nutrition status is likely to regress without continued provision of supplemental foods.

[a] A breastfeeding mother and her infant shall be placed in the highest priority level for which either is qualified.

SOURCE: 7 CRF Subpart C, Section 246.7(d)(4), and *Federal Register*, April 19, 1995, 60(75):19, 487–419, 491.

biologically measurable indicators of risk that respond to the WIC program intervention and that are in the causal pathway from the determinant to the undesirable outcome.

Several issues need to be considered in interpreting the nutrition risks used in the WIC priority system. First, most biologically measurable indicators (e.g., low hemoglobin concentration) that respond to WIC program benefits (e.g., iron-fortified foods) are evidence of pathology (e.g., anemia) and are therefore indicators for a curative and not a preventive program. The high priority that the WIC program gives these indicators is in concert with the policy that curing the present ill is generally to be given a higher priority than preventing a future ill. However, the WIC program also is supposed to be preventive so that it is not faced with curing problems that it could have prevented. If a high percentage of the WIC program resources is taken up in curing problems, the WIC program will be unable to fulfill its preventive role.

Second, there may be different degrees of risk within a priority category. Many states recognize this and set subpriority levels within any given priority category. For example, hemoglobin or hematocrit measurements may serve to assign subpriority risk levels that differentiate among individuals with varying risks of anemia. The WIC priority system generally does not operate such that a high subpriority condition in priority level VI, for example, would be served in preference to a low subpriority condition in priority level V.

A final issue to consider in the context of the WIC priority system is the dual objective of a preventive and curative program. Some state WIC agencies have set nutrition risk criteria with the intent of selecting both those who have the condition and those who might develop the condition if not given WIC program benefits. Criteria for anemia fall in this category. However, generous cutoff points do not necessarily achieve this goal. The committee affirms the importance of primary prevention and suitable methods to identify those at risk of developing health and nutrition problems. However, it believes that more work is needed to find the best methods for achieving this.

When resources are limited and not all individuals eligible for participation can be served, it is important that the criteria in the highest priority levels have the highest overall yields possible. That is, the overall yield in Priority I should be higher than the overall yield in Priority II, and so on. It is likely that some of the predisposing nutrition risk indicators at current low priority levels—e.g., homelessness—may have higher overall yields than some medical risk indicators in Priority I—for example, asymptomatic bacteriuria as a renal medical risk for pregnant woman. With the current priority system, an overweight child who may not actually benefit would be served in preference to a homeless child who would be more likely to benefit from participation in the WIC program.

SUMMARY AND IMPLICATIONS

In summary, the best criteria for targeting WIC program benefits are those that most closely predict a potential nutrition and health benefit from these interventions. Theoretical considerations in choosing indicators, such as how close they are in the causal pathway to the outcome to be prevented, are less important than how well the indicator actually targets those who will benefit from the intervention. However, very few indicators used in the WIC program or elsewhere have been examined for this characteristic. In the meantime, the decision of which criteria to use must be based on the degree to which the criterion is both an indicator of risk and, theoretically, also an indicator of potential benefit. The risk criteria—that is, the risk indicators and their cutoff points—should be chosen and prioritized such that a high percentage of those truly at risk will be selected and a high percentage of those selected can benefit.

In the discussion in the subsequent chapters of this report, the committee examines the association between the risk indicators and nutrition and health outcomes in situations similar to those encountered by WIC program participants. Then, the committee examines why, in theory, these risk indicators might be indicators of potential benefit. In addition, empirical evidence of the ability to predict a benefit, if such evidence exists, is presented. In many cases, the discussion focuses on evidence of efficacy of the WIC program only since no information about yield of benefit is available. Based on this framework, the committee makes recommendations for each of the nutrition risk criteria reviewed. The following decision process underlies these recommendations:

- For nutrition risk criteria for which there is good evidence of both nutrition and health risk and benefit from the WIC program, the committee recommends use of these criteria by all state WIC programs.
- For nutrition risk criteria for which the risk indicator is a predictor of both nutrition and health risk and benefit from the WIC program but for which cutoffs have been set so that many individuals selected are not truly at risk, the committee recommends using the risk indicator with more stringent cutoff values.
- For risk criteria for which there is strong evidence of nutrition and health risk but uncertain evidence of benefit, the committee recommends using the nutrition risk criteria and conducting further research on the benefit from the WIC program.
- For risk criteria for which there is good evidence of nutrition and health risk and benefit from the WIC program but poor ability to identify those with the condition, the committee recommends that action be taken to develop better assessment tools. Pending this assessment, the committee recommends using the best available methods to identify the condition, using scientifically justifiable cutoff values.
- For risk criteria for which there is strong evidence of nutrition and health risk but no direct or indirect evidence of benefit, either theoretical or empirical, the committee recommends discontinuing use of these criteria.
- For risk indicators with weak evidence of risk or benefit, the committee recommends discontinuing use of these criteria.

The WIC program is a broad-based and comprehensive food and nutrition program with three main components: (1) supplemental foods, (2) nutrition education, and (3) referrals to health care and social service providers. Thus, evidence of benefit from the WIC program, either theoretical or empirical, could be from any of the three program components. In making its recommendations for each nutrition risk criterion, however, the committee decided that evidence of benefit from the WIC program should reflect the ability of an individual with that risk to benefit from the WIC food package or, in some cases, from nutrition education.

Benefit from only the referral services of the WIC program was not considered sufficient to justify the use of a nutrition risk criterion. Three main reasons for this decision follow: (1) the provision of supplemental foods and nutrition education account for nearly all the WIC program costs; (2) it is difficult to justify the provision of a monthly food package worth approximately $30 per WIC participant unless there is evidence that the individual can benefit from the food package or the nutrition education that accompanies the provision of food; and (3) the WIC program is designed to be only an adjunct to good health care and is not itself a health program.

REFERENCES

COMMIT Research Group. 1995. Community Intervention Trial for Smoking Cessation (COMMIT). I. Cohort results from a four-year community intervention. Am. J. Public Health 85:183–192.

Gorstein, J., K. Sullivan, R. Yip, M. de Onis, F. Trowbridge, P. Fajans, and G. Clugston. 1994. Issues in the assessment of nutritional status using anthropometry. Bull World Health Organ. 72:273–283.

Habicht, J-P., and D.L. Pelletier. 1990. The importance or context in choosing nutritional indicators. J. Nutr. 120:1519–1524.

Last, J.M. 1988. A Dictionary of Epidemiology. London: Oxford University Press.

Ruel, M.T., J-P. Habicht, K. Rasmussen, and R. Martorell. In press. Screening for interventions: The risk or benefit approach? Am. J. Clin. Nutr.

Winkvist, A. 1992. Maternal Depletion Among Pakistani and Guatemalan Women. Ph.D. Dissertation, Cornell University, Ithaca, N.Y..

Yip, R., I. Parvanta, K. Scanlon, E.W. Borland, C.M. Russell, and F.L. Trowbridge. 1992. Pediatric nutrition surveillance system—United States, 1980–1991. Morbid. Mortal. Weekly Rep. 41(SS-7):1–24.

4

Anthropometric Risk Criteria

This chapter provides information about anthropometric characteristics of women, infants, and children that are used to place them in Priorities I through III in the WIC program (biochemical and other medical risk criteria in Priorities I through III are in Chapter 5). It begins with a consideration of the use of reference anthropometric measures. Then, it covers anthropometric criteria used for pregnant or postpartum women, followed by risk criteria used for infants and children. For each risk criterion, available information is provided about the prevalence of the condition in the population eligible for participation in the WIC program, use of each criterion as an indicator of risk and a predictor of benefit, and cutoff points in use in WIC programs nationwide. A summary of anthropometric risk criteria used by state WIC agencies appears in Table 4-1.

USE OF ANTHROPOMETRIC MEASURES IN THE WIC PROGRAM

The major uses of anthropometric measures in the WIC program are twofold: (1) to screen women, infants, and children with nutrition risks for certification to participate in the program and (2) to assess their responses to interventions over time. Their use to assess individuals has several implications for interpreting results and choosing cutoff points.

First, a woman or child's position relative to the reference standard for the anthropometric measure being evaluated, whether it is expressed as a percentile or a z-score, represents a statement of the probability that the individual is part of the healthy distribution (also called specificity). It is not a statement about the probability that the mother or child is unhealthy. The farther away a

TABLE 4-1 Summary of Anthropometric Risk Criteria in the WIC Program and Use by States

	States Using Pregnant Women	Postpartum Women Lactating	Postpartum Women Nonlactating	Infants	Children
Women					
Prepregnancy underweight	54	18	15	—	—
Low maternal weight gain	53	—	—	—	—
Maternal weight loss during pregnancy	33	—	—	—	—
Prepregnancy overweight	53	17	12	—	—
High gestational weight gain	37	38	15	—	—
Maternal short stature	0	1	1	—	—
Postpartum underweight	—	43	43	—	—
Postpartum overweight	—	42	39	—	—
Infants and Children					
Low birth weight	—	—	—	53	8
Small for gestational age	—	—	—	10	—
Short stature	—	—	—	48	50
Underweight	—	—	—	53	52
Low head circumference	—	—	—	7	—
Large for gestational age	—	—	—	14	—
Overweight	—	—	—	53	49
Failure to thrive	—	—	—	30	27

NOTE: Dashes indicate criterion was not used for that subgroup.

SOURCE: Adapted from USDA (1994).

measurement is from the central part of the distribution of healthy individuals, the greater the likelihood that it indicates health and nutrition disorders. As described in Chapter 3, yield for a given cutoff point increases with prevalence. If the assessed population were exactly the same as the healthy reference population, then one would expect, for example, that 5 percent of children would have heights at or below the 5th percentile. If a screened population has an excess of children with height-for-age below a cutoff point (e.g., 10 percent below the 5th percentile), one could assume that at least the difference (10 minus 5 equals 5 percent) represents short stature resulting from environmental causes, including diet.

Most anthropometric measurements that are below the 5th or the 10th percentile or above the 95th percentile are considered abnormal. These statistical cutoffs define the central 85 or 90 percent of the reference distribution as the normality range. For some anthropometric measures, such as maternal weight gain, recommended cutoffs reflect an even smaller portion of the distribution. These cutoffs do not truly define the normal range from a health or nutrition point of view; rather, they are used as a guide to facilitate clinical assessment (IOM, 1990).

It is impossible to find a cutoff that has both the highest sensitivity and the highest yield (Rasmussen and Habicht, 1989), as discussed in Chapter 3. When interventions have no adverse effects, the choice of cutoff points for defining risk depends mainly on the available resources and the priorities to be addressed.

However, if factors causing decreased nutrition status tend to affect all mothers or children in the population, *all* individuals can be assumed to be malnourished (Keller, 1988; Yip, 1993), and selection of a specific cutoff point may be irrelevant. Experience shows that in populations with high prevalences of both short stature and underweight children, major causes of such abnormalities are usually health and nutrition. Likewise, low maternal prepregnancy weight or weight gain in pregnancy may result from a variety of factors, but populations with high prevalences of both are often malnourished.

Although anthropometry has widely been used as a measure of or proxy for various conditions related to health and nutrition, abnormal anthropometric measures themselves do not provide specific etiologic information. For example, a child may be abnormally short because of infection, inadequate food intake, psychological disorders, endocrine or metabolic diseases, or simply normal variation in a population.

Finally, although most anthropometric criteria are able to predict some present or future risk, they may not be indicative of a possible response to or benefit from participating in the WIC program. Indicators of risk and indicators of benefit are not always identical. As discussed in Chapter 3, for the best use of WIC program resources, one should use benefit indicators and cutoff points to target services to those individuals who are likely to benefit. For most anthropometric criteria, a positive response can be viewed as a benefit from participation in the WIC program.

All the anthropometric measurements covered in this chapter are practical and can be obtained with reliability in the WIC program setting with adequate training of personnel, periodic quality assurance reviews, and use of appropriate equipment that is calibrated regularly.

MATERNAL ANTHROPOMETRIC RISK CRITERIA

A summary of anthropometric risk criteria as predictors of risk and benefit for pregnant and postpartum women appears in Table 4-2.

Prepregnancy Underweight

Prepregnancy underweight is defined as a prepregnant weight below a certain cutoff point based on reference data of desirable weights for nonpregnant women of the same height. Weight alone is not a very sensitive measure of maternal body size: at the same weight, a tall woman may be underweight, while a short woman, overweight (IOM, 1990). Thus, weight-for-height status is a better way of assessing women for poor health and nutritional status, although still crude and indirect. The lower a woman's weight-for-height, the more likely it is that she is undernourished (IOM, 1990).

Maternal prepregnancy weight-for-height is usually defined in one of two ways: (1) weight below a designated percentage of a reference standard or (2) body mass index (BMI = kg/m^2) below a specified cutoff. Although reference standards for women have not been validated specifically in relation to reproduction, prepregnancy underweight has been defined as less than 90 percent of the 1959 Metropolitan Life Insurance weight value for a given height

TABLE 4-2 Summary of Anthropometric Risk Criteria as Predictive of Risk or Benefit Among Pregnant and Postpartum Women

			Postpartum Women			
	Pregnant Women		Lactating		Nonlactating	
Risk Criterion	Risk	Benefit	Risk	Benefit	Risk	Benefit
Prepregnancy underweight	✓	✓	?	?	?	?
Low maternal weight gain	✓	✓	✓	✓	?	?
Maternal weight loss during pregnancy	✓	✓				
Prepregnancy overweight	✓	✓	?	?	?	?
High gestational weight gain	✓	✓	?	?	✓	✓
Maternal short stature	✓	0	?	?	?	?
Postpartum underweight			✓	✓	?	?
Postpartum overweight			✓	✓	✓	✓
Abnormal postpartum weight change	?	?	?	?	?	?

NOTE: ✓ = predictive of risk or benefit; ? = evidence unclear; 0 = evidence but no effect; blank = not applicable to that group.

(ideal body weight, or IBW), which is equivalent to a BMI of less than 19.8 (IOM, 1990). This definition has been widely adopted in the United States (e.g., ACOG, 1993; Wilcox and Marks, 1995) and is used in this chapter unless otherwise noted.

Prevalence of and Factors Associated with Prepregnancy Underweight

Underweight may be associated with poverty, substandard living conditions, inadequate food intake, chronic or infectious diseases, or conditions that induce malabsorption of nutrients (IOM, 1990). Using the above cutoff value, 20 percent of the low-income women included in the 1990 Pregnancy Nutrition Surveillance System (PNSS) data set were underweight, and 6 percent of these PNSS women were classified as being very underweight (BMI < 18.0) (Wilcox and Marks, 1995). The percentage of underweight women decreased as age increased, with the highest prevalence of underweight observed among Asian women (Wilcox and Marks, 1995). White adolescents, in particular, may routinely attempt to limit their body weights by restricting their dietary intakes and exercising excessively (Larson, 1991). Substance abuse is also associated with low prepregnancy weight-for-height (Johnson et al., 1994). However, some women may be healthy and well nourished, but simply lean.

In a study of about 600 WIC program participants in California who were followed through two consecutive pregnancies, the most important factor predicting a low prepregnancy weight-for-height at the beginning of the second pregnancy was low prepregnancy weight in the first pregnancy (Caan et al., 1987). As household size increased, the risk of prepregnancy underweight decreased. Maternal age was inversely associated with prepregnancy underweight, and black race was associated with increased risk, but these findings did not quite reach statistical significance ($p < .07$ and $p < .09$, respectively).

Prepregnancy Underweight as an Indicator of Nutrition and Health Risk

Compared with women with normal weight-for-height, women with low prepregnancy weight-for-height are at higher risk for low-birth-weight (LBW) infants (Brown and Schloesser, 1990; Elkblad and Grenman, 1992; IOM, 1990; Nandi and Nelson, 1992; WHO, 1995), retarded fetal growth (Abrams, 1991; Elkblad and Grenman, 1992; Kramer, 1987a, b), and perinatal mortality (Hogberg et al., 1990; IOM, 1990).

Some studies have found that prepregnancy underweight is associated with a higher incidence of various pregnancy complications, such as antepartum hemorrhage, premature rupture of membranes, anemia, endometritis (IOM, 1992b), and cesarean delivery (Elkblad and Grenman, 1992), but the small number of studies examining this question limits the ability to draw inferences.

The relationship between maternal underweight and preterm delivery (delivery before 37 weeks' gestation) is controversial, with some reports concluding that the relationship is strong and others finding no significant association (Berkowitz and Papiernik, 1993).

The committee could find no studies assessing whether prepregnancy underweight is associated with increased risk for poor lactational performance or poor health during the postpartum period. This is a complicated question to address, because it is also necessary to consider the potential mediating influence of gestational weight gain.

Prepregnancy Underweight as an Indicator of Nutrition and Health Benefit

Data from several food supplementation trials have demonstrated that intervention to improve nutrition can increase birth weight in underweight women (Edozien et al., 1979; IOM, 1990). Two evaluations of the Missouri WIC program separately examined the impact of WIC program participation in underweight women. Schramm (1986) reported that participants who were at least 15 percent underweight before pregnancy had significantly lower Medicaid paid claims for newborn medical services than did nonparticipants. However, using another sample of Missouri WIC participants, Stockbauer (1987) reported that WIC program participation was not associated with significantly lower rates of LBW in women who began pregnancy at least 10 percent underweight. Neither of these studies adjusted for gestational weight gain. Providing WIC program benefits to underweight women is likely to reduce the rate of LBW even if only a subset of underweight women respond, because prepregnancy underweight is a prevalent condition among low-income American women.

In the study by Caan and colleagues (1987), receiving WIC program benefits after the first pregnancy was associated with a decreased risk of maternal underweight, but this finding was not statistically significant.

Results of recent studies suggest that maternal underweight may be associated with poor fetal growth because of poor plasma volume expansion early in pregnancy (Rosso et al., 1992) or because of interaction among low prepregnancy weight, psychosocial stress, and cigarette smoking (Cliver et al., 1992). With improved understanding of the complex mechanisms by which maternal underweight influences fetal growth, it may become possible to target those underweight women who will readily benefit from WIC program participation.

The committee identified no data addressing the efficacy of maternal prepregnancy underweight as a nutrition risk indicator for either breastfeeding or postpartum nonlactating women. Since gestational weight gain may change a woman's weight category after delivery, postpartum weight-for-height is a more relevant indicator of maternal nutritional status for lactating or postpartum women.

ANTHROPOMETRIC RISK CRITERIA 73

Use of Prepregnancy Underweight as a Nutrition Risk Criterion in the WIC Setting

Table 4-1 summarizes the extent to which prepregnancy underweight is used as a nutrition risk criterion by the WIC program. The ideal weight-for-height cutoffs ranged from 85 to 95 percent.

Recommendations for Prepregnancy Underweight

The risk of *prepregnancy underweight* is well documented for pregnant women but not for postpartum women. There is both empirical evidence and a theoretical basis for benefit from participation in the WIC program. Therefore, the committee recommends use of *maternal prepregnancy underweight* as a nutrition risk criterion for pregnant women by the WIC program, with a cutoff value of 90 percent of IBW or a BMI less than 19.8. The committee recommends discontinuation of the use of *maternal prepregnancy underweight* as a nutrition risk criterion for postpartum women by the WIC program.

The committee recommends research to determine the cutoffs for underweight that would produce the highest yield for reproductive outcomes and to improve the ability to distinguish healthy, well-nourished, slender women from women who are underweight because of poor nutrition or other factors that could be ameliorated through WIC program participation.

The committee also recommends studies to examine interventions aimed at improving maternal health, lactation performance, or other postpartum outcomes for women who had low prepregnancy weight-for-height.

Low Maternal Weight Gain

Low maternal weight gain is often defined in relation to the lower limits of the Institute of Medicine's (IOM) BMI-specific total weight gain recommendations: less than 12.5 kg for women who begin pregnancy with a low BMI (< 19.8), less than 11.5 kg for women with a normal BMI (19.8–26.0), and less than 7 kg for those with a high BMI (> 26.0 to 29.0) or obese BMI (> 29.0) (IOM, 1990). Because total gain is not known until delivery, weight gain during the second and third trimesters is substituted. The IOM (1990) recommended cutoffs of less than 0.45 kg/month in obese women and less than 0.9 kg/month in nonobese women. These recommendations, as well as "provisional" weight gain grids, were provided with the acknowledgment that validated data on which to provide confident recommendations were not available. A slightly lower than recommended gain is not necessarily a problem, provided that weight gain appears to progress toward the BMI-specific target (IOM, 1990). Before intervening, further evaluation is recommended to rule out measurement error, assess health and nutrition status, and consider other possible explanations for the low gain.

Little is known about the prevalence of a low maternal weight gain assessed during gestation, but approximately 39 percent of the women included in the 1990 PNSS had a total gain that was less than the lower limit recommended for their prepregnant BMI category (Wilcox and Marks, 1995).

Prevalence of and Factors Associated with Low Maternal Weight Gain

The published literature consistently shows that maternal weight gain is highly variable. A low gestational weight gain occurs most commonly among women with a high prepregnancy BMI, especially those who are obese (IOM, 1990). This lower gain may reflect intentional weight restriction on the part of the mother, but low rates of weight gain also occur in settings in which *all* women were encouraged to gain weight (Taffel et al., 1993). Conversely, many other obese women experience high rates of gestational weight gain.

Among married mothers delivering live singleton infants who participated in the 1980 National Natality Survey, a total maternal weight gain of less than 6.8 kg was associated with maternal short stature, cigarette smoking, black race, Hispanic ethnicity, low levels of maternal education, and high maternal BMI (IOM, 1990; Kleinman, 1990).

Southeast Asian background, young maternal age (within 2 years of menarche), multiparity, unmarried status, and low income have also been associated with an increased risk of low total maternal weight gain in U.S. women (IOM, 1990). Physical activity, work outside the home, stress, or moderate alcohol use appear to have little effect on gestational weight gain in U.S. women (IOM, 1990), but data are limited. The 1990 PNSS reported that Asian and American-Indian women were the ethnic/racial groups most likely to have a low total gestational weight gain, but maternal age was not a risk factor for a low weight gain (Wilcox and Marks, 1995).

The use of illegal drugs, especially cocaine, is associated with low maternal weight gain (Petitti and Coleman, 1990). The literature does not give a clear answer as to whether cigarette smokers tend to gain less weight than nonsmokers during pregnancy (Johnston, 1991).

Data are not available to assess whether older age (> 35 years) affects weight gain beyond the contributions of increased parity or BMI. One report on the determinants of weight gain in a small group of black adolescents concluded that delayed enrollment in the WIC program (late in pregnancy) and consumption of less than three snacks per day were significant predictors of a slow gestational weight gain (Stevens-Simon and McAnarney, 1992).

Recent results from a multiethnic cohort study of about 10,000 pregnancies concluded that maternal height, hypertension, cesarean delivery, and fetal size were positively associated with the maternal weight gain in each of the three trimesters. However, association with weight gain differed by trimester for prepregnancy body size, age, parity, smoking status, race/ethnicity, and diabetes mellitus (Abrams et al., 1995). The most important predictors of weight gain were maternal age and Asian race or ethnicity in the first trimester; prepregnant body mass, parity, and height in the second trimester; and hypertension, age, and parity in the third trimester.

Low Maternal Weight Gain as an Indicator of Nutrition and Health Risk

The IOM (1990) concluded that low maternal weight gain during the second and third trimester is a determinant of fetal growth, and that low maternal gain is associated with smaller average birth weights and an increased risk of delivering an infant with fetal growth restriction. Studies published since that report confirm this finding (Hickey et al., 1993; Parker and Abrams, 1992; Scholl et al., 1990a). In the recently conducted World Health Organization (WHO) collaborative meta-analysis of studies from populations around the world, low maternal weight gain or low maternal attained weight at 20, 28, or 36 weeks' gestation was associated with increased risk of fetal growth restriction or an infant small for gestational age (SGA). Odds ratios were especially high for women with low prepregnancy weights (WHO, 1995). Attained weights at 20, 28, and 36 weeks predicted LBW and SGA with reasonable sensitivity (at least 35 percent) and odds ratios of about 2.5 (WHO, 1995). However, two studies of presumably well-nourished clinic populations reported that low total maternal weekly weight gain (Dawes and Grudzinskas, 1991a) or deviation from an "optimal curve" (Theron and Thompson, 1993) had relatively low specificity and yields as predictors of SGA. Low yields are not surprising given that fetal growth is multifactorial, and total maternal weight gain by healthy pregnant women with good pregnancy outcome is highly variable (Abrams and Parker, 1990).

The relationship between low maternal weight gain and small fetal size is modified by maternal prepregnancy BMI. At high BMIs, a low maternal weight gain has less impact. However, there is also evidence that a low maternal weight gain (< 6.8 kg) is associated with an increased risk of delivering infants who are SGA (Parker and Abrams, 1992). Thus, low rates of gestational weight gain remain a concern, even among obese women. Overall, women with both a low gestational weight gain and a low prepregnancy BMI are at highest risk for delivering a low-birth-weight infant.

Studies of preterm delivery usually express total weight gain as a rate of weight gain (total gain/gestational age) to adjust for gestation. Although several studies suggested that a low weekly rate of maternal weight gain throughout pregnancy is associated with early spontaneous delivery, the data could be considered only suggestive, especially given difficulties in accurately determining gestational age (IOM, 1990). Studies published in the 1990s tend to support a relationship between low rate of maternal weight gain and preterm birth (Hickey et al., 1995; Kramer et al., 1992; Siega-Riz et al., 1994; Wen et al., 1990; WHO, 1995).

Effects of the specific pattern of maternal weight gain on fetal size or preterm delivery are under study. Some investigators provide evidence that a low maternal weight gain early in pregnancy is significantly related to low-birth-weight infants (Scholl et al., 1990a) and infants who are SGA (Abrams and Newman, 1991); others do not agree (Dawes and Grudzinskas, 1991b; Petitti et al., 1991). A recent study of almost 3,000 white women concluded that, after controlling for total maternal weight gain and other factors, a low gestational weight gain during the second trimester was associated with decreased birth weight (Abrams and Selvin, 1995). At least three studies suggest that a low rate of maternal weight gain late, but not early, in pregnancy is associated with spontaneous preterm delivery (Abrams et al., 1989; Hediger et al., 1989; Hickey et al., 1995).

Some studies have also found associations of a low maternal weight gain with neonatal complications. A study of low-income, black adolescents reported that a slow rate of maternal weight gain (< 0.23 kg per week) was associated with longer infant hospital stays, more admissions to the neonatal intensive care units, and more antibiotic treatments (Stevens-Simon and McAnarney, 1992). Fetal or infant mortality appears to be higher in women with low rates of weight gain (Hogberg et al., 1990), and the relationship is particularly strong in women with low prepregnancy weights-for-height (IOM, 1992b; Johnson, 1991).

It is postulated that nutrition during pregnancy may play a role in the development of long-term health conditions in the offspring during childhood or adulthood. In support of this, Godfrey and co-workers (1994) found that a low maternal triceps skinfold thickness at 15 weeks of gestation and a low weight gain from 15 to 35 weeks of gestation were associated with higher blood pressure in the offspring at about 11 years of age. This is an area of active investigation.

Maternal weight gain may relate to other health outcomes in pregnancy or postpartum, but few data have been published. A Finnish study reported that women with low gestational weight gain (< 5 kg) had fewer deliveries requiring surgery and a shorter second stage of labor (Elkblad and Grenman, 1992). Little is known about the effects of low rates of gestational weight gain on spontaneous abortion, congenital malformations, maternal complications, or the long-term health of the mothers. Gestational weight gain does not appear to be associated with the volume or composition of breast milk for women residing in industrialized countries (Dewey et al., 1991a; IOM, 1990). However, a recent study of well-nourished lactating Danish women reported that women who gained more than 17 kg produced milk with a much higher fat concentration than did women with a low (< 11 kg) prenatal weight gain (Michaelson et al., 1994).

Low Maternal Weight Gain as an Indicator of Nutrition and Health Benefit

Studies to examine whether low maternal weight gain is a useful indicator of nutrition and health benefit are hindered by problems in study methodology, difficulties in estimating dietary intake accurately, and low statistical power (IOM, 1990). The great variability among women in such characteristics as energy requirements, physical activity, body size, and health practices also complicates understanding of the relationship.

Most experimentally designed studies have been conducted in developing countries and have demonstrated that dietary supplementation can improve infant birth weight, especially in women with the poorest nutritional status (IOM, 1990). However, relatively few experimental nutrition supplementation trials have specifically examined effects of such supplementation on maternal weight gain. Although the results of those studies tend to show that supplementation improves both maternal weight gain and infant birth weight, results have been inconclusive. Furthermore, the link between energy supplements and gestational weight gain is weaker among women in industrialized countries, presumably because of lesser degrees of malnutrition before and during pregnancy.

Observational studies have reported on the relationship between dietary intake and maternal weight gain, with conflicting results (IOM, 1990). Gestational weight gain, but not dietary intake, was strongly associated with birth weight in a study of 529 primarily white, middle-class women (Aaronson and Macnee, 1989). No statistically significant relationships between dietary intake and birth weight were detected in a recent study of black inner-city women (the relationship between diet and weight gain was not reported) (Johnson et al., 1994). In pregnant adolescents, Scholl and colleagues (1991) reported a significant association between energy intake early in pregnancy and total weight gain. They also reported a relationship between gestational weight gain and infant birth weight, but the relationship between energy intake and birth weight was not significant. Kramer (1993) reported only slight effects of protein and energy intake on maternal weight gain. However, Susser's review of data from the Dutch famine and supplementation trials concluded that dietary influences on birth weight appear to bypass gestational weight gain (Susser, 1991).

Of the three WIC program evaluations that have reported on the program's impact on maternal weight gain, two suggest a positive effect. The first National WIC Evaluation (Edozien et al., 1979) showed associations between food supplementation of more than 3 months and increases in both maternal weight gain and birth weight. Results of the second National WIC Evaluation (Rush et al., 1988c) suggested that WIC supplemented mothers consumed more energy and gained more weight; although birth weight was not improved overall, fetal head circumference was greater. Of special note is the significant finding in this study that WIC program participation reversed initial low maternal weight gain identified at the time of the first visit to the WIC program. WIC program participation was also associated with lower maternal fat stores late in pregnancy. Newer evidence suggests that maternal fat mobilization in late pregnancy reflects improved fetal growth (Hediger et al., 1994). The single randomized controlled trial of the WIC program, which has been criticized for its small sample size (Kramer, 1993), did not show improvements in either maternal weight gain or birth weight with WIC program participation overall, but improvements were observed in smokers and members of other higher-risk subgroups (Metcoff et al., 1985).

In addition to providing food supplements, the WIC program also provides education with the objective of improving maternal anthropometric status and infant outcomes. Observational studies have correlated advice about weight gain with actual prenatal weight gain (Taffel et al., 1993) and dietary counseling and milk vouchers with improved dietary scores (Mendelson et al., 1991). A recent meta-analysis identified only three experimental trials assessing the impact of providing maternal education or counseling with the goal of increasing maternal energy or protein intake (Kramer, 1993). The single study that specifically evaluated gestational weight gain as an outcome reported that those who received nutrition education gained on average 1 kg more than those who did not. There was not a significant increase in birth weight in this study, possibly because the study subjects were not at nutritional risk. In another critical review of the experimental studies of nutrition education during pregnancy, it was determined that the literature was so sparse and poorly designed that it was difficult to determine whether interventions were effective (Boyd and Windsor, 1993).

Nonetheless, increases in the official recommendations for weight gain during pregnancy in the United States have been accompanied by a 50 percent increase in the average amount of weight gained by pregnant women (IOM, 1990). Thus, practical experience suggests that pregnant women respond to the advice that they are given.

Use of Low Maternal Weight Gain as a Nutrition Risk Criterion in the WIC Setting

Definitions of inadequate weight gain during pregnancy vary widely among the 53 state WIC agencies (see Table 4-1) that use this risk criterion. Specified cutoff values for rate of weight gain range from 0.7 kg per month to 1.8 kg per month in the last two trimesters. Some states compare pattern of gain against a weight gain chart (presumably similar to that recommended by the IOM).

Recommendations for Low Maternal Weight Gain

The risk of *low maternal weight gain* is well documented in pregnant women. There is both empirical evidence and a theoretical basis for benefit from participation in the WIC program. Therefore, the committee recommends use of *low maternal weight gain* as a nutrition risk criterion for pregnant women by the WIC program, with the IOM cutoff values of < 0.9 kg/month in nonobese women and < 0.45 kg/month in obese women.

The committee also recommends research to define low weight gain throughout gestation in relation to reproductive and longer-term outcomes, its yield as a indicator of risk, and its response to WIC program intervention.

Maternal Weight Loss During Pregnancy

Weight loss can occur any time during a pregnancy. A woman can have a net loss by the time she delivers, or her weight can fluctuate up and down periodically.

Prevalence of and Factors Associated with Maternal Weight Loss During Pregnancy

Although it is uncommon for a woman to experience a net loss in weight by the time that she delivers, it is not uncommon for a woman to lose some weight, especially during the first trimester. No data are available on the prevalence of this occurrence.

Maternal Weight Loss During Pregnancy as an Indicator of Nutrition and Health Risk

Most of the studies that examine weight loss during pregnancy do so in women experiencing hyperemesis gravidarum (severe nausea and vomiting of pregnancy). Gross and colleagues (1989) found that women who lost more than

5 percent of their prepregnancy weight in the first trimester had lower total weight gains, were more likely to deliver by cesarean section, and had infants who had lower mean birth weights and more growth retardation. The study's findings are interesting but should be viewed with caution because the sample size was small (64) and the analyses were bivariate.

Maternal Weight Loss During Pregnancy as an Indicator of Nutrition and Health Benefit

The committee could identify no studies examining interventions to address maternal weight loss. Weight loss may indicate underlying dietary or health practices or health or social conditions that could be improved by the supplemental food, nutrition education, and referrals provided by the WIC program.

Use of Maternal Weight Loss During Pregnancy as a Nutrition Risk Criterion in the WIC Setting

Of the 33 state WIC agencies that reported using weight loss as a nutrition risk criterion (see Table 4-1), the most common cutoff values were any weight loss or weight falling below the self-reported prepregnancy weight.

Recommendation for Maternal Weight Loss During Pregnancy

The risk of *weight loss during pregnancy* is documented. There is a theoretical basis for pregnant women to benefit from participation in the WIC program. Therefore, the committee recommends use of *weight loss during pregnancy* as a risk criterion for pregnant women by the WIC program, with a cutoff value of greater than 2 kg during the first trimester and greater than 1 kg during the second or third trimesters.

Prepregnancy Overweight

The definitions used to define excess body weight vary substantially throughout the scientific literature and in clinical and public health practice. The terms *obesity* and *overweight* are often used interchangeably to describe a high weight-for-height. The IOM (1990) defined overweight as a BMI range of 26 to 29 kg/m^2 (consistent with 120 to 135 percent of the 1959 Metropolitan Life Insurance Company weight-specific tables) and obesity as a BMI of > 29 kg/m^2 (consistent with > 135 percent of IBW on the basis of the same reference).

Prevalence of and Factors Associated with Prepregnancy Overweight

Data from the third National Health and Nutrition Examination Survey (NHANES III; 1988–1991) indicate that with a BMI cutoff of 27.3 kg/m^2, 20 and 34 percent of women age 20 to 29 and 30 to 39 years, respectively, were overweight (Kuczmarski et al., 1994). Furthermore, comparison of these data with findings from previous national surveys showed a dramatic trend upward. For example, by using the same definition of overweight for all surveys, the prevalence of overweight among women 20 to 29 years of age was only 10 percent in 1960–1962, but it increased to 13 percent in 1971–1974 and then to 15 percent in 1976–1980.

Obesity is especially common among minority women and is associated with lower levels of education, lower income, and increasing age (Flegal et al., 1988). Data from the 1990 PNSS indicate that 29 percent of the low-income women had a prepregnancy BMI greater than 26.0 kg/m^2, and 19 percent were classified as very overweight (BMI > 29.0 kg/m^2) (Wilcox and Marks, 1995). Older women and American-Indian women were most likely to be overweight. Another report of PNSS data from 1990 and 1991 indicated that very overweight (BMI > 29 kg/m^2) women were more likely to be black and older than 35 years and were less likely to report smoking or alcohol use than women who were of normal weight or overweight (Cogswell et al., 1995).

In a study of about 600 WIC program participants in California who were followed through two consecutive pregnancies, the following characteristics were significantly associated with increased risk of beginning the second pregnancy with a high maternal prepregnancy weight-for-height (> 120 percent of IBW): high prepregnancy weight-for-height during the first pregnancy, high birth weight of the first infant, and large number of individuals in the household. In that multiethnic study, Southeast Asian and black mothers were at lower risk of high second prepregnancy weight (Caan et al., 1987).

Prepregnancy Overweight as an Indicator of Nutrition and Health Risk

Although consistent evidence indicates that, on average, obese women have larger babies than women of lower weight-for-height, they are at substantially increased risk of delivering macrosomic infants (Larsen et al., 1990), a condition accompanied by higher risks of shoulder dystocia and morbidity in the mother or fetus (Elkblad and Grenman, 1992; IOM, 1990; Issacs et al., 1994; Perlow et al., 1992). The risk of delivering LBW infants is controversial for obese women. Some studies suggest that obesity is protective against LBW (Johnson et al., 1992); others report risks comparable to those in nonobese women; and still others suggest that obesity is associated with increased risk for delivering growth-retarded infants (Perlow et al., 1992), especially if gestational weight gain is low (Hickey et al., 1993; Parker and Abrams, 1992).

Relatively few studies have assessed the relationship between maternal obesity and the risk of spontaneous preterm delivery. Siega-Riz and colleagues (1994) noted a clear but nonsignificant trend toward a decreased risk of preterm delivery with increasing BMI. However, in the Collaborative Perinatal Project, Naeye (1990) found obese women to be at increased risk for preterm delivery and for higher perinatal mortality rates. Other investigators (Abrams and Parker, 1988; Lucas et al., 1988; Rahaman et al., 1990; Taffel, 1986) also reported higher perinatal mortality rates among obese mothers. Using data from the National Natality Survey, Little and Weinberg (1993) found that obesity was more strongly related to stillbirth in the intrapartum period (during labor and delivery) than in the antenatal period (before labor), perhaps because of the mechanical problems of delivery.

Gestational diabetes, non-insulin-dependent diabetes mellitus, and hypertension are significantly more likely in obese women (Issacs et al., 1994; Perlow et al., 1992; Ratner et al., 1991). Obese women may also be at increased risk for developing preeclampsia (Eskenazi et al., 1991; Sibai et al., 1995). Labor and delivery complications are more common among overweight women than among their normal weight counterparts (Elkblad and Grenman, 1992; IOM 1990, 1992b). Most studies report a two- to threefold risk for cesarean delivery among overweight women (Elkblad and Grenman, 1992; Issacs et al., 1994; Perlow et al., 1992; Ratner et al., 1991; Witter et al., 1995), and several studies have reported a statistically significant increase in the number of infections such as endometritis (Issacs et al., 1994; Perlow et al., 1992).

Maternal obesity may be associated with an increased risk for major congenital malformations (undefined, in aggregate) (Naeye, 1990). A recent study also suggested that obese women had twice the risk of delivering children with neural tube defects and certain other major birth defects (Waller et al., 1994).

Prepregnancy overweight is thought to be a risk factor for postpartum retention of prenatal weight gain (Parker, 1994). In the 1988 National Maternal and Infant Health Survey, 20 percent of women with normal prepregnancy weight-for-height reported that they retained the weight they gained during pregnancy (defined as > 4 kg at 10 to 18 months postpartum), whereas 38 percent of the women whose prepregnancy weight-for-height was classified as overweight reported retaining their prenatal weight gain (Keppel and Taffel, 1993).

Prepregnancy Overweight as an Indicator of Nutrition and Health Benefit

Although several dietary intervention studies have been conducted with the goal of restricting maternal food intake and minimizing weight gain and excessive fetal size, the safety and effectiveness of this approach are questionable (Abrams, 1988). Clinical trials of energy and protein restriction among women who have either a high weight-for-height or a high gestational weight gain have produced nonsignificant results, in opposite directions (Kramer, 1993). Two small studies have demonstrated that overweight women can be motivated to change their diets, but neither study had a control group (Dornhurst et al., 1991; Mendelson et al., 1991).

Participation in the WIC program has been associated with significantly lower rates of LBW in overweight women (> 120 percent IBW) (Stockbauer, 1987). However, Schramm (1986) reported that WIC program participation was not associated with significantly lower Medicaid claims for newborns among women who began pregnancy at > 120 percent of their IBW.

Virtually no studies have been published with the explicit objective of evaluating how WIC program participation affects maternal obesity. However, a study in California comparing women participating in the WIC program who received food supplementation during two consecutive pregnancies found that women who received supplementation for 5 to 7 months postpartum had half the risk of being overweight of those who received supplementation only briefly (Caan et al., 1987). Although the study was observational rather than experimental, it was very well designed. The investigators attributed the finding to supplementation with more nutrient-rich foods from the WIC program—an action that might reduce the consumption of inexpensive, high-calorie, low nutrient foods.

A technology assessment panel for the National Institutes of Health concluded that most people desiring to lose and control weight need to make a lifelong commitment to changes in lifestyle, dietary practices, and behavioral responses (NIH Technology Assessment Conference Panel, 1992). Current guidelines for prenatal care call for individualized nutrition counseling for obese mothers. The objective is to promote adequate nutrient intake and maternal weight gain to meet the needs of the growing fetus while minimizing the risk of increasing obesity in the mother (IOM, 1992a). The receipt of nutritious foods, counseling, and education through the WIC program both before and after delivery, with or without lactation, has the potential to modify diet and activity patterns and thereby to reduce long-term obesity.

Use of Prepregnancy Overweight as a Nutrition Risk Criterion in the WIC Setting

Table 4-1 summarizes the extent to which prepregnancy overweight is used as a nutrition risk criterion. Most states used a cutoff point of 120 percent of IBW for height, but the range for cutoff points went from a low of 110 percent to a high of 150 percent of IBW.

Recommendations for Prepregnancy Overweight

The risk of *prepregnancy overweight* is well documented for pregnant and postpartum women. There is both empirical evidence and a theoretical basis for benefit from WIC program participation. Therefore, the committee recommends use of *prepregnancy overweight* as a nutrition risk criterion for pregnant and postpartum women by the WIC program, with the cutoff values of BMI greater than 26. To improve potential for benefit from WIC program participation, the committee recommends research on culturally appropriate methods of effective intervention for obese women.

High Gestational Weight Gain

Definitions of *excessive gestational weight gain* that depend on knowledge of total weight gain are not practical in the WIC setting. There are no scientifically determined definitions of high weight gain at various points of pregnancy that are linked to reproductive or other health outcomes. The IOM (1990) recommended that a gain of more than 3 kg per month be considered potentially excessive, especially if it occurs during the second half of pregnancy. However, it is important to rule out other explanations (e.g., measurement error, fluid changes, multiple gestation) before concluding that excessive weight gain resulted from problems related to nutrient intake and energy balance.

Prevalence of and Factors Associated with High Gestational Weight Gain

Data from the 1990 PNSS indicate that 33 percent of these low-income women had total gestational weight gains that surpassed the upper limit of that recommended for their prepregnancy BMI category (Wilcox and Marks, 1995). Thus, high maternal weight gain is one of the most common nutritional problems occurring in U.S. pregnant women today. The committee could find no reports of the prevalence of excessive weight gain identified during pregnancy.

Compared to research on the determinants of low gestational weight gain, little is known about the women with high gestational gain. Data on married women in the 1980 National Natality Survey suggest that white women were more likely than black women to gain > 16 kg, which is the upper limit advised for normal weight women (IOM, 1990); however, among participants in the 1990 PNSS, black and Hispanic women were more likely to have a high total gestational weight gain than were Asian women (Wilcox and Marks, 1995).

High Gestational Weight Gain as an Indicator of Nutrition and Health Risk

Very high gestational weight gain is associated with increased rates of high birth weight or macrosomia (Cogswell et al., 1995; IOM, 1990). In adolescents, high maternal weight gain at 16 weeks of gestation or later was associated with a doubled risk of macrosomia (Scholl et al., 1990b). An increased risk for cesarean deliveries among women with large gestational weight gains (Elkblad and Grenman, 1992; Johnson et al., 1992; Parker and Abrams, 1992) is seen even after adjusting for birth weight. However, in adolescents, Stevens-Simon and McAnarney (1992) found that high weight gain was associated with complications in the newborn rather than the mother. These investigators reported that fetal distress, meconium aspiration, antibiotic use, and stays in the neonatal intensive care unit were more likely among the infants of mothers with high rates of weight gain (> 0.59 kg/week). After adjusting for several other risk factors, Johnson and co-workers (1992) noted that meconium staining (but no other neonatal complications) was more common among the offspring of mothers with high rates of weight gain. A very high rate of maternal weight gain may be associated with spontaneous preterm delivery (Siega-Riz et al., 1994; Wen et al., 1990).

Although a high maternal weight gain is a hallmark of developing preeclampsia, evidence suggests that it results from rather than causes this condition (IOM, 1990).

Postpartum weight retention is probably the most frequently studied outcome related to excessive weight gain. Evidence reviewed by the IOM (1990) and from the 1988 National Maternal and Infant Health Survey (NMIHS) suggests that women who exceed the upper limit of IOM weight gain recommendations are significantly more likely to retain weight after delivery, with black women twice as likely as white women to retain excess weight (Keppel and Taffel, 1993; Parker and Abrams, 1993). Among low-income black adolescents (who are at increased risk of obesity), those with high gestational weight gain were more likely than those with low weight gain to retain extra weight early in the postpartum period (Stevens-Simon and McAnarney, 1992).

High Gestational Weight Gain as an Indicator of Nutrition and Health Benefit

An observational study by Cogswell and co-workers (1995) suggests that limiting total gestational weight gain for very overweight women to 11 kg might reduce the risk of delivering infants with macrosomia. Few data are available to assess whether interventions to reduce excessive maternal weight gain are effective. Two clinical trials of energy and protein restriction among women who either had a high weight-for-height or a high gestational weight gain had nonsignificant results, but in opposite directions (Kramer, 1993). In a third study, a small group of pregnant women with gestational diabetes were able to follow the controlled energy (1,200- to 1,800-kcal) diet that was prescribed for them during late pregnancy. That intervention led to lower maternal weight gain and fewer macrosomic infants (Dornhurst et al., 1991). However, the study had no control group, and it is not known whether women without diabetes would be as willing to change their behaviors.

Evidence that women who participated in the WIC program postpartum began their subsequent pregnancies less overweight suggests that women with high prenatal weight gains may benefit from WIC program participation during the postpartum period especially (Caan et al., 1987). The WIC program provides highly nutritious food, counseling, and education to postpartum women with the objective of supporting behaviors that can produce a healthy weight over the long term. This is especially important for women who seek to reduce their weight while maintaining successful lactation.

Use of High Gestational Weight Gain as a Nutrition Risk Criterion in the WIC Setting

Table 4-1 summarizes the extent to which high gestational weight gain is used as a nutrition risk criterion. There is little consistency in the cutoff points, which range from a low of 1.8 kg/month to a high of 4.5 kg/month.

Recommendations for High Gestational Weight Gain

The risk of *high gestational weight gain* is well documented for pregnant and postpartum women. There is a theoretical basis and limited empirical evidence for benefit from WIC program participation. Therefore, the committee recommends use of *high maternal weight gain* as a nutrition risk criterion for pregnant and postpartum women by the WIC program, with the IOM cutoff values of greater than 3 kg per month during pregnancy and the BMI-specific upper limits for total weight gain for postpartum women.

The committee also strongly recommends research to identify valid cutoff values for high weight gain during pregnancy. It further recommends testing interventions to protect fetal growth while preventing excessive maternal weight gain, as well as strategies to address excessive weight gain in the postpartum period.

Maternal Short Stature

Maternal short stature may be primarily genetically determined, but it also may reflect nutrition deprivation that occurred during the mother's growth when she was in utero or during childhood (e.g., stunting). No methods are available to differentiate these two etiologies, but a social, medical, and family history may be instructive. A cutoff point of 157 cm has been recommended to define maternal short stature (IOM, 1990).

Prevalence of and Factors Associated with Maternal Short Stature

Data from national surveys indicate that the proportion of U.S. women ages 18 to 24 years with short stature decreased from about 25 percent in the early 1960s to about 17 percent in the early 1970s. In the late 1970s, the prevalence increased to 18 percent (IOM, 1990). Current estimates were not available.

A history of low socioeconomic status, large family size, exposure to malnutrition, chronic disease, and exposure to emotional or psychological stresses are factors associated with short stature in adults (Mascie-Taylor, 1991). Short stature is more prevalent in women of Asian and Hispanic background and among recent immigrants to the United States (Rimoin et al., 1986).

Maternal Short Stature as an Indicator of Nutrition and Health Risk

Some studies suggest that maternal height is positively associated with the birth weight of the offspring, even after considering maternal weight (Abrams, 1991; Luke et al., 1993), but other investigators report that the relationship of maternal height and birth weight is mediated through maternal weight (Krasovec and Anderson, 1991). Women with short stature are at increased risk of delivering infants who are SGA or growth-retarded (Abrams and Newman, 1991; Kramer, 1987b; Wen et al., 1990). In some populations, a statistically significant association between short stature and increased risk of spontaneous preterm delivery has been reported (Kramer et al., 1992; Wen et al., 1990) but not consistently (Abrams et al., 1989; Kramer, 1987b). Data from developing and industrialized countries suggest that maternal short stature is associated with increased perinatal mortality (Krasovec and Anderson, 1991). Analysis of data from the 1980 National Natality Survey and National Fetal Mortality Survey found no association between maternal height and stillbirth (Little and Weinberg, 1993).

Although women with short stature in the 1980 National Natality Survey gained about 1 kg less than taller women during pregnancy, after controlling for other variables, short stature was not associated with an increased risk of a low maternal weight gain (Kleinman, 1990).

Women with short stature appear to be at increased risk for labor abnormalities and cesarean delivery because of cephalopelvic disproportion (IOM, 1990; Johnson et al., 1992).

Maternal Short Stature as an Indicator of Health and Nutrition Benefit

Although it is not possible to affect maternal short stature, interventions may still affect the outcomes of pregnancy.

The environmental disadvantages that caused stunting in a woman with short stature during her own development may also limit fetal growth during her pregnancies (Baird, 1977; Luke et al., 1993; Ounsted and Ounsted, 1968). If transfer of nutritional stress across generations actually exists, then interventions designed to improve fetal growth as much as possible, such as improved nutrition through food supplementation during pregnancy, might break the cycle. However, the effect of food supplementation on birth weight did not differ by maternal stature in a Guatemalan women study (Habicht and Yarbrough, 1980), and the committee identified no WIC program evaluations that examined women with short stature in particular.

Even if an intervention were shown to increase birth weight in the pregnancies of women who are stunted, appropriate application of the intervention would be a challenge. It would be difficult to target those women whose short stature resulted from stunting rather than genetics. Also, because short stature is associated with an increased risk of cephalopelvic disproportion, the benefits of increased birth weight must be counterbalanced against the potential for increased morbidity to mother and infant caused by difficulties during labor and delivery.

Use of Maternal Short Stature as a Nutrition Risk Criterion in the WIC Program

In 1992, no state WIC agency used maternal short stature as a nutrition risk criterion for pregnant women (see Table 4-1). One of 45 state agencies used short stature in combination with low prepregnancy weight as a nutrition risk criterion for breastfeeding and nonlactating, postpartum women.

Recommendations for Maternal Short Stature

The risk of *maternal short stature* is well documented for pregnant women. There is no empirical evidence or theoretical basis for benefit from participation in the WIC program on the basis of short stature alone. Thus, until there is evidence that the adverse outcomes associated with short stature can be alleviated through intervention during pregnancy, the committee does not recommend that *maternal short stature* be used as a nutrition risk criterion for pregnant women by the WIC program.

Nonetheless, evaluating short stature among women has clinical utility for both assessment for increased risk of poor intrauterine growth and individualizing maternal weight gain recommendations (short pregnant women are advised to gain at the lower end of the recommended weight gain range [IOM, 1990]). Height in combination with a social and nutrition history may be useful in identifying women who were stunted as children, and this information may be useful in tailoring specific educational or social service interventions for WIC program participants. This may be especially true for subgroups of women who were at risk for malnutrition earlier in their lives, such as recent immigrants.

Postpartum Underweight

Reference standards that take time since delivery into consideration are not available for identifying whether breastfeeding or nonlactating, postpartum women are underweight. It has been estimated that on average, a woman will lose about 5 kg immediately after delivery of the infant and the products of conception and another 2 to 3 kg during the next few weeks postpartum, primarily because of diuresis (Prichard et al., 1985). The pattern of weight loss after this interval depends on how much weight was gained during pregnancy, the composition of the gestational weight gain (for example, whether there was a higher proportion of fluid or fat), maternal diet, exercise, and method of infant feeding. Maternal weight loss after delivery varies greatly, with some women falling well below their prepregnancy weights shortly after birth and others never losing much of the weight they gained.

Prevalence of and Factors Associated with Postpartum Underweight

Virtually nothing is known about the prevalence of low maternal weight-for-height in either lactating or nonlactating U.S. mothers after delivery. In a study of women who were not obese before pregnancy and who delivered living, singleton, term infants, about 25 percent of the respondents reported weights 10 to 18 months postpartum that were below the prepregnancy weights that they reported at the same time (Keppel and Taffel, 1993). The extent to which these postpartum weights would qualify as underweight was not reported.

Predictors of low postpartum weight-for-height have not been reported. On a theoretical basis, the following factors might be associated with low weight-for-height status in a postpartum woman, regardless of infant feeding method: inadequate diet during pregnancy, low prenatal weight gain, low prepregnancy weight-for-height, infections including human immunodeficiency virus infection, inadequate food availability or intentional dieting after pregnancy, excessive energy expenditure, and psychological conditions that impair appetite or food behaviors, including eating disorders and depression.

Postpartum Underweight as an Indicator of Nutrition and Health Risk

Low maternal weight-for-height during the postpartum period is of concern because it may indicate poor energy stores or the lack of replenishment of maternal nutrient stores that were mobilized during pregnancy. Low maternal weight-for-height may also indicate that a mother is not consuming an adequate amount of food to meet her energy needs.

Breastfeeding is a robust process, even in seriously malnourished women. The major predictor of successful lactation is the infant's demand for milk (IOM, 1991). Although some studies in developing countries suggest that underweight women may produce a lower volume of milk, the findings are complex to interpret and are not consistent (IOM, 1991). The nutrition risk of postpartum underweight is greater to the breastfeeding mother than to the infant if the mother consumes less energy than required to cover her increased needs.

In a study of well-nourished women in the United States, Nommsen and co-workers (1991) reported that the lipid content of human milk was positively associated with increased maternal weight-for-height, but only during the second 6 months of lactation. They suggested that the underlying relationship between percentage of IBW and the fat content of human milk becomes apparent only after women have depleted the fat that they stored during pregnancy (Nommsen et al., 1991).

Postpartum Underweight as an Indicator of Health and Nutrition Benefit

It is assumed that adequate nutrition during the postpartum period helps the mother to cope with intense physical and emotional demands as she recovers from pregnancy and delivery, breastfeeds her infant, adapts to new motherhood, and provides infant care.

For breastfeeding mothers, the nutrition needs of lactation require special consideration. Because women with a low weight-for-height probably have low fat stores, which are ordinarily mobilized to help meet the extra energy costs of lactation, it is reasonable to expect them to benefit from the supplemental foods provided by the WIC program.

Studies of chronically undernourished Guatemalan women suggest that energy supplements offered during the postpartum period can buffer maternal nutrition stresses associated with concurrent lactation and pregnancy or short interconceptional periods (Marchant et al., 1990). Furthermore, provision of supplemental energy to this population throughout two consecutive pregnancies and the period of lactation between them was associated with large increases in birth weight not seen when supplements were provided only during pregnancy. Although maternal underweight per se was not the focus of those studies, it is likely that the majority of women included in the studies had low postpartum weight-for-height (Villar and Rivera, 1988).

No studies have been reported addressing the efficacy of postpartum interventions to improve the maternal or infant health or nutrition specifically in underweight postpartum women and their infants living in the United States. However, a well-designed evaluation of the postpartum component of the WIC program suggests that the provision of WIC program benefits during the postpartum period is associated with better maternal and infant health (Caan et al., 1987). Circumstances at that time created a natural experiment in which postpartum participants were either served or not served by the WIC program on the basis of geographic, policy, and agency factors rather than individual maternal factors. The extended feeding group received WIC program benefits for 5 to 7 postpartum months, whereas the comparison group's benefits were terminated within 2 months after delivery. Both groups participated in the WIC program during both a first pregnancy and a subsequent pregnancy and delivered within 3 years of the first one.

After adjusting for differences between the groups, extended feeding was associated with significantly improved fetal size at the end of the second pregnancy: weight at birth was increased by 131 g and length at birth was extended by 0.3 cm. The increased risk of delivering a low-birth-weight infant in the comparison group versus that in the extended feeding group approached statistical significance. Extended postpartum feeding was associated with improved prepregnancy weight at the beginning of the second pregnancy among women who began their first pregnancy underweight (< 90 percent IBW), suggesting that postpartum supplementation may have improved or protected postpartum energy stores, although the finding was not statistically significant.

It is not known if women who are underweight after delivery are less likely to initiate or succeed at breastfeeding. In developing countries, studies examining whether it is possible to improve lactational performance by feeding undernourished mothers, who are almost always underweight, have yielded mixed results and have been subject to methodologic difficulties (Abrams, 1991; IOM, 1991). Overall, these studies suggest that providing food supplements to lactating mothers may increase maternal postpartum weight and improve maternal health (IOM, 1991). Well-designed supplementation studies of women with a high degree of malnutrition show an adverse effect of malnutrition on milk volume (Gonzalez-Cossio et al., 1991; Khin-Maung-Naing, 1987), but most studies of less malnourished women do not (IOM, 1991). It is also possible that maternal dietary supplementation contributes to decreased duration of lactational amenorrhea in malnourished women (IOM, 1991), but this may have only minor importance to actual health outcomes (Kurz, 1993).

Because maternal underweight after delivery or throughout the first year postpartum can be a marker of poor maternal health or environmental stress, identification of these women and assessment of their social, nutrition, and medical risk factors have the potential to identify interventions that can improve maternal and fetal health.

Use of Postpartum Underweight as a Nutrition Risk Criterion in the WIC Setting

Table 4-1 summarizes use of maternal postpartum underweight as a nutrition risk criterion. The majority of WIC state agencies defined underweight at < 90 percent ideal weight-for-height or a BMI of < 19.8, but cutoff values vary widely.

Recommendations for Postpartum Underweight

The risk of *maternal postpartum underweight* is documented in postpartum women. There is empirical evidence and a theoretical basis for benefit from participation in the WIC program. Therefore, the committee recommends use of *maternal postpartum underweight* as a nutrition risk criterion for postpartum women by the WIC program, with the IOM cutoff value of a BMI of 19. It also recommends research to determine the most valid postpartum cutoff points for lactating and nonlactating women.

Postpartum Overweight

Recent data indicate that, depending on age, the prevalence of overweight among U.S. women of childbearing age ranges from about 20 to 30 percent (Kuczmarski et al., 1994). Given that the median gestational weight gain in the United States was almost 14 kg in 1989 (CDC, 1992), it is important to know the extent to which postpartum weight retention contributes to this public health problem.

No standard definition exits for postpartum weight retention or postpartum obesity. Women can be classified as overweight by comparing their postpartum weight-for-height with the reference for nonpregnant women. Postpartum weight retention is often defined as postpartum weight minus prepregnancy weight. By 6 weeks postpartum, much of the weight retained is likely to be maternal fat (Prichard et al., 1985).

Review of older studies, when the average gestational weight gain was much lower than it is currently, indicates that women with an average prenatal weight gain retained about 1 kg more than the expected weight increase with age (IOM, 1990).

Results from studies of postpartum weight retention vary according to study population, the follow-up periods after delivery, and definitions or observations of infant feeding practices. Methodologic problems include bias from inaccurate recall of prepregnancy weight, failure to adjust for the expected increase in body weight with age, and lack of information on energy intake and exercise patterns. In the absence of reference standards specific to postpartum lactating or nonlactating women, the IOM (1992a) recommended application of the nonpregnant BMI cutoff values to these populations: 120 to 135 percent IBW (BMI 26 to 29 kg/m^2) to define overweight, and greater than 135 percent IBW or BMI > 29 kg/m^2 to define obesity.

Prevalence of and Factors Associated with Postpartum Overweight

Using nationally representative data on postpartum weight retention of 2,845 U.S. women whose pregnancies resulted in term, live, singleton births, the 1988 NMIHS reported the median weight retention of 1.5 kg at 10 to 18 months after delivery. However, 25 percent of the white women and 45 percent of black women retained more than 4 kg. These data suggest that it is possible that pregnancy contributes to postpartum overweight or obesity (IOM, 1990; Keppel and Taffel, 1993; Parker, 1994; Parker and Abrams, 1993).

Data from the 1988 NMIHS suggest that median weight retention was 0.7 kg for white mothers and 3.2 kg for black mothers among women whose gestational weight gains were in accordance with their recommended BMI-specific ranges (Keppel and Taffel, 1993). In another analysis of the same data set that focused on women whose prepregnancy weight-for-height was in the normal range and that controlled for other factors, black women were more than twice as likely as white women to retain 9 kg or more postpartum (Parker and Abrams, 1993). This racial differential is extremely important because cross-sectional studies have shown that black women are already at a high risk for obesity (Flegal et al., 1988; Kuczmarski et al., 1994). Studies of postpartum overweight for women of other racial/ethnic groups have not been reported.

Overall, the bulk of the evidence does not support the view that lactation promotes increased weight loss (IOM, 1991; Parker, 1994). However, a study comparing postpartum weight loss between breastfeeders (defined as nursing for at least 12 months) and bottle feeders (who weaned their infants to the bottle by age 3 months) reported highly significant differences at between 6 and 12 months after birth, but not earlier (Dewey et al., 1993). Among the breastfeeders, high feeding frequency and milk energy output were associated with less weight loss between 3 and 6 months after birth but more rapid weight loss between 9 and 12 months after birth. These results underscore the need for studies that precisely classify women by infant feeding method and follow them for an extended period of time.

Other risk factors for postpartum weight retention include a high prepregnancy weight-for-height (such women have wide variations in postpartum weight loss) and low income (Parker, 1994). Cigarette smoking is associated with less weight retention. The influences of maternal age, parity, and length of interconceptional periods are interrelated and complex. Segel and McAnarney (1994) followed 30 black, low-income adolescents for about 3 years after pregnancy and concluded that high gestational weight gain as well as prepregnancy obesity were risk factors for postpartum obesity in this group.

Postpartum Overweight as an Indicator of Nutrition and Health Risk

There is little question that overweight is a serious health problem. Obese women are at increased risk of heart disease, diabetes mellitus, hypertension, and some types of cancer (Abrams and Berman, 1993; NRC, 1989). Furthermore, obese postpartum women are at increased risk for maternal complications and poor perinatal outcomes during subsequent pregnancy. Evidence from a study of more than 700 primiparous Australian women suggests that a high postpartum weight-for-height (BMI > 26 kg/cm^2) at 1 month postpartum is associated with a statistically significant increased risk of discontinuing breastfeeding by 6 months (Rutishauser and Carlin, 1992). Other studies are needed to examine the influence of postpartum obesity on lactation success.

A recent study of 121 white and 224 black women (7 to 12 months postpartum) who participated in a South Carolina WIC program concluded that the most important variables in predicting postpartum weight loss were prepregnancy weight, prenatal weight gain, parity, and prenatal exercise. After these factors were controlled, race predicted that black women retained 6.4 pounds more than white women. Black women reported significantly higher mean energy and fat intake and significantly lower amounts of prenatal and postpartum activity. The authors concluded that the weight differential between black and white mothers might be explained by higher energy intake and lower activity levels in black women postpartum (Boardley et al., 1995).

Postpartum Overweight as an Indicator of Nutrition and Health Benefit

No studies have specifically described the health effects of dieting among nonlactating mothers during the postpartum period (Parker, 1994). It has been proposed that weight losses of less than 2 kg/month for normal-weight women and 3 kg/month for overweight or obese women after the first month postpartum are consistent with successful lactation (Dewey and McCrory, 1994; IOM, 1991). A recent uncontrolled study demonstrated that lactating women can lose weight and maintain adequate milk quantity and quality by following a moderately restricted diet over a 10-week postpartum period; however, one-third of the original subjects dropped out of the study (Dusdieker et al., 1994).

The single evaluation of postpartum intervention by participation in the WIC program suggested that women who participated in the WIC program for 5 to 7 months after birth had half the odds of being overweight at the beginning of their next pregnancy (Caan et al., 1987). The investigators hypothesized that WIC program participants who already have adequate energy intakes may have substituted the more nutrient-dense WIC foods for less expensive foods that provided more calories but fewer nutrients.

By assessing maternal postpartum overweight, the WIC program is in a position to identify women who are retaining excess postpartum weight, women whose overweight status continues, and women who have become overweight because of weight gain during the postpartum period. The WIC program's assessment and follow-up of women's weight during the postpartum period may provide the only possibility of intervention, because in contrast to the intensive monitoring of health status that occurs during pregnancy, most women receive relatively little medical care during the postpartum period.

Use of Postpartum Overweight as a Nutrition Risk Criterion in the WIC Setting

In 1992, most of the agencies that used postpartum overweight as a risk criterion for breastfeeding and nonlactating women (see Table 4-1) used the cutoff point of 120 percent of IBW. Cutoff values ranged from 110 to 135 percent of IBW and included several categories of overweight.

Recommendations for Postpartum Overweight

The risk of *postpartum overweight* is documented in postpartum women. There is empirical evidence and a theoretical basis for benefit from participation in the WIC program. Therefore, the committee recommends use of *postpartum overweight* as a nutrition risk criterion for postpartum women by state WIC agencies, using cutoff values of > 120 percent of IBW or a BMI of > 26.0 kg/m^2

after 6 weeks postpartum. The committee also recommends research to determine the most valid cutoff points.

The committee recommends the design and testing of culturally appropriate interventions to reduce maternal overweight after delivery or to prevent further gain.

Abnormal Postpartum Weight Change

Theoretically, the criterion *abnormal postpartum weight change* has the potential to identify a group of women who are at special and acute nutrition risk, especially when it is related to weight loss. However, there is no standard definition for *abnormal postpartum weight change* in either lactating or postpartum women. Weight loss that exceeds suggested rates of maternal weight loss consistent with adequate lactation has been proposed (IOM, 1991, 1992a).

Prevalence of and Factors Associated with Abnormal Postpartum Weight Change

Abnormal postpartum weight change has not been described in the literature; therefore, nothing is known about its epidemiology or factors associated with its occurrence.

Abnormal Postpartum Weight Change as an Indicator of Health and Nutrition Risk

A recent review concluded that if a woman has adequate fat reserves, it is probably safe to restrict energy intake moderately to enhance weight loss during lactation (Dewey and McCrory, 1994), and a subsequent study supports this view of no increased risk (Dusdieker et al., 1994).

Abnormal Postpartum Weight Change as an Indicator of Health and Nutrition Benefit

No studies have examined the possible health benefits of intervening for women with high rates of weight loss or gain after delivery. Common sense suggests that when a rapid weight loss or gain over a short period of time is observed in a postpartum woman, additional assessments of maternal health and psychological, social, and economic status are warranted to determine the cause and that the food and/or nutrition education provided by the WIC program can help remedy the problem.

Use of Abnormal Maternal Weight Change as a Nutrition Risk Criterion in the WIC Setting

The few state WIC agencies that used abnormal postpartum weight change as a nutrition risk criterion for postpartum women (see Table 4-1) used cutoff points that ranged from maternal weight loss of greater than 0.9 kg/month to a 6-month postpartum weight of 18 kg less than the postpartum weight at 6 weeks, or an increase in weight of at least 10 percent in women who were at desirable weight at 6 weeks postpartum.

Detection of abnormal maternal postpartum weight change requires repeated measurements of maternal weight over a relevant time period, which may sometimes not be possible in WIC program settings.

Recommendation for Abnormal Postpartum Weight Change

Although there is a theoretical basis for benefit from participation in the WIC program, no risks have been documented, and there is no standard definition for this change in either lactating or postpartum women. Therefore, the committee recommends discontinuation of use of *abnormal postpartum weight change* as a nutrition risk criterion for postpartum women by the WIC program.

ANTHROPOMETRIC RISK CRITERIA FOR INFANTS AND CHILDREN

A summary of anthropometric risk criteria as predictors of risk and benefit for infants and children appears in Table 4-3.

Low Birth Weight

The term *low birth weight* (LBW) is used to describe a weight of less than 2,500 g at birth. Infants and children with LBWs can be broadly categorized into two subgroups: (1) those who are born preterm, that is, at less than 37 weeks of gestation and (2) those who are growth retarded in utero and who are born SGA (see the section Small for Gestational Age). Because weight at birth is a function of both duration of gestation and interuterine growth of the fetus, an LBW infant can be both preterm and SGA.

TABLE 4-3 Summary of Anthropometric Risk Criteria as Predictive of Risk or Benefit Among Infants and Children

	Infants		Children	
Risk Criterion	Risk	Benefit	Risk	Benefit
Low birth weight	✓	✓	✓	✓
Small for gestational age	✓	✓		
Short stature	✓	✓	✓	✓
Underweight	✓	✓	✓	✓
Low head circumference	✓	✓		
Large for gestational age	✓	0		
Overweight	✓	✓	✓	✓
Slow growth	✓	✓	✓	✓

NOTE: ✓ = predictive of risk or benefit; 0 = evidence but no effect; blank = not applicable to that group.

Prevalence of and Factors Associated with LBW

The national prevalence of LBW in 1991 was 70.8 per 1,000 live-born infants (CDC, 1994). Across ethnic groups, the prevalence of LBW was substantially higher among infants of black mothers (135 per 1,000 live births) than among white, Hispanic, Native American, and Asian groups. Similar ethnic differences were observed among infants of low-income families (Yip et al., 1992a).

LBW is caused by a short gestational period, intrauterine growth retardation (IUGR), or both. In general, factors related to IUGR and preterm delivery are not identical (see SGA following and Chapter 5 for specifics). For example, poor maternal nutrition status is one of the major causes of SGA, but it is not an important determinant of prematurity (Kramer et al., 1992). On the other hand, infections (Taha et al., 1993; Villar et al., 1989), maternal cocaine use (Petitti and Coleman, 1990), and prepregnancy and gestational hypertension (particularly severe preeclampsia) (Kramer et al., 1990a, 1992) are related to both SGA and preterm delivery. The causes of LBW vary for different populations, as does the nature of LBW (WHO, 1995). In developing countries, most LBW infants are SGA or had IUGR. In contrast, in industrialized countries, the majority of LBW infants were delivered preterm (Ashworth and Feachem, 1985; CDC, 1994; IOM, 1990).

LBW as an Indicator of Nutrition and Health Risk

LBW is one of the most important biologic predictors of infant death and deficiencies in physical and mental development during childhood among those babies who survive (IOM, 1985). The consequences of LBW caused by IUGR differ from those of LBW caused by prematurity.

Premature LBW infants generally exhibit higher neonatal, perinatal, and postnatal mortalities than their full-term counterparts of the same birth weight, primarily because immunologic immaturity is more pronounced in preterm infants (Meyer and Comstock, 1972; Read et al., 1994; Sappenfield et al., 1987; Starfield et al., 1982). A recent study comparing perinatal weight-specific mortality in the United States and Norway found that, after adjustment for the mean birth weight in each country, the higher rate of perinatal death among U.S. infants could be entirely attributed to a small excess of preterm deliveries (Wilcox and Marks, 1995). Despite their earlier disadvantage, premature infants, if they survive, experience a lower risk of infections such as diarrhea and exhibit more growth during childhood than infants with IUGR (Barros et al., 1992).

The associations of LBW with poor health, growth, and development may persist throughout childhood, but the magnitudes of these associations may weaken as a child becomes older. LBW continues to be a strong predictor of growth in early childhood (Binkin et al., 1988). It has been reported that 20 to 40 percent of the prevalence of low length-for-age in the first 2 years of life can be attributed to LBW (Gayle et al., 1987). A recent study has shown that children with extreme LBWs (i.e., below 750 g) are at very high risk for long-term neurobehavioral dysfunction and poor school performance (Hack et al., 1994; Klebanov et al., 1994; McCormick et al., 1992).

LBW as an Indicator of Nutrition and Health Benefit

Infants and children born with LBW, particularly LBW caused by IUGR, must receive an optimal nutrient intake to survive, meet the needs of an extended period of relatively rapid postnatal growth, and complete their growth and development. They therefore have the potential to benefit from the WIC program. Interventions that support breastfeeding and that provide nutrient-dense food, nutrition education, and health referrals help to assure that this will occur. Little information is available on potential benefits relative to different WIC program components and different types of LBW.

Use of LBW as a Nutrition Risk in the WIC Setting

Low birth weight was used as a nutrition risk criterion for infants by 53 state WIC agencies in 1992 (see Table 4-1). The cutoff point was set universally as 2,499 or 2,500 g in all state WIC agencies. One of eight agencies that used LBW as a criterion for children ages 1 to 5 years used 1,500 g as the cutoff point. Birth-weight data are routinely collected in most hospitals and perinatal clinics, and the information is readily available to the WIC program.

Recommendations for LBW

The risk of *LBW* is well documented in infants and also is documented in children. There is empirical evidence and a theoretical basis for benefit from participation in the WIC program. Therefore, the committee recommends use of *LBW* as a nutrition risk criterion for infants and children by the WIC program, with the conventional cutoff value of less than 2,500 g. However, priority should be given to using the SGA and prematurity criteria (see subsequent section and "Prematurity" in Chapter 5) over the LBW criterion for infants. If LBW is used as the sole nutrition risk criterion for infants, a cutoff value of 2,500 g may be too low, because some heavier newborns also have elevated nutrition and health risks. However, there is no need to increase the LBW cutoff value in the WIC program for infants if the SGA and prematurity criteria are followed.

In addition, the committee recommends research to assess the effectiveness of interventions used to improve health and nutrition outcomes for LBW infants.

Small for Gestational Age

Small for gestational age (SGA) is defined as an infant's weight at birth below a certain cutoff point compared with some reference point for infants of comparable gestational age. Because weight at birth is a function of both the duration of gestation and the intrauterine growth of the fetus, assessment of birth weight on the basis of gestational age has a great advantage in that it differentiates LBW that results from poor fetal growth from LBW that results from prematurity. SGA implies intrauterine growth retardation (IUGR) and as such, the two terms are often used interchangeably. Strictly speaking, however, SGA and IUGR are not synonymous (Altman and Hytten, 1989). Some infants who are SGA (e.g., those born to short mothers) may merely represent the lower tail of the normal fetal growth distribution, but the growth of some infants who are not identified as SGA may have actually been restricted in utero (e.g., infants born to tall cigarette smokers). In individual cases, however, it is very difficult to know whether the observed birth weight is the result of true IUGR. The likelihood that the SGA is due to IUGR increases as the prevalence of IUGR increases in the population.

For infants born after 26 weeks of gestation, WHO (1995) recommends the use of William's Birth Weight Curve, which was derived from a large, multiracial population in California (Williams et al., 1982). The most frequently used cutoff point for diagnosing SGA is the 10th percentile. For full-term infants, this value (corresponding to 2,900 g in William's Birth Weight Curve) is greater than the conventional cutoff point of 2,500 g for LBW. Mounting evidence indicates that infants with birth weights above 2,500 g but below some predefined cutoff point around the 10th percentile still carry significantly higher health and nutrition risks than infants with birth weights above the 10th percentile (Balcazar and Haas, 1991; Kimball et al., 1982; Kramer, 1987a; Lester et al., 1986).

Prevalence of and Factors Associated with SGA

The national prevalence of full-term ($\geq$ 37 weeks of gestation) LBW infants was 26.5 per 1,000 live-born infants in 1991 (CDC, 1994). The prevalence was much higher among black infants than white infants (47.2 versus 22.0 per 1,000 live births, respectively).

The determinants of fetal growth have been the subject of considerable research (e.g., Abrams, 1994; Abrams and Newman, 1991; Barros et al., 1992; IOM, 1990; Kramer, 1987b; Kramer et al., 1990a; Stein and Susser, 1984; Wen et al., 1990). In general, maternal stature, prepregnancy weight, weight gain during gestation, gestational energy intake and expenditure during pregnancy, and maternal health all have important and independent influences on the rate of fetal growth. These factors are also related to underlying socioeconomic deprivation (IOM, 1985).

Gestational nutrition status is affected by maternal energy and nutrient intakes, weight gain, and fat deposition during pregnancy (Villar et al., 1992). Consequently, research has focused on nutrition interventions to improve maternal nutrition status as a means of reducing SGA. The consistently positive, although sometimes modest, effect of food supplementation and the negative effect of increased energy needs during pregnancy on birth weight have been demonstrated both in developing countries and in low-income populations of industrialized countries (Adair and Pollitt, 1985; Chavéz and Martínez, 1980; Habicht and Yarbrough, 1980; Kramer, 1993; Lechtig and Klein, 1981; Prentice et al., 1983; Rush et al., 1988c). Maternal height and weight may be influenced by the mother's past nutritional status; and they, in turn, can affect fetal growth.

Other factors affecting fetal growth include maternal health (such as the presence of infection and prepregnancy and gestational hypertension—particularly severe preeclampsia), cigarette smoking, and alcohol consumption (Jacobson et al., 1994; Kramer et al., 1990a; Plouin et al., 1983; Shu et al., 1995). The use of certain pharmacologic substances (including cocaine) adversely affects birth weight (Ashworth and Feachem, 1985; Dolan-Mullen et al., 1994). Teenage mothers have a higher frequency of LBW infants for any given parity, and a short interconceptional interval is associated with an increased risk of SGA and prematurity (Lieberman, 1995; Rawling et al., 1995). A greater percentage of LBW babies is born to blacks and Asians than to whites of similar socioeconomic status (James, 1992; Wang et al., 1994). High altitude is also related to a higher prevalence of LBW (Yip et al., 1993). Many of these factors influence both fetal growth and gestational duration (WHO, 1995). Some risk factors are amenable to appropriate health interventions (e.g., maternal health, cigarette smoking), but others are not (e.g., altitude, race).

SGA as an Indicator of Nutrition and Health Risk

Overwhelming evidence indicates that impairment of fetal growth can have adverse effects on the nutrition and health of children during infancy and childhood, including higher mortality and morbidity, slower physical growth, and possibly slower mental development (Ashworth and Feachem, 1985; Binkin et al., 1988; Fancourt et al., 1976; Harvey et al., 1982; IOM, 1990; McCormick, 1985; Parkinson et al., 1981; Teberg et al., 1988; Villar et al., 1984). Infants who are SGA are more likely to have congenital abnormalities (Khoury et al., 1988). Severely growth-retarded infants are at markedly increased risk for fetal and neonatal death, hypoglycemia, hypocalcemia, polycythemia, and neuro-cognitive complications of pre- and intrapartum hypoxia (IOM, 1990; Kramer et al., 1990b). Over the long term, growth-retarded infants may have permanent mild deficits in growth and neurocognitive development (Binkin et al., 1988; Dunn et al., 1986; IOM, 1991; Teberg et al., 1988). Some studies have even suggested that the restriction of fetal growth may increase the risk of ischemic heart disease, hypertension, obstructive lung disease, diabetes mellitus, and death from cardiovascular disease in adulthood (Barker et al., 1993a, b; 1989; Valdez et al., 1994). When infants who are SGA are also preterm, their health risks also include those associated with prematurity (WHO, 1995) (see Chapter 5).

Body proportionality may be related to different outcomes of babies who are SGA. The most commonly used proportionality index is Rohrer's ponderal index, which is defined as $(100 \times \text{weight in grams})/(\text{crown-heel length in centimeters})^3$ (Khoury et al., 1990). An infant with a high ponderal index has a relatively high weight-for-length, whereas an infant with a low ponderal index is thin, with low weight-for-length. Infants who are SGA and who have an adequate ponderal index exhibit less catch-up growth than their counterparts with a low ponderal index (Kramer, 1987a). In contrast, infants who are SGA and who have a low ponderal index have an increased risk for postnatal morbidity compared with those with an adequate ponderal index (Caulfield et al., 1991; Villar et al., 1990).

Conlisk (1993) studied the risk in the United States of neonatal mortality among infants with proportionate weight-for-length and those with dispropor-tionate weight-for-length (decreased weight-for-length). The results showed that, in both blacks and whites, disproportionate infants with lower birth weights had a higher risk of mortality. Those with birth weights greater than 2,400 g (black) and 2,800 g (white) had a lower risk of mortality than proportionate infants. The effect of birth weight on mortality was significantly greater for the disproportionate versus the proportionate infants with birth weights of less than 2,200 g (black) or less than 2,600 g (white). Several studies report that SGA and low ponderal index are related to increased insulin resistance during infancy and a higher risk of mortality from cardiovascular disease during adulthood (Barker et al., 1993b; Phillips et al., 1994).

SGA as an Indicator of Nutrition and Health Benefit

Appropriate nutrition and health interventions for infants who are SGA can help minimize the adverse health and nutrition consequences associated with SGA as well as maximize the potential for subsequent catch-up growth and development among these infants.

Infants who are SGA can benefit from breastfeeding, which is promoted by the WIC program. Human milk is the most appropriate food for young infants because it is nutritious and confers immunity and because it is fed in a manner that avoids bacterial contamination (Atkinson et al., 1990; IOM, 1991). The beneficial effects of human milk on reducing morbidity and mortality and promoting optimal growth have been demonstrated in both developing and industrialized countries (DaVanzo et al., 1983; Habicht et al., 1986; IOM, 1991; Launer et al., 1990). When breastfeeding is not possible or feasible, infants who are SGA need formula that is tailored to their special needs (IOM, 1992b), and this can be provided through the WIC program.

The WIC program may also benefit infants by leading to regular surveillance, early prevention, and referral for treatment of health complications related to SGA. Among infants and children admitted to the WIC program on the basis of the presence of LBW and SGA (among other criteria), Rush and colleagues (1988b) observed better immunization levels, a more frequent regular source of health care, better digit memory, and more advantageous child behavior than among infants in control groups.

Use of SGA as a Nutrition Risk Criterion in the WIC Setting

Of the 10 state WIC agencies using the small for gestational age nutrition risk criterion in 1992 (USDA, 1994) (see Table 4-1), the reference data used for evaluating SGA differed from state to state. Measuring SGA can easily be implemented in the WIC program setting.

Recommendations for SGA

The risk of *SGA* is well documented in infants and children. There is empirical evidence and a theoretical basis for benefit from participation in the WIC program. Therefore, the committee recommends the use of *SGA* as a nutrition risk criterion for infants and children by the WIC program, with a cutoff value of less than the 10th percentile because it includes full-term infants who are SGA with birth weights of greater than 2,500 g.

In addition, the committee recommends further studies to relate body proportionality to risks and also to potential benefits from interventions.

Short Stature

Short stature is defined by an infant's length-for-age or a child's height-for-age below some cutoff point compared with the National Center for Health Statistics-U.S. Centers for Disease Control and Prevention (NCHS-CDC) reference data. The term *length* is used for infants and children under 2 years of age when their body height is measured in a recumbent position. For older children, standing height is measured and the term *height* applies. For simplicity, the word *stature* is used in this section when either measure might apply. Stature represents the amount of linear growth that has been achieved. Short stature may result from normal variation or from health and nutrition inadequacies that are usually long term in nature. In the latter case, the term *stunting* is used to indicate that shortness is pathologic. In contrast to older children, in whom stunting may be a past event, stunting in infants and younger children (i.e., under 3 to 4 years of age) represents an ongoing process of failing to grow.

Prevalence of and Factors Associated with Short Stature

The prevalence of short stature among infants and children targeted by the WIC program in 1991 (defined as below the 5th percentile of the NCHS-CDC reference standard) was 5 percent or higher. The highest prevalence, about 12 percent, was observed in Asian children (USDA, 1991; Yip et al., 1992a).

Abnormal short stature in infants and children is widely recognized as a response to a limited nutrient supply at the cellular level. The maintenance of basic metabolic functions takes precedence, and resources are diverted from linear growth. Unavailability of nutrients for cells results directly from inadequate food intake and frequent diseases, particularly infectious diseases. Short stature is related to the lack of total dietary energy and to a poor quality of diet, namely, a diet that provides inadequate protein, particularly animal protein, and inadequate amounts of such micronutrients as zinc, vitamin A, iron, copper, iodine, calcium, and phosphorus. However, the mechanisms by which these factors affect bone growth are poorly understood (Allen, 1994; Chwang et al., 1988; Golden, 1994; Golden and Golden, 1981; Prentice and Bates, 1994; Waterlow, 1994b; West et al., 1988).

The negative effect of diseases, most commonly infectious diseases, on the growth of children is well-known, and the magnitude of the effect depends on infection management practices, feeding practices, and food adequacy and quality (Tomkins and Watson, 1989). Insufficient amounts of growth hormone and a lack of physical exercise, either as a result of inadequate nutrient intake or poor health, may also contribute to some cases of stunting (Karlberg et al., 1994; Torun and Viteri, 1994). Food inadequacy and infection are often synergistically related to each other in their effects on child growth. Stature deficits are significantly greater when both food inadequacy and infection occur together than when these two conditions occur separately over the same period Lutter et al., 1992). This indicates the importance of offering interventions that combine both food and health components.

The impact of inadequate food and frequent episodes of infectious disease on short stature is especially pronounced in the first few years of life. During early infancy, breastfeeding reduces morbidity and mortality, especially in developing countries, and promotes and maintains normal growth (Feachem and Koblinsky, 1984; Habicht et al., 1986; Seward and Serdula, 1984). Exclusive and frequent breastfeeding is recommended to promote health and well-being in industrialized countries as well as in developing countries (IOM, 1991; WHO, 1988, 1991). The first 2 to 3 years is a time of vulnerability: linear growth is very rapid; young children are highly dependent on others for care; they are susceptible to infectious disease; their nutritional requirements, expressed as the amounts of energy or nutrients received per kilogram per day, are greater than at any subsequent time of life; and most adverse factors will have significant and lasting effects. Consequently, stature deficits are more likely to accrue actively before 3 years of age and ease in later childhood. In general, later growth cannot completely compensate for previous losses (Martorell et al., 1994).

The impact of poverty on nutrition status varies from place to place, depending in part on the existence of public health and nutrition programs (Dreze and Sen, 1991). In general, strong associations between short stature and poverty exist in the developing world; and of all commonly used anthropometric indices, short stature is generally regarded as the best summary indicator of general deprivation and poor environment in developing countries (ACC/SCN, 1992; Beaton et al., 1990; WHO, 1995). Similar associations, albeit less strong, can also be found in the industrialized world. In the United States, income-related short stature in children is consistently observed in large surveys (Abraham et al., 1975; CDC, 1972; Hamill et al., 1972; Kerr et al., 1982; Owen and Lubin, 1973; Owen et al., 1974). An examination of poverty-related height differences in U.S. children using the first and second National Health and

Nutrition Examination Surveys (NHANES I) and (NHANES II) data found that children from families living above the poverty level were about 1 to 2 cm taller than children living below the poverty level (Jones et al., 1985). Differentials in short stature are more strongly associated with long-term than with single-year measures of income (Miller and Korenman, 1994).

A child's height-for-age is also affected by mode of feeding and other factors. After the third month of exclusive breastfeeding, infants may have median lengths of 0.1 to 0.2 z-scores (about 4 to 8 percentiles) less than the NCHS-CDC reference median (Dewey et al., 1991b). (These reference data are based on the length of predominantly bottle-fed infants.) Breastfed infants may remain slightly shorter during the ensuing period of ad libitum mixed feeding of human milk and solid foods (WHO, 1995). Parents' size, particularly height, influences a child's stature through genetic endowment and fetal growth. Birth weight, even in the range commonly accepted as normal (2.5 to 4.0 kg), is a powerful predictor of linear growth during both infancy and childhood (Binkin et al., 1988).

The fact that some of the variation in birth weight and subsequent infant linear growth is determined by maternal health and nutrition status indicates the importance of targeting interventions to pregnant women and mothers. Demonstrable differences in stature exist among children of different ethnic and racial groups. Black infants, for example, tend to be shorter during infancy (Yip et al., 1993). Insufficient evidence is available to indicate that the shorter stature of Asian children is not influenced by nutrition, because many Asian children in the United States have a refugee background, and there has been a clear upward secular trend in the growth of these children (Yip et al., 1992b). Ethnic and racial differences, however, are relatively minor compared with the differences associated with environmental factors (Habicht et al., 1974; WHO, 1995).

Higher altitude or a lower partial pressure of oxygen is associated with shorter statures, with the difference between 500 and 2,000 m being 0.4 z-scores (about a 1.0-cm difference for 3-year-old children) (Yip et al., 1988).

Short Stature as an Indicator of Nutrition and Health Risk

Short stature because of inadequate dietary intake combined with high rates of infection is a strong predictor of nutrition and health risk, but short stature because of normal variations in a population is not.

Stunted infants are likely to become stunted children, and stunted children are likely to be stunted adolescents and adults, especially if there are no improvements in health and nutrition. Stunting early in life leads to reduced maximal physical working capacity and capacity for sustained work (endurance) and probably a reduced level of intellectual capacity (Martorell et al., 1994; Waterlow, 1994b). In a Guatemalan study, childhood stature at 3 years of age was highly related to adult height, grip strength of the right hand, and fat-free mass—all of which are key determinants of adult work capacity. Size at 3 years of age also predicted nonverbal intelligence, numeracy, literacy, and school attainment when analyses controlled for village characteristics and characteristics of the home environment (Martorell et al., 1992).

Stunted infants and children are also likely to become severely ill when they develop infections and are more likely to die than normal individuals (Martorell and Ho, 1984). A consistent finding in studies of the relationship between malnutrition and mortality has been that stunting in infants and young children has a greater ability than severe underweight of recent origin to predict subsequent (e.g., 6 to 24 months of follow-up) mortality, but low weight-for-age is usually the best predictor of all (Pelletier, 1994). Relationships between stunting and mortality are influenced by age, gender, seasonality, socioeconomic status, and burden of infectious disease, which vary from population to population (Pelletier et al., 1993). Short stature has been consistently associated with comparatively low performance in developmental scales among infants and toddlers, and with poor intelligence quotient and other cognitive test scores among children. In economically impoverished populations where children are nutritionally at risk, it seems likely that this association is partly explained by environmental factors, including poor nutrition.

Short Stature as an Indicator of Nutrition and Health Benefit

The effects of food supplementation on the stature of malnourished infants and children have been mixed. A review of more than 200 supplementary feeding programs in developing countries concluded that the effect of supplementation on nutrition status, as assessed by growth performance, was surprisingly small (Beaton and Ghassemi, 1982). It was suggested that the small effect might simply reflect a low level of improvement in the diet. Alternatively, the small effect could be due to the fact that few studies were adequately designed to infer causality, and thus the expected effect may have been diminished by confounding (Pinstrup-Anderson et al., 1993). When supplementary feeding is demonstrated to be given in adequate amounts to malnourished young children, stature has improved (Habicht and Butz, 1979).

Benefits have resulted from a number of food supplementation and health interventions that have produced demonstrable changes in food intake. Some interventions that supported improved growth and development started at early stages of life, even as early as the prenatal period (Heikens et al., 1993; Martorell and Habicht, 1986; Martorell et al., 1982; Mora et al., 1981; Walker et al., 1991).

After 14 months of food supplementation, 1- to 5-year-old children who had heights-for-age below the 3rd percentile of U.S. heights-for-age gained, on average, 1.5 cm more in stature than children who were above the 3rd percentile (Rao and Naidu, 1977). Early supplementary feeding also has been shown to improve cognition in adolescence (Pollitt et al., 1993).

Compared with results from developing countries, benefits in terms of improved linear growth from nutrition and health interventions, including the WIC program, are much smaller and often statistically insignificant in industrialized countries. Edozien et al. (1979) found that the WIC program had a significant impact on the linear growth of infants and children (± 0.23–0.56 cm) after 6 to 11 months of program participation. However, because short stature was used as a criterion for eligibility for participation in the WIC program, the increase in average length after WIC program participation might be due to regression to the mean: those whose values were low tend to rise and those whose values were high tend to fall independent of any treatment effect (Rush et al., 1988a). In one study that made more than one follow-up measurement after enrollment in the WIC program, a decrease in the prevalence of short stature (defined as below the 10th percentile) was seen between follow-up visits only in children ages 6–23 months (CDC, 1978). Hick and colleagues (1982) reported that children who had received WIC program benefits prenatally were less likely to be below the 10th percentile of height for their age group. Rush and colleagues (1988b) found statistically significant increases in the heights of infants and children who participated in the WIC program either prenatally or within 3 months of birth, once differences in birth weight were taken into account in their analyses. Furthermore, these investigators showed effects of the WIC program specific to some minority children enrolled in the program early in life. In comparison with controls, for example, Hispanic children enrolled before their first birthday had smaller discrepancies in stature than white or black children enrolled later.

Among the many factors that explain the varying effectiveness of food supplementation and health intervention in improving linear growth, age and infectious disease are now being reemphasized. Increased age tends to decrease the responsiveness of growth to food supplementation. Other things being equal, food supplementation of infants generates a greater response than food supplementation of children (Martorell et al., 1994). Within the period of infancy, the greatest response of stature to nutrition supplementation coincides with weaning (ages 3–6 months) and the peak incidence and duration of infectious diseases (ages 9–12 months) (Lutter et al., 1990). In a Guatemalan food supplementation study, each 100 kcal of supplement received per day was associated with approximately 5 mm in additional gains in stature in children age 2 years and 4 mm in those age 3 years. Similar age differences in impact have been noted in India (Gopalan et al., 1973) and in Jamaica (Walker et al., 1991).

A high frequency of infections increases nutrition requirements, and dietary intakes that would otherwise be sufficient become inadequate. Food supplementation benefits not only children who have inadequate dietary intakes, but also those who have high rates of infections, in that supplementation protects children from the negative effects of infections on growth (Lutter et al., 1989). Food supplementation combined with treatment of infections often results in a height response greater than that from either food supplementation or treating the infection alone (Heikens et al., 1993; Lutter et al., 1989).

Despite the improved linear growth demonstrated by many food supplementation studies, the mean stature of children, particularly older children, was often less than that of children in higher socioeconomic groups and less than the 50th percentile of the NCHS-CDC reference standard. This indicates that the interventions overcome only part of the height deficits incurred by stunted children (Lutter et al., 1989; Martorell and Habicht, 1986; Mora et al., 1981; Walker et al., 1991). Complete reversal of stunting may take several generations and may involve broad improvements in socioeconomic status and general living conditions. In this sense, mean height-for-age among older children at population levels is a useful indicator of health and nutrition benefit from long-term socioeconomic development.

Use of Short Stature as a Nutrition Risk Criterion in the WIC Setting

Use of short stature as a risk criterion by state WIC agencies is summarized in Table 4-1. Cutoff points ranged from the 5th to 25th (infants) and the 5th to 30th (children) percentiles, with the median values being the 5th (infants) and 10th (children) percentiles (USDA, 1994). Measuring an infant's length is difficult compared with measuring a child's standing height, but it still easier and less expensive and invasive than many biochemical and clinical assessments.

Recommendation for Short Stature

The risk of *short stature* that is caused by inadequate nutrition and poor health is well documented for infants and children, and the anthropometric measurement is practical in the WIC setting. There is clear evidence that short stature that resulted from malnutrition may respond to appropriate health and nutrition interventions Therefore, the committee recommends use of *short stature* as a nutrition risk criterion for infants and children by the WIC program, with a cutoff value of below the 5th percentile.

Underweight

Underweight is defined by a weight-for-height below a certain cutoff in comparison with the reference standard of the NCHS and the CDC. Underweight reflects the body's thinness, but the term does not necessarily imply the nature and causes of underweight. The term *wasting* applies to underweight that results from a recent abnormal process leading to significant failure to gain weight or to the loss of weight (WHO, 1995). Differentiation between underweight and wasting therefore requires understanding of the process that leads to underweight.

Prevalence of and Factors Associated with Underweight

The prevalence of underweight, defined as weight-for-height below the 5th percentile of the reference standard in the general U.S. population, was less than 5 percent in 1991 (Yip et al., 1992a). A similar prevalence of underweight was seen in each of five racial/ethnic groups: white, black, Hispanic, Indian, and Asian.

Poverty, infectious disease, and inadequate energy intake, especially occurring recently, are major factors that contribute to a higher than expected prevalence of underweight. The effect of diet on a body's thinness has been suggested to be related more to a total energy deficit than to deficits of any specific nutrients (Malcolm, 1978; Waterlow, 1978). Sudden disasters or seasonal food shortages increase the prevalence of underweight in affected areas (Brown et al., 1982; Yip and Sharp, 1993). In the United States, where the overall prevalence of underweight is low, relatively little underweight can be attributed to nutrition and health problems at the population level. This does not mean, however, that underweight reflecting poor nutrition status is not present among some subgroups of the population, especially low-income subgroups. Low-income U.S. infants and children have a higher than expected prevalence of underweight, and the degree of underweight is often serious (CDC, 1987; Jones et al., 1985; Miller and Korenman, 1994; Miller et al., 1989; Owen et al., 1974). Infectious disease, as well as reduced dietary intake, may contribute. Severely wasted infants with no evidence of medical causes for their wasting but who respond to feeding treatment have been reported among low-income families and teenage mothers (Listernick et al., 1985).

For infants, especially during their first 6 months, formula feeding does not afford the same protection against common infectious diseases, and food-borne illness, as does breastfeeding (IOM, 1990). During late infancy, inappropriate weaning and feeding practices also contribute to the development of underweight (IOM, 1991). During the entire period of infancy and childhood, birth weight has a strong influence on weight-for-height values. Infants with lower birth weights, even if they are within the normal range, are more likely to be thinner (Binkin et al., 1988). Given the same birth weights, premature infants have higher weights-for-height than infants with fetal growth restriction (Binkin et al., 1988).

Among the nonpathologic factors affecting an infant's weight-for-height, a notable one is feeding practice. Breastfed infants living under favorable conditions and infants studied in various geographic areas have been reported to grow faster than the NCHS weight-for-height norm during the first 6 months and then slower than this norm after the recommended exclusive breastfeeding period (WHO, 1995). The absolute deviation from the reference median in each period was a z-score of about 0.2 (a change of 8 percentiles). The reasons for and consequences of this marked difference are not yet understood. Other nonpathologic factors that reduce weight-for-height of infants include high altitude (Yip et al., 1988), health and nutrition problems of the parents, parental short stature, and certain racial and ethnic backgrounds. The influence of parents' stature and race is generally minor.

Underweight as an Indicator of Nutrition and Health Risk

To study the relationship of underweight to mortality, 2,019 Bangladesh children ages 13 to 23 months were followed for 24 months (Chen et al., 1980). Severe, but not mild to moderate, underweight was related to higher rates of mortality. However, compared with other anthropometric predictors (e.g., arm circumference, height-for-age, and weight-for-age), weight-for-height had the lowest ability to predict subsequent mortality. Similar studies have since been conducted in other developing countries. In most of those studies, weight-for-height was indeed a weak predictor of subsequent child mortality (Alam et al., 1989; Bairagi, 1981; Bagenholm and Nasher, 1989; Briend et al., 1986, 1987; Heywood, 1982; Kasango Project Team, 1983; Katz et al., 1989; Smedman et al., 1987; Vella et al., 1994). Analysis of some of these studies with a multiplicative model that incorporated both disease burden and nutrition status showed something different from previous investigations: a substantial proportion of mortality could be explained by mild to moderate malnutrition, and there was no threshold in the relationship between malnutrition and death at the population level (Pelletier et al., 1993). Thus, even mild to moderate malnutrition, the kind more commonly seen in low-income populations in industrialized countries, is of concern.

Underweight is also a poor correlate of short stature at either an individual or a population level (Gorstein et al., 1994; Haaga, 1986; Victora, 1992), but new approaches to examining this relationship may be needed (Brown et al., 1982; Martorell, 1989; Waterlow, 1994a).

Underweight and other health and nutrition risks may share common determinants, or they may be causally related to one another; but other factors may affect the way in which they are related. Underweight and short stature, for example, are two different dimensions of poor growth, and each may be related to different aspects of diet (Garrow et al., 1994; Victora, 1992). Compared with height-for-age and weight-for-age, weight-for-height is an equally good or even better predictor of subsequent respiratory infections and diarrhea in some developing countries (Black et al., 1984; Delgado et al., 1983; Schelp et al., 1990; Tomkins, 1981). Across different communities, wasting was also a more consistent predictor of infections than was stunting (Lindtjorn et al., 1993).

Underweight as an Indicator of Nutrition and Health Benefit

Although underweight is in general a poor indicator of risk, many studies show that it is a fairly good indicator that a severely wasted infant or child being treated for malnutrition would benefit from participation in a feeding program. Positive responses might take the form of increases in weight-for-height for age, and decreases in morbidity and mortality. Significant responses in weight-for-height were reported in infants and children attending nutrition-rehabilitation centers, and the extent of the response was hypothesized to be related to initial levels of malnutrition (Beaudry-Darismé and Latham, 1973; Beghin and Viteri, 1973; Rivera, 1988). In areas with a high rate of malnutrition, a common practice of feeding programs is that one uses weight-for-height to select individuals for enrollment.

Review of some of the early food supplementation studies reveals that, in general, supplementary feeding, when given in adequate amounts to malnourished infants, had a positive effect on weights-for-height (Habicht and Butz, 1979; Rivera, 1988). No significant improvement in weight was found when there was no clear evidence of dietary improvement. On the other hand, in studies that noted an improvement in total dietary intake after supplementation, positive changes in body weight were consistently found among children with low weights-for-height or weights-for-age.

Two common difficulties in evaluating the response of weight-for-height in intervention studies were noted. One is the absence of an appropriate comparison group; this lack may bias the response in either direction. The other difficulty is the presence of regression to the mean, which is especially relevant to weight-for-height, because measurements involve both height and weight. If a child is admitted to an intervention program only because he or she suffered from a temporary deficiency in weight-for-height or a measurement error, he or she is more likely to have a higher weight-for-height some time later, even in the absence of any program effect. However, in studies that adopted appropriate designs and analytical methods to reduce such problems, weight-for-height was still responsive to interventions for malnourished children in developing countries (Heikens et al. 1989, 1993; Rivera et al. 1991).

Positive changes in weight-for-height as a response to nutrition and health interventions have also been observed in some populations in industrialized countries, but they have been much smaller and often statistically insignificant. Such evidence can be found with the WIC program (Edozien et al., 1979; Heimendinger et al., 1984; Hick et al., 1982). The prevalence of underweight (defined as less than the 10th percentile) among infants enrolled in the WIC program, for example, was negatively related to the number of follow-up visits (a proxy for duration in the program) (CDC, 1978). Participation in the WIC program had no significant impact on weight but had a positive effect on weight-for-height for infants and children who had participated in the program either prenatally or within 3 months of birth (Rush et al., 1986).

Changes in weight-for-height are associated negatively with the initial level of wasting, which cannot be attributed to the effect of regression to the mean (Rivera, 1988). This explains why in developing countries the benefit from food supplementation in terms of weight changes is usually small or even indiscernible. Although weight-for-height can be calculated without knowing the age, changes in weight-for-height as a response to food supplementation usually increase with an infant's age and peak between the ages of 6 and 24 months, which coincides with weaning and the peak incidence and duration of diarrhea and other infectious diseases (Heimendinger et al., 1984; Lutter et al., 1990; Martorell and Habicht, 1986). The presence of infections or other diseases may offset the positive effect of food supplementation on weight changes.

Weight-for-height has also been shown to be an indicator of benefit of nutrition intervention when defined as improvements in linear growth and survival. A recent study in Guatemala indicated that weight-for-height, but not height-for-age, at 3 and 6 months of infancy were significant determinants of benefit from supplementation as measured by height-for-age at 3 years of age (Ruel et al., 1995). The study suggested that lower weight-for-height increased the effect of food supplementation on height. In addition, although weight-for-height may decrease when interventions are removed, lasting improvements in linear growth and survival can be achieved by targeting interventions to wasted children. Using weight changes as an indicator of benefit, Rao and Naidu (1977) indicated that Indian children who were wasted gained more weight following food supplementation than did children who were stunted.

In famine-prone areas of Africa, cutoff values of weight-for-height in a population have been used successfully to trigger emergency food relief efforts to reduce mortality in young children (Lawrence et al., 1994).

Use of Underweight as a Nutrition Risk Criterion in the WIC Setting

Underweight is widely used as a criterion of nutrition risk in infants and children, respectively (see Table 4-1). Specific cutoff points ranged from the 5th to the 25th percentiles for infants, and the 5th to the 30th percentiles for children, with the median value for both infants and children being the 10th percentile (USDA, 1994). Measurement of underweight is relatively easy to implement and highly feasible in the WIC program.

Recommendation for Underweight

The risk of *underweight* that results from nutrition and health problems is documented in infants and children, and a practical method to identify this risk is available. There is indirect evidence from supplementation trials that underweight infants and children can benefit from participation in the WIC program. Therefore, the committee recommends the use of *underweight* as a nutrition risk criterion for infants and children, with a cutoff value of the 5th percentile.

Low Head Circumference

Low head circumference (LHC) is diagnosed when an infant's head circumference (occipital frontal circumference) is below a specified cutoff point using NCHS-CDC reference data for comparable age. Head circumference during infancy and early childhood relates directly to brain weight and volume (Bray et al., 1969; Cooke et al., 1977), and LHC is widely used in clinical settings to screen for potential developmental or neurologic disabilities in infants and children (Avery et al., 1972; Babson and Henderson, 1974). However, LHC alone does not necessarily indicate an abnormal head size. The diagnosis of abnormal LHC (microcephaly) must also be based on the presence of other evidence and knowledge of the causes of LHC.

Prevalence of and Factors Associated with LHC

Some evidence indicates that the mean head circumference is increasing among healthy populations in industrialized countries (Gerver et al., 1989; Lindgren et al., 1994; Ounsted et al., 1985; Paul et al., 1986; Tsuzaki et al., 1990). This positive secular trend should be taken into account in estimating and comparing the prevalence of LHC. No specific information is available regarding the prevalence of LHC in low-income U.S. populations, except that head circumference is in general lower in children of lower socioeconomic status (see below).

LHC is related to a variety of genetic, nutrition, and health factors. Although some LHCs are normal, some result directly from impaired brain development during pregnancy and the perinatal or postnatal period. Abnormal LHCs can be caused by genetic disorders such as autosomal and sex chromosome abnormalities (Palmer et al., 1992; Ratcliffe et al., 1994). Health factors related to LHC include phenylketonuria, exposure to neurotoxic substances, cocaine and alcohol use during pregnancy, intracranial hemorrhages, perinatal asphyxia, ischemic brain injury, and other major congenital central nervous system abnormalities (Eckerman et al., 1985; Ikenoue et al., 1993; Levy et al., 1994; Little and Snell, 1991; Nulman et al., 1994; Regev and Dubowitz, 1988; Verkerk et al., 1994).

Malnutrition during critical stages of brain development (i.e., from early fetal life through approximately 3 months following delivery) can result in reduced numbers of brain cells (Manser, 1984; Dobbing, 1973; Winick, 1969; Winick and Rosso, 1969), which may correlate with diminished growth of the head and other dimensions of growth (Dobbing, 1974; Stein et al., 1975). Thus, maternal prepregnancy weight, fat stores, and weight gain during pregnancy positively predict the head circumferences of newborn infants (Crawford et al., 1993; Miller and Merritt, 1979), and infants with fetal growth restriction tend to have smaller heads than infants with normal weight-for-gestational age (Kramer et al., 1989).

Ample evidence indicates that head size is related to socioeconomic status, and the relationship is mediated in part by nutrition factors. The head circumference of children in developing countries is significantly lower than that of children in industrialized countries (Hamill et al., 1979; Malina et al., 1975). In industrialized countries, children of low socioeconomic status usually have mean head circumferences less than those of children of higher socioeconomic status (CDC, 1972; Cook et al., 1976; Niswander and Gordon, 1972; Wright et al., 1992).

LHC as an Indicator of Nutrition and Health Risk

Abnormal LHC because of pathologic processes is indicative of future risk. The most common risk is poor neurocognitive abilities. Compared with infants of very low birth weight (VLBW) who have larger head circumferences, infants with very low birth weights (< 1.5 kg) who have a smaller head circumference have more motor abnormalities at 12 months of age (Simon et al., 1993), lower IQs at 3 years (Hack and Breslau, 1986), and poorer cognitive function, academic achievement, and behavior at 8 years (Hack et al., 1991). Because

LHC is associated with LBW and poor growth, LHC is also a strong marker of growth retardation and other dimensions of growth and development.

Among infants who are SGA, those with LHC have neonatal mortalities significantly greater than those without LHC (Lubchenco, 1981). These infants with both SGA and LHC, termed proportionally small, also have higher rates of morbidity such as birth asphyxia, respiratory distress, and neonatal infections but less hyperbilirubinaemia than disproportionally small infants (i.e., infants with SGA but not LHC) (Cuttini et al., 1991). A small head circumference during infancy is even hypothesized to be a contributing factor to death from cardiovascular disease in adult life (Barker et al., 1993b).

LHC as an Indicator of Nutrition and Health Benefit

In contrast to many studies examining head circumference as a pregnancy outcome, only a few have linked head circumference changes to nutrition and health interventions directed to infants and children. Stunted Jamaican children ages 9 to 24 months were randomly assigned to four groups: control, milk-based formula supplementation, psychosocial stimulation, and both interventions (Walker et al., 1991). After 12 months, supplemented children had an average increase of 0.3 cm in head circumference, along with other improvements in growth. No changes were observed with stimulation. Most effects from food supplementation occurred in the first 6 months. A positive but statistically insignificant association was demonstrated between head circumference and WIC program participation among infants and children (Rush et al., 1988b). The association was stronger in children who were black, boys, or living alone with their mothers. In neither the Jamaican nor the U.S. study was LHC used as a major criterion to select children for supplementation interventions.

Although more data are needed, increases in head circumference associated with postnatal nutrition intervention are plausible because they are parallel to the changes associated with prenatal interventions. Furthermore, the brain grows rapidly during infancy: the rate of head growth exceeds the rate of length and weight gain during the first 6 months of life. Thus, nutrition factors can be expected to have an important effect during this critical period (Dobbing, 1970, 1973).

Use of LHC as a Nutrition Risk Criterion in the WIC Setting

Few state WIC agencies presently use low head circumference as a nutrition risk criterion (USDA, 1994) (see Table 4-1). A head circumference can be measured more easily than length or height (Bhushan and Paneth, 1991; Kramer et al., 1989), but efforts should be made to avoid the influence of scalp edema or head molding (particularly after a difficult vaginal or forceps-assisted delivery) on head circumference measurements in infants. A head circumference measurement should be compared with reference values for infants of comparable age rather than comparable length or height.

Recommendation for LHC

The risk of *LHC* is well documented in infants, and a practical method to identify this risk is available. There is indirect scientific evidence, suggestive evidence from a WIC program evaluation, and a theoretical basis for concluding that infants with LHC benefit from participation in the WIC program. Therefore, the committee recommends use of *LHC* as a nutrition risk criterion for infants by the WIC program, with a cutoff value of below the 5th percentile of increments in head circumference for age (Roche and Himes, 1980).

Large for Gestational Age

Large for gestational age (LGA) is defined as a birth weight above a specified cutoff point using reference data for comparable gestational age. LGA is sometimes termed high birth weight for full-term and postterm infants, but LGA may also occur with preterm birth. LGA represents the upper end of the birth weight distribution.

Prevalence of and Factors Associated with LGA

In the United States, 12.7 percent of white infants and 5.5 percent of black infants weighed 4,000 g or more at birth in 1985 (IOM, 1990). The prevalence of infants who weighed 4,500 g or more is estimated to be less than 2 percent (Puffer and Serrano, 1987).

Maternal obesity, high prepregnancy weights, and large gestational weight gains contribute significantly to LGA (IOM, 1990). Many newborn babies who are LGA are born to women with diabetes mellitus, which may or may not have been diagnosed before or during pregnancy (Lubchenco, 1981). LGA can also be genetically determined (WHO, 1995).

LGA as an Indicator of Nutrition and Health Risk

Infant mortality rates are higher among full-term infants who weigh more than 4,000 g than for infants weighing between 3,000 and 4,000 g (IOM, 1973; Puffer and Serrano, 1987). However, the likelihood of dying because of a birth weight above 4,000 g is much less than that of infants with LBW (i.e., those weighing less than 2,500 g) (IOM, 1990) and the number of infant deaths attributed to LGA is small. When LGA occurs with preterm birth, the mortality risk is higher than that when either condition exists alone (Battaglia et al., 1966) (see also Chapter 5).

One study suggests that infants with a history of LGA are likely to remain taller and heavier and to have a higher risk of overweight during childhood than infants without LGA (Binkin et al., 1988). The committee found no other evidence that LGA indicates nutritional risk.

LGA as an Indicator of Health and Nutrition Benefit

When treated appropriately, LGA infants usually have a good prognosis (Lubchenco, 1981). LGA infants may benefit from the WIC program in the same ways that other newborns do: support from promoting breastfeeding and healthy infant feeding practices, the provision of nutrient-dense supplemental foods to the mother or formula for the infants, and health referrals from the program to detect or treat medical complications that may accompany LGA.

Use of the LGA as a Nutrition Risk Criterion in the WIC Setting

For the 14 state WIC agencies using high birth weight as a risk criterion for determining WIC program eligibility for infants in 1992, cutoff points ranged from 4,000 to 5,000 g, and the median cutoff point was 4,500 g (USDA, 1994). Birth weight data are routinely collected in most hospitals and are readily available to the WIC program.

Recommendations for LGA

The nutrition risk of *LGA* is low in infants. The benefit of the WIC program to infants who are LGA is no greater than that to any other newborn. Therefore, the use of LGA as a risk criterion for WIC program participation is not recommended. However, if *LGA* continues to be used, the committee recommends that the cutoff point be above the 90th percentile on William's Birth Weight Curve (Williams et al., 1982). For infants born at 40 weeks of gestation, the 90th percentile corresponds to a birth weight of approximately 4,000 g.

Overweight

Overweight is defined by weight-for-height above a specified cutoff point using NCHS-CDC reference data (Kanders, 1995). The term *overweight* is preferred over *obesity* to describe high weight-for-height because high weights-for-height can be a result of either greater lean body mass or adiposity. A distinction between overweight and obesity cannot be made just by measuring weight-for-height. The term *obesity* implies excessive fatness.

Prevalence of and Factors Associated with Overweight

The prevalence of overweight among infants and children in low-income U.S. families, defined as weight-for-height above the 95th percentile of the NCHS-CDC reference standard, was about 9 percent in 1991—higher than the expected 5 percent in a normal distribution (Yip et al., 1992a). The prevalence was higher in Hispanic, Native American, and black children than in white or Asian children.

In humans, overweight because of excess body fat can result from excessive energy intake, decreased energy expenditure, or impaired regulation of energy metabolism. Obesity therefore reflects an imbalance between energy intake and energy expenditure and is related to environmental and genetic factors (Kanders, 1995).

One probable environmental factor is prolonged overfeeding. Bottle feeding and early introduction of solid food may contribute to this practice, but overfeeding has not been confirmed as a major cause of obesity in studies that compared the food intakes of lean and obese infants and young children (Dietz, 1983). In fact, studies indicate that obese infants do not eat significantly more than their lean peers (Mumford and Morgan, 1982; Vobecky et al., 1983). Similar conclusions were also reached by studies of older children and adolescents (Dietz, 1983; Frank et al., 1978; Keen et al., 1979; Kromhout, 1983; Rolland-Cachera and Bellisle, 1986). However, most studies used recall data to estimate energy intakes, and such data are subject to a number of errors (see Chapter 6).

The results of a few studies have suggested that dietary composition may play a role in obesity. It has long been known that a high-fat, low-protein diet increases body fat content in animals (Filer, 1993). In humans, a high-fat, low-carbohydrate diet induces slightly greater levels of energy storage compared with a low-fat, high-carbohydrate diet with an equal energy content (Pi-Sunyer, 1993). A study of 48 children ages 9 to 11 years examined the relationship of percentage of body fat (measured by triceps skinfold thickness) and total fat intake (Gazzaniga and Burns, 1993). After adjusting for energy intake, resting energy expenditure, and physical activity, the percentage of body fat correlated positively with intake of total, saturated, monounsaturated, and polyunsaturated fatty acids and negatively with carbohydrate and total energy. In a cohort study of 146 children ages 3 to 5 years, an increase in BMI over a 3-year period was associated with an increased intake of energy from fat but not an increased total energy intake (Klesges et al., 1995). These findings indicate the importance of an appropriately balanced diet for preventing and treating obesity.

Some evidence indicates that low energy expenditure contributes to the development of obesity. In a study by Roberts and colleagues (1988), total energy expenditure and metabolizable energy intake were measured by the doubly labeled water method and by indirect calorimetry at 3 months of age. Total energy expenditure was about 20 percent lower in the infants who became overweight by the age of 1 year than in the infants who did not. There was no significant difference in postprandial metabolic rates, suggesting that physical activity, not thermogenesis, was reduced in the overweight infants.

Fontvieille and Ravussin (1993) compared the resting metabolic rates of Pima Indian children ages 3 to 5 years with those of white children. Although the Pima Indian children were taller, heavier, and fatter than the white children, the resting metabolic rate adjusted for body size, composition, and sex was similar in the two groups. Also, Pima Indian girls spent little time playing sports and considerable time watching television. In boys, the more time spent in sports activity, the leaner the child. Dietz and Gortmaker (1985) reported a direct association between television viewing and obesity in children.

Genetic factors have long been hypothesized to be associated with obesity (Garn and Clark, 1976; Garn et al., 1989). The correlation between obesity in the parents and obesity in their children is often strong (Burns et al., 1993; Garn, 1985; Klesges et al., 1995). The risk of obesity among children is lowest when neither parent is obese, higher when one parent is obese, and highest when both parents are obese (Dietz, 1983). The children of obese parents are also more likely to develop persistent obesity than other children (Price et al., 1990). Genetic studies in animals have shown that mutations at loci on six different chromosomes produce the obese phenotype in mice (Friedman and Leibel, 1990; Leiter, 1993). Recently, an obese (*ob*) gene was identified in mice that, when mutated, causes profound obesity and type II diabetes resembling morbid obesity in humans (Zhang et al., 1994).

Overweight as an Indicator of Nutrition and Health Risk

Just as infantile fatness (as measured by subcutaneous fat) predicts fatness during childhood (Leung and Robson, 1990), weight-for-height during early infancy predicts weight-for-height during late infancy and childhood (Binkin et al., 1988). Similarly, children who are overweight are more likely than other children to become overweight adolescents and adults (Mossberg, 1989; Sorensen and Sonne-Holm, 1988; Stark et al., 1981). Rolland-Cachera and co-workers (1987, 1989) followed more than 100 French children from age 1 year to adulthood. They showed that BMI in childhood significantly predicted BMI at 18 to 25 years in both sexes; the prediction became stronger as the children became older. Associations between obesity in childhood and obesity in adulthood were consistently positive in a review of studies published between

1970 and 1992 (Serdula et al., 1993). About one-third of obese preschool-age children and about half of obese school-age children were obese as adults. The risk of adult obesity was at least twice as high for obese children as for nonobese children and was even greater for children who were obese at older ages. Studies have shown that obesity in adulthood is an important risk factor for hypertension, diabetes, heart disease, gall bladder disease, certain cancers, and premature mortality (NIH, 1985).

Direct relationships between obesity and adverse health consequences are not as extensively documented in children as in adults. Among a few early studies that suggested a more frequent occurrence of illness in obese infants than in nonobese infants, methodologic problems such as inappropriate controls and diagnoses tend to invalidate their conclusions (Mallick, 1983). One study suggested that obese children may manifest many of the same disturbances as obese adults, including hyperinsulinism, hyperlipidemia, and hypertension (Rosenbaum and Leibel, 1989). Javier-Nieto and co-workers (1992) linked weight and height measures for children ages 5 to 18 years from 1933 to 1945 with follow-up mortality data over 30 to 40 years for both sexes combined. They found a statistically significant linear trend in the odds of adult mortality by quintile of childhood relative weight. However, because the measurements were obtained in the 1930s and 1940s from children who had relatively low weights-for-height by current standards, it is not clear how applicable the results are to children today.

The censure of overweight people in modern industrial societies may lead to social and psychological problems, including feelings of inadequacy and poor self-esteem (Gortmaker, 1993; Wadden et al., 1984).

Misclassification of a normal child as obese may have adverse consequences (Mallick, 1983). Unjustified and medically unsupervised dietary restriction based on such a misclassification may result in permanent stunting of growth and delayed development in infants and children (Lifshitz and Moses, 1989; Pugliese et al., 1983; Taitz, 1977). Even modest energy restriction in children with increased adiposity has been associated with a significant reduction in rate of increase in height (Dietz and Hartung, 1985). Because of these well-recognized health risks, the Committee on Nutrition of the American Academy of Pediatrics (1981) has recommended that dietary energy restriction not be used as a means to induce weight loss in infants and children.

Overweight as an Indicator of Nutrition and Health Benefit

Inasmuch as obesity during infancy and childhood is related to obesity during adulthood and adult obesity is associated with a number of adverse health consequences, it is assumed but not verified that treatment of excess adiposity in young children will be more effective than treatment of adiposity in adults. This is because behavioral patterns and social environments can be strongly influenced by the caregiver, and reducing potential risk factors (e.g., hyperlipidemia and hypertension) as early as possible may maximize beneficial effects for preventing long-term morbidity and mortality.

A 5- and 10-year follow-up of children from a family-based behavioral treatment program showed that weight reductions were significant compared with those for controls, but even in the best performing group, 30 to 40 percent of children were still overweight at 10 years (Epstein et al., 1990). Little information is available with regard to other long-term health consequences.

Commonly accepted weight control regimens emphasize sufficient energy content and adequate vitamins, minerals, and proteins in the diet to meet requirements for normal growth, along with increased physical activity and behavior modification (CN-AAP, 1981; Epstein and Wing, 1987). More data are needed to identify optimal treatments for obesity as judged by their impacts on health outcomes, and the preventive roles of nutrition and health interventions require further investigation (Flegal, 1993; Robinson, 1993).

Overweight infants and children may benefit from participation in the WIC program by receiving foods that are rich in such nutrients as protein, iron, calcium, vitamin A, and vitamin C. A food package modified to be low in fat might be especially beneficial. For those who are overweight because of obesity, the nutrient-dense WIC food package together with sensible eating plans provided by the WIC program may help to improve dietary quality and establish healthy eating habits. These interventions may place participants in a better position for future success of weight control and help them avoid the risks of unwarranted and self-imposed weight loss activities. Also, through its health referral function, the WIC program can help obese individuals with clinical complications to obtain early diagnosis and treatment by health professionals.

Use of the Overweight as a Nutrition Risk Criterion in the WIC Setting

Table 4-1 summarizes use of overweight as a nutrition risk criterion by state WIC agencies. The cutoff points used for overweight ranged from the 89th to 95th percentiles for the infants and 75th to 95th percentiles for children.

Recommendation for Overweight

The risk of *overweight* is documented in infants and children, and the method for identifying overweight is straightforward. There is a theoretical basis for benefit from participation in the WIC program. Therefore, the committee recommends the use of *overweight* as a nutrition risk criterion for infants and children in the WIC program, with a cutoff value at above the 95th percentile of NCHS-CDC references.

Slow Growth

Assessing gain or loss of weight and growth involves repeated anthropometric measurements over time. Multiple measurements provide confirmatory information about attained growth and a dynamic picture of growth changes (velocity) that permit the early detection of slow growth. However, identification of abnormal growth cannot rely on measuring growth changes alone. A lack of weight gain may be a result of a successful weight control program. The diagnosis of slow growth must consider other evidence including previous growth conditions and possible causes of growth changes. Failure to thrive (FTT), a condition in which growth is abnormally slow, is a medical diagnosis and is covered in Chapter 5. Anthropometric assessment in the WIC program may identify the need for referral for the diagnosis and treatment of FTT of any origin. Nonorganic failure to thrive is a medical term for poor growth without apparent medical cause.

Weight change is the anthropometric measurement that is most indicative of slow growth, especially in infants and young children. Two types of weight criteria are used in the literature: those based on weight loss and those based on attained growth below a specified percentile on the NCHS-CDC reference curve. An easy and common approach to identifying weight loss in a clinical setting is to plot a child's weights measured over time on the NCHS-CDC reference curve and examine if the plotted points cross major percentile lines more than once or fall from the lowest percentile.

Prevalence of and Factors Associated with Slow Growth

Undereating, for any number of reasons, and disease conditions are the main causes of abnormally slow growth. However, some infants who apparently have a genotype for a smaller size have a normal downward shift in growth rate between 3 and 18 months of age (Smith et al., 1976), which may be mistaken for growth faltering. Factors that are associated with undereating by an infant or child include lack of social support for the caregiver; an adverse social and psychological environment; a disorganized family; depressed parents or caregivers; and the caregiver's lack of education, health and nutrition knowledge, mental and physical abilities, and responsibility for child care (Lifshitz et al., 1991; McCrae et al., 1978).

Slow Growth as an Indicator of Nutrition and Health Risk

Infants and children who have slow growth may be malnourished and likely to remain so over an extended period (Oates et al., 1985). Persistent malnutrition may be translated into elevated morbidity and mortality risks, especially when diseases secondary to nonorganic FTT occur. If an infant or child has FFT, he or she may remain developmentally delayed despite weight gain (see also Chapter 5) (Drotar and Sturm, 1992; Wolke et al., 1990).

Slow Growth as an Indicator of Nutrition and Health Benefit

Otherwise healthy infants and children with abnormally slow growth can certainly benefit from nutrition and health interventions to improve weight and height gain. Indeed, such a benefit has been recognized as so plausible and unique that a formal diagnosis of nonorganic FTT must be based on a positive response of weight gain to nutrition rehabilitation (Lifshitz et al., 1991; McCrae et al., 1978). Interventions promote compensatory catch-up growth that restores deficits in weight and other dimensions of growth (Casey and Arnold, 1985). Although nutrition and health interventions may restore physical growth, they may only partially correct any developmental delays (Frank and Zeisel, 1988). An actual diagnosis of FFT should be made by a physician.

Use of Slow Growth as a Nutrition Risk in the WIC Setting

Table 4-1 summarizes use of abnormal growth as a nutrition risk criterion by state WIC agencies. The method of measurement (i.e., attained growth versus growth velocity) and cutoff points varied greatly. Identifying poor growth requires repeated measurements, which is sometimes impossible in the WIC setting. For recent immigrants especially, longitudinal data may be unavailable for identifying abnormally slow growth.

Recommendation for Slow Growth

The risk of *slow growth* is well documented in infants and children, and repeated visits make its identification possible for some infants and children. There is an empirical and theoretical basis for infants and children with slow growth to benefit from participation in the WIC program. The committee recommends the use of *slow growth* as a nutrition risk criterion for infants and children, with a cutoff value of below the 3rd percentile of change in weight, stature, or head circumference for age (Roche and Himes, 1980).

SUMMARY AND CONCLUSIONS

Conclusions

Anthropometric measurements are objective, nonintrusive, and easy to obtain; and they have been used as major nutrition risk criteria in the WIC program. However, there are no clear cutoff points for distinguishing an abnormal from a normal state, and the measurements provide no specific information about the cause of a problem. In spite of this, the current emphasis on these risk criteria is justified and should be continued because most anthropometric criteria have reasonably close relationships with risks, benefits, or both. Improvements in measurements lead to program benefits.

Anthropometric measurements are useful nutrition risk criteria for a number of conditions affecting pregnant or postpartum women, infants, and children. Their usefulness for women may improve if separate reference standards can be developed and tested for subgroups, such as adolescents and lactating women.

Different cutoff points may be needed for setting the specific criteria for different groups or for different outcomes. The anthropometric criteria discussed here are at best weak predictors of health and nutrition outcomes. Given the multifactorial nature of pregnancy and lactational outcomes, it is likely that the use of combinations of anthropometric with other criteria may be more useful for predictive purposes than the use of a single criterion.

Table 4-4 summarizes the committee's recommendations concerning the use of nutrition risk criteria for anthropometric measures.

Research Needs

1. Establish reference standards for pregnant, breastfeeding, and postpartum weight-for-height. The most important gaps relate to cutoffs to assess inadequate and excessive maternal weight gain during pregnancy, and body weight status of postpartum lactating and nonlactating women. Studies are urgently needed to describe the distribution of these measures in normative populations, to validate cutoff values against health outcomes, and, using the principles described in Chapter 3, to establish cutoffs with the highest yield.

2. Establish reference standards for maternal weight gain during pregnancy and maternal weight change after delivery.

3. Determine the impact of WIC program participation on health outcomes for pregnant and lactating and nonlactating postpartum women who have specific risk factors. For example, it is important to understand whether WIC program participation increases maternal weight gain and thus birth weight,

TABLE 4-4 Summary of Anthropometric Risk Criteria and Committee Recommendations for the Specific WIC Population

Risk Criterion	Committee Recommendation	Pregnant Women	Postpartum Women Lactating	Postpartum Women Nonlactating	Infants	Children
Women						
Prepregnancy underweight	Use with cutoff value of IBW <90% or BMI <19.8	✓				
Low maternal weight gain	Use with cutoff value of <0.9 kg/mo for nonobese and <0.45 kg/mo for obese	✓				
Maternal weight loss during pregnancy	Use with cutoff value of >2 kg first trimester, >1 kg 2nd or 3rd trimesters	✓				
Prepregnancy overweight	Use with cutoff value of IBW >120% or BMI >26	✓	✓	✓		
High gestational weight gain	Use with cutoff value of >3 kg/mo	✓	✓	✓		
Maternal short stature	Do not use					
Postpartum underweight	Use with cutoff value of IBW <90% or BMI <19		✓	✓		
Postpartum overweight	Use with cutoff value of IBW >120% or BMI >26 after 6 weeks postpartum		✓	✓		
Abnormal postpartum weight change	Do not use					

Infants and Children

Low birth weight	Use with cutoff value of <2,500 g	✓ ✓
Small for gestational age	Use with cutoff value of <10th percentile	✓ ✓
Short stature	Use with cutoff value of <5th percentile	✓ ✓
Underweight	Use with interim cutoff of 5th percentile	✓ ✓
Low head circumference	Use with cutoff value of <3rd percentile	✓
Large for gestational age	Do not use	
Overweight	Use with cutoff value of >95th percentile	✓
Slow growth	Use with cutoff value of <3rd percentile	✓

NOTE: ✓ = subgroup to which the recommendation applies; IBW = ideal body weight; BMI = body mass index.

whether WIC program participation has special benefit for women with prepregnancy underweight or short stature, and how the WIC program can affect long-term obesity in women.

4. Assess the effectiveness of interventions used to improve health and nutrition outcomes for LBW infants.

5. Relate body proportionality of SGA infants to risks and to potential benefits from interventions.

6. To ensure maximum benefit from the program, establish a priority system by comparing anthropometric criteria for their ability to predict the benefit intended by the program.

7. Examine the benefits of the WIC program relative to individual anthropometric criteria. Available data from the WIC program could be used for this purpose, or collection and analysis of these data could be organized. Such analysis would permit more accurate evaluation of the WIC program.

8. Compare populations with different distributions of an anthropometric measure (WHO, 1995) to determine the relative effects of different cutoff points on detection of nutrition and health risks and predictions of benefit. Results of this research will be useful for relating group attributes (e.g., low income, lack of education, and minority background) to benefits from participation in the WIC program.

REFERENCES

Aaronson, L.S., and C.L. Macnee. 1989. The relationship between weight gain and nutrition in pregnancy. Nurs. Res. 38:223–227.

Abraham, S., F.W. Lowenstein, and D.E. O'Connell. 1975. Preliminary Findings of the First Health and Nutrition Examination Survey, United States, 1971–1972: Anthropometric and Clinical Findings. DHEW Pub. No. (HRA) 75-1229. Rockville, MD: U.S. Department of Health, Education, and Welfare, National Center for Health Statistics.

Abrams, B. 1988. Maternal weight gain and pregnancy outcome in overweight women. Clin. Nutr. 7:197–204.

Abrams, B. 1991. Maternal undernutrition and reproductive performance. Pp. 31–60 in Infant and Child Nutrition Worldwide: Issues and Perspectives, F. Falkner, ed. Boca Raton, Fla.: CRC Press.

Abrams, B. 1994. Weight gain and energy intake during pregnancy. Clin. Obstet. Gynecol. 37:515–527.

Abrams, B., and C. Berman. 1993. Women, nutrition and health. Curr. Probl. Obstet. Gynecol. Fertil. 16:3–61.

Abrams, B., and V. Newman. 1991. Small-for-gestational-age birth: Maternal predictors and comparison with risk factors of spontaneous preterm delivery in the same cohort. Am. J. Obstet. Gynecol. 164:785–790.

Abrams, B., and J. Parker. 1988. Overweight and pregnancy complications. Int. J. Obes. 12:293–303.

Abrams, B., and J.D. Parker 1990. Maternal weight gain in women with good pregnancy outcome. Obstet. Gynecol. 76:1–7.

Abrams, B., and S. Selvin. 1995. Maternal weight gain pattern and birth weight. Obstet. Gynecol. 86:163–169.

Abrams, B., V. Newman, T. Key, and J. Parker. 1989. Maternal weight gain and preterm delivery. Obstet. Gynecol. 74:577–583.

Abrams, B., S. Carmichael, and S. Selvin. 1995. Factors associated with the pattern of maternal weight gain during pregnancy. Obstet. Gynecol. 86:170–176.

ACC/SCN (United Nations Administrative Committee on Coordination/Subcommittee on Nutrition). 1992. Second Report on the World Nutrition Situation, Vol. 1. Global and Regional Results. Geneva: ACC/SCN.

ACOG (American College of Obstetricians and Gynecologists). 1993. Nutrition during pregnancy: ACOG Technical Bulletin No. 179. Int. J. Gynecol. Obstet. 43:67–74.

Adair, L.S., and E. Pollitt. 1985. Outcome of maternal nutritional supplementation: A comprehensive review of the Bacon Chow study. Am. J. Clin. Nutr. 41:948–978.

Alam, N., B. Wojtyniak, and M.M. Rahaman. 1989. Anthropometric indicators and risk of death. Am. J. Clin. Nutr. 49:884–888.

Allen, L.H. 1994. Nutritional influences on linear growth: A general review. Eur. J. Clin. Nutr. 48(suppl. 1):75–89.

Altman, D.G., and F.E. Hytten. 1989. Intrauterine growth retardation: Let's be clear about it. Br. J. Obstet. Gynaecol. 96:1127–1132.

Ashworth, A., and R.G. Feachem. 1985. Interventions for the control of diarrheal diseases among young children: Prevention of low birth weight. Bull. WHO 63:165–184.

Atkinson, S.A., L.A. Hanson, and R.K. Chandra, eds. 1990. Human Lactation 4: Breastfeeding, Nutrition, Infection and Infant Growth in Developing and Emerging Countries. St. Johns, Newfoundland: ARTS Biomedical Publishers.

Avery, G.B., L. Meneses, and A. Lodge. 1972. The clinical significance of "measurement microcephaly". Am. J. Dis. Child. 123:214–217.

Babson, S.G., and N.B. Henderson. 1974. Fetal undergrowth: Relation of head growth to later intellectual performance. Pediatrics. 53:890–894.

Bagenholm, G.C., and A.A. Nasher. 1989. Mortality among children in rural areas of the People's Democratic Republic of Yemen. Ann. Trop. Paediatr. 9:75–81.

Bairagi, R. 1981. On validity of some anthropometric indicators as predictors of mortality. Am. J. Clin. Nutr. 34:2592–2594.

Baird, D. 1977. Epidemiological patterns over time. Pp. 5–15 in the Epidemiology of Prematurity, D.M. Reed and F.J. Stanley, eds. Baltimore, Md.: Urban and Shwarzenberg.

Balcazar, H., and J.D. Haas. 1991. Retarded fetal growth patterns and early neonatal mortality in a Mexico City population. Bull. Pan. Am. Health Org. 25:55–63.

Barker, D.J., P.D. Winter, C. Osmond, B. Margetts, and S.J. Simmonds. 1989. Weight in infancy and death from ischaemic heart disease. Lancet 2:577–580.

Barker, D.J., P.D. Gluckman, K.M. Godfrey, J.E. Harding, J.A. Owens, and J.S. Robinson. 1993a. Fetal nutrition and cardiovascular disease in adult life. Lancet 341:938–941.

Barker, D.J., C. Osmond, S.J. Simmonds, and G.A. Wield. 1993b. The relation of small head circumference and thinness at birth to death from cardiovascular disease in adult life. Br. Med. J. 306:422–426.

Barros, F.C., S. R. Huttly, C.G. Victora, B.R. Kirkwood, and J.P. Vaughan. 1992. Comparison of the causes and consequences of prematurity and intrauterine growth retardation: A longitudinal study in southern Brazil. Pediatrics 90:238–244.

Battaglia, F.C., T.M. Frazier, and A.E. Hellegers. 1966. Birth weight, gestational age, and pregnancy outcome with special reference to high birth weight-low gestational age infant. Pediatrics 37:417–422.

Beaton, G.H., and H. Ghassemi. 1982. Supplementary feeding programs for young children in developing countries. Am. J. Clin. Nutr. 35:863–916.

Beaton, G.H., A. Kelly, J. Kevany, R. Martorell, and J. Mason. 1990. Appropriate Uses of Anthropometric Indices in Children. ACC/SCN State of the Art Series, Nutrition Policy Discussion Paper. No. 7. Geneva: Administrative Committee on Coordination/Subcommittee on Nutrition.

Beaudry-Darismé, M., and M.C. Latham. 1973. Nutrition rehabilitation centers: An evaluation of their performance. J. Trop. Pediatr. Environ. Child Health 19:299–332.

Beghin, I.D., and F.E. Viteri. 1973. Nutrition rehabilitation centers: An evaluation of their performance. J. Trop. Pediatr. Environ. Child Health 19:403–416.

Berkowitz, G.S., and E. Papiernik. 1993. Epidemiology of preterm birth. Epidemiol. Rev. 15:414–443.

Bhushan, V., and N. Paneth. 1991. The reliability of neonatal head circumference measurement. J. Clin. Epidemiol. 44:1027–1035.

Binkin, N.J., R. Yip, L. Fleshood, and F.L. Trowbridge. 1988. Birth weight and childhood growth. Pediatrics 82:828–834.

Black, R.E., K.H. Brown, and S. Becker. 1984. Malnutrition is a determining factor in diarrhea duration, but not incidence, among young children in a longitudinal study in rural Bangladesh. Am. J. Clin. Nutr. 39:87–94.

Boardley, D.J. R.G. Sargent, A.L. Coker, J.R. Hussey, and P.A. Sharpe. 1995. The relationship between diet, activity, and other factors, and postpartum weight change by race. Obstet. Gynecol. 86:834–838.

Boyd, N.R., Jr., and R. Windsor. 1993. A meta-evaluation of nutrition education intervention research among pregnant women. Health Educ. Q. 20:327–345.

Bray, P.F., W.D. Shields, G.J. Wolcott, and J.A. Madsen. 1969. Occipitofrontal head circumference—an accurate measure of intracranial volume. J. Pediatr. 75:303–305.

Briend, A., C. Dykewicz, K. Graven, R.N. Mazumder, B. Wojtyniak, and M. Bennish. 1986. Usefulness of nutritional indices and classifications in predicting death of malnourished children. Br. Med. J. Clin. Res. Ed. 293:373–375.

Briend, A., B. Wojtyniak, and M.G. Rowland. 1987. Arm circumference and other factors in children at high risk of death in rural Bangladesh. Lancet 2:725–728.

Brown, J.E., and P.T. Schloesser. 1990. Prepregnancy weight status, prenatal weight gain, and the outcome of term twin gestations. Am. J. Obstet. Gynecol. 162:182–186.

Brown, K.H., R.E. Black, and S. Becker. 1982. Seasonal changes in nutritional status and the prevalence of malnutrition in a longitudinal study of young children in rural Bangladesh. Am. J. Clin. Nutr. 36:303–313.

Burns, T.L., P.P. Moll, and R.M. Lauer. 1993. Genetic models of human obesity—family studies. Crit. Rev. Food Sci. Nutr. 33:339–343.

Caan, B., D.M. Horgen, S. Margen, J.C. King, and N.P. Jewell. 1987. Benefits associated with WIC supplemental feeding during the interpregnancy interval. Am. J. Clin. Nutr. 45:29–41.

Casey, P.H., and W.C. Arnold. 1985. Compensatory growth in infants with severe failure to thrive. South. Med. J. 78:1057–1060.

Caulfield, L.E., J.D. Haas, J.M. Belizán, K.M. Rasmussen, and B. Edmonston. 1991. Differences in early postnatal morbidity risk by pattern of fetal growth in Argentina. Paediat. Perinat. Epidemiol. 5:263–275.

CDC (Center for Disease Control). 1972. Ten-State Nutrition Survey 1968–1970. III. Clinical, Anthropometry, Dental. DHEW Pub. No. (HSM) 72–8131. Atlanta: CDC.

CDC (Centers for Disease Control). 1978. CDC analysis of nutritional indices for selected WIC participants. Washington, D.C.: U.S. Food and Nutrition Service.

CDC (Centers for Disease Control). 1987. Nutritional status of minority children: United States 1986. Morbid. Mortal. Weekly Rep. 36:366–369.

CDC (Centers for Disease Control) 1992. Pregnancy risks determined from birth certificate data—United States, 1989. Morbid. Mortal. Weekly Rep. 41(30):556–563.

CDC (Centers for Disease Control). 1994. Increasing incidence of low birthweight: United States, 1981–1991. Morbid. Mortal. Weekly Rep. 43(18):335–339.

Chavéz, A., and C. Martínez. 1980. Effects of maternal undernutrition and dietary supplementation on milk production. Pp. 274–284 in Maternal Nutrition During Pregnancy and Lactation, H. Aebi and R. G. Whitehead, eds. Bern: Hans Huber.

Chen, L.C., A. Chowdhury, and S.L. Huffman. 1980. Anthropometric assessment of energy-protein malnutrition and subsequent risk of mortality among preschool aged children. Am. J. Clin. Nutr. 33:1836–1845.

Chwang, L.C., A.G. Soemantri, and E. Pollitt. 1988. Iron supplementation and physical growth of rural Indonesian children. Am. J. Clin. Nutr. 47:496–501.

Cliver, S.P., R.L. Goldenberg, G.R. Cutter, H.J. Hoffman, R.L. Copper, S.J. Gotlieb, and R.O. Davis. 1992. The relationships among psychosocial profile, maternal size, and smoking in predicting fetal growth retardation. Obstet. Gynecol. 80:262–267.

CN-AAP (Committee on Nutrition, American Academy of Pediatrics) 1981. Nutritional aspects of obesity in infancy and childhood. Pediatrics 68:880–883.

Cogswell, M.E., M.K. Serdula, D.W., Hungerford, and R. Yip. 1995. Gestational weight gain among average-weight and overweight women-what is excessive? Am. J. Obstet. Gynecol. 172:705–712.

Conlisk, E.A. 1993. The Heterogeneity of Low Birth Weight as it Relates to the Black-White Gap in Birthweight Specific Neonatal Mortality. Ph.D. Dissertation. Cornell University, Ithaca, N.Y.

Cook, R.A., S.B. Davis, F.H. Radke, and M.E. Thornbury. 1976. Nutritional status of Head Start and nursery school children. I. Food intake and anthropometric measurements. J. Am. Diet. Assoc. 68:120–126.

Cooke, R.W.I., A. Lucas, P.L.N. Yudkin, and J. Pryse-Davies. 1977. Head circumference as an index of brain weight in the fetus and newborn. Early Hum. Dev. 1:145–149.

Crawford, M.A., W. Doyle, A. Leaf, M. Leighfield, K. Ghebremeskel, and A. Phylactos. 1993. Nutrition and neurodevelopmental disorders. Nutr. Health. 9:219–235.

Cuttini, M., I. Cortinovis, A. Bossi, and U. de Vonderweid. 1991. Proportionality of small for gestational age babies as a predictor of neonatal mortality and morbidity. Paediatr. Perinat. Epidemiol. 5:56–63.

DaVanzo, J., W.P. Butz, and J-P. Habicht. 1983. How biological and behavioural influences on mortality in Malaysia vary during the first year of life. Population Studies 37:381–402.

Dawes, M.G., and J.G. Grudzinskas. 1991a. Repeated measurement of maternal weight gain during pregnancy: Is this a useful practice? Br. J. Obstet. Gynaecol. 98:189–194.

Dawes, M.G., and J.G. Grudzinskas. 1991b. Patterns of maternal weight gain in pregnancy. Br. J. Obstet. Gynaecol. 98:195–201.

Delgado, H.L., V. Valverde, J.M. Belizan, and R.E. Klein. 1983. Diarrheal disease, nutritional status and health care: Analysis of their interrelationships. Ecol. Food Nutr. 12:229–234.

Dewey, K.G., and M. McCrory. 1994. Effects of dieting and physical activity on pregnancy and lactation. Am. J. Clin. Nutr. 59:446S–453S.

Dewey, K.G., M.J. Heinig, L.A. Nommsen, and B. Lonnerdal. 1991a. Maternal versus infant factors related to breast milk intake and residual milk volume: The DARLING study. Pediatrics 87:829–837.

Dewey, K.G., M.J. Heinig, L.A. Nommsen, and B. Lonnerdal. 1991b. Adequacy of energy intake among breast-fed infants in the DARLING study: Relationships to growth velocity, morbidity, and activity levels. Davis Area Research on Lactation, Infant Nutrition and Growth. J. Pediatr. 119:538–547.

Dewey, K.G., M.J. Heinig, and L.A. Nommsen. 1993. Maternal weight-loss patterns during prolonged lactation. Am. J. Clin. Nutr. 58:162–166.

Dietz, W.H., Jr. 1983. Childhood obesity: Susceptibility, cause, and management. J. Pediatr. 103:676–686.

Dietz, W.H., Jr., and S.L. Gortmaker. 1985. Do we fatten our children at the television set? Obesity and television viewing in children and adolescents. Pediatrics 75:807–812.

Dietz, W.H., Jr., and R. Hartung. 1985. Changes in height velocity of obese preadolescents during weight reduction. Am. J. Dis. Child. 139:705–707.

Dobbing, J. 1970. Undernutrition and the developing brain. The relevance of animal models to the human problem. Am. J. Dis. Child. 120:411–415.

Dobbing, J. 1973. Quantitative growth and development of human brain. Arch. Dis. Child. 48:757–767.

Dobbing, J. 1974. The later growth of the brain and its vulnerability. Pediatrics. 53:2–6.

Dolan-Mullen, P., G. Ramirez, and J.Y. Groff. 1994. A meta-analysis of randomized trials of prenatal smoking cessation interventions. Am. J. Obstet. Gynecol. 171:1328–1334.

Dornhorst, A., J.S. Nicholls, F. Probst, C.M. Paterson, K.L. Hollier, R.S. Elkeles, and R.W. Beard. 1991. Calorie restriction for treatment of gestational diabetes. Diabetes 40(suppl. 2):161–164.

Dreze, J., and A. Sen. 1991. Hunger and Public Action. London: Oxford University Press.

Drotar, D., and L. Sturm. 1992. Personality development, problem solving, and behavior problems among preschool children with early histories of nonorganic failure-to-thrive: A controlled study. J. Dev. Behav. Pediatr. 4:266–273.

Dunn, H.G., C. J. Hughes, and M. Schulzer. 1986. Physical growth. Pp. 35–53 in Sequelae of Low Birthweight: The Vancouver Study, H.G. Dunn, ed. London: Mac Keith Press.

Dusdieker, L.B., D.L. Hemingway, and P.J. Stumbo. 1994. Is milk production impaired by dieting during lactation? Am. J. Clin. Nutr. 59:833–840.

Eckerman, C.O., L.A. Sturm, and S.J. Gross. 1985. Different developmental courses for very-low-birthweight infants differing in early head growth. Dev. Psychol. 21:813–827.

Edozien, J.C., B.R. Switzer, and R.B. Bryan. 1979. Medical evaluation of the Special Supplemental Food Program for Women, Infants, and Children. Am. J. Clin. Nutr. 32:677–692.

Ekblad, U., and S. Grenman. 1992. Maternal weight, weight gain during pregnancy and pregnancy outcomes. Int. J. Gynaecol. Obstet. 39:277–283.

Epstein, L.H., and R.R. Wing. 1987. Behavioral treatment of childhood obesity. Psychol. Bull. 101:331–342.

Epstein, L.H., A. Valoski, R.R. Wing, and J. McCurley. 1990. Ten-year follow-up of behavioral family-based treatment for obese children. J. Am. Med. Assoc. 264:2519–2523.

Eskenazi, B., L. Fenster, and S. Sidney. 1991. A multivariate analysis of risk factors for preeclampsia. J. Am. Med. Assoc. 266:237–241.

Fancourt, R., S. Campbell, D. Harvey, and A.P. Normal. 1976. Follow-up study of small-for-dates babies. Br. Med. J. 1:1435–1437.

Feachem, R.G., and M.A. Koblinsky. 1984. Interventions for the control of diarrhoeal diseases among young children: Promotion of breastfeeding. Bull. World Health Organ. 62:271–291.

Filer, L.J., Jr. 1993. A summary of the workshop on child and adolescent obesity: What, how, and who? Crit. Rev. Food Sci. Nutr. 33:287–305.

Flegal, K.M. 1993. Defining obesity in children and adolescents: Epidemiological approaches. Crit. Rev. Food Sci. Nutr. 33:307–312.

Flegal, K.M., W.R. Harlan, and J.R. Landis. 1988. Secular trends in body mass index and skinfold thickness with socioeconomic factors in young adult women. Am. J. Clin. Nutr. 48:535–543.

Fontvieille, A.M., and E. Ravussin. 1993. Metabolic rate and body composition of Pima Indian and Caucasian children. Crit. Rev. Food. Sci. Nutr. 33:363–368.

Frank, D.A., and S.H. Zeisel. 1988. Failure to thrive. Pediatr. Clin. North Am. 35:1187–1206.

Frank, G.C., G.S. Berenson, and L. S. Webber. 1978. Dietary studies and the relationship of diet to cardiovascular disease risk factor variables in 10-year-old children: The Bogalusa Heart Study. Am. J. Clin. Nutr. 31:328–340.

Friedman, J.M., and R.L. Leibel. 1990. Tackling a weighty problem. Cell 69:217–220.

Garn, S.M. 1985. Continuities and changes in fatness from infancy through adulthood. Curr. Probl. Pediatr. 15:1–47.

Garn, S.M., and D.C. Clark. 1976. Trends in fatness and origin of obesity. Ad Hoc Committee to Review the Ten-State Nutrition Survey. Pediatrics 57:443–456.

Garn, S.M., T.V. Sullivan, and V.M. Hawthorne. 1989. Fatness and obesity of the parents of obese individuals. Am. J. Clin. Nutr. 50:1308–1313.

Garrow, J.S., J.C. Waterlow, and B. Schürch. 1994. Causes and mechanisms of linear growth retardation. Proceeding of an IDECG Workshop. London, January 15–18, 1993. Eur. J. Clin. Nutr. 48: S2–S216.

Gayle, H.D., M.J. Dibley, J.S. Marks, and F.L. Trowbridge. 1987. Malnutrition in the first two years of life: The contribution of low birth weight to population estimates in the United States. Am. J. Dis. Child. 141:531–534.

Gazzaniga, J.M., and T.L. Burns. 1993. Relationship between diet composition and body fatness, with adjustment for resting energy expenditure and physical activity, in preadolescent children. Am. J. Clin. Nutr. 58:21–28.

Gerver, W.J.M., N.M. Drayer, and W. Schaafsma. 1989. Reference values of anthropometric measurements in Dutch children. The Oosterwolde Study. Acta. Paediatr. Scand. 78:307–313.

Godfrey, K.M., T. Forrester, D.J. Barker, A.A. Jackson, J.P. Landman, J.S. Hall, V. Cox, and C. Osmond. 1994. Maternal nutritional status in pregnancy and blood pressure in childhood. Br. J. Obstet. Gynaecol. 101:398–403.

Golden, M.H. 1994. Is complete catch-up possible for stunted malnourished children? Eur. J. Clin. Nutr. 48:S58–S71.

Golden, M.H.N., and B.E. Golden. 1981. Effect of zinc supplementation on the dietary intake, rate of weight gain, and energy cost of tissue deposition in children recovering from severe malnutrition. Am. J. Clin. Nutr. 34:900–908.

González-Cossio, T., J-P. Habicht, H. Delgado, and K.M. Rasmussen. 1991. Food supplementation during lactation increases infant milk intake and the proportion of exclusive breast feeding. FASEB J 5:A917.

Gopalan, C., M.C. Swaninathan, V.K. Kumari, D.H. Rao, and K. Vijayaraghavan. 1973. Effect of calorie supplementation on growth of under nourished children. Am. J. Clin. Nutr. 26:563–566.

Gorstein, J., K. Sullivan, R. Yip, M. de Onis, F. Trowbridge, P. Fajans, and G. Clugston. 1994. Issues in the assessment of nutritional status using anthropometry. Bull. World Health Organ. 72:273–283.

Gortmaker, S.L., A. Must, J.M. Perrin, A.M. Sobol, and W.H. Dietz. 1993. Social and economic consequences of overweight in adolescence and young adulthood. N. Engl. J. Med. 329:1008–1012.

Gross, S., C. Librach, and A. Cecutti. 1989. Maternal weight loss associated with hyperemesis gravidarum: A predictor of fetal outcome. Am. J. Obstet. Gynecol. 160:906–909.

Haaga, J.G. 1986. Negative bias in estimates of the correlation between children's weight-for-height and height-for-age. Growth 50:147–154.

Habicht, J-P., and W.P. Butz. 1979. Measurement of health and nutrition effects of large scale nutrition intervention projects. Pp. 133–182 in Evaluating the Impact of Nutrition and Health Programs, R.E. Klein, ed. New York: Plenum Press.

Habicht, J-P., and C. Yarbrough. 1980. Efficiency in selecting pregnant women for food supplementation during pregnancy. Pp. 314–336 in Maternal Nutrition During Pregnancy and Lactation, H. Aebi and R. G. Whitehead, eds. Bern: Hans Huber.

Habicht, J-P., R. Martorell, C. Yarbrough, R.M. Malina, and R.E. Klein. 1974. Height and weight standards for pre-school children: How relevant are ethnic differences in growth potential? Lancet 1:611–614.
Habicht, J-P., J. DaVanzo, and W.P. Butz. 1986. Does breastfeeding really save lives, or are apparent benefits due to biases? Am. J. Epidemiol. 123:279–290.
Hack, M., and N. Breslau. 1986. Very low birth weight infants: Effects of brain growth during infancy on intelligence quotient at 3 years of age. Pediatrics. 77:196–202.
Hack, M., N. Breslau, B. Weissman, D. Aram, N. Klein, and E. Borawski. 1991. Effect of very low birth weight and subnormal head size on cognitive abilities at school age. N. Engl. J. Med. 325:231–237.
Hack, M., H.G. Taylor, N. Klein, R. Eiben, C. Schatschneider, and N. Mercuri-Minich. 1994. School-age outcomes in children birth weights under 750 g. N. Engl. J. Med. 331:753–759.
Hamill, P.V.V., F.E. Johnston, and S. Lemeshow. 1972. Height and Weight of Children: Socioeconomic Status, United States. DHEW Pub. No. (HSM) 73-1601. National Centers for the Health Statistics. Vital Health Stat. 11(119).
Hamill, P.V.V., T.A. Drizd, C.L. Johnson, R.B. Reed, A.F. Roche, and W.M. Moore. 1979. Physical growth: National Center for Health Statistics percentiles. Am. J. Clin. Nutr. 32:607–629.
Harvey, D., J. Prince, J. Bunton, C. Parkinson, and S. Campbell. 1982. Abilities of children who were small-for-gestational-age babies. Pediatrics 69:296–300.
Hediger, M.L., T.O. Scholl, D.H. Belsky, I.G Ances, and R.W. Salmon. 1989. Patterns of weight gain in adolescent pregnancy: Effects on birth weight and preterm delivery. Obstet. Gynecol. 74:6–12.
Hediger, M.L., T.O. Scholl, J.I. Schall, M.F. Healey, and R.L. Fischer. 1994. Changes in maternal upper arm fat stores are predictors of variation in infant birth weight. J. Nutr. 124:24–30.
Heikens, G.T., W.N. Schofield, S. Dawson, and S.Grantham-McGregor. 1989. The Kingston Project. I. Growth of malnourished children during rehabilitation in the community, given a high energy supplement. Eur. J. Clin. Nutr. 43:145–160.
Heikens, G.T., W.N. Schofield, and S. Dawson. 1993. The Kingston Project. II. The effects of high energy supplement and metronidazole on malnourished children rehabilitated in the community: Anthropometry. Eur. J. Clin. Nutr. 47:160–173.
Heimendinger, J., N. Laird, J.E. Austin, P. Timmer, and S. Gershoff. 1984. The effects of the WIC program on the growth of infants. Am. J. Clin. Nutr. 40:1250–1257.
Heywood, P. 1982. The functional significance of malnutrition: Growth and prospective risk of death in the highlands of Papua New Guinea. J. Food Nutr. 39:13–19.
Hick, L.E., R.A. Langham, and J. Takenaka. 1982. Cognitive and health measures following early nutritional supplementation: A sibling study. Am. J. Public Health 72:1110–1118.
Hickey, C.A., S.P. Cliver, R.L. Goldenberg, J. Kohatsu, and H.J. Hoffman. 1993. Prenatal weight gain, term birth weight, and fetal growth retardation among high-risk multiparous black and white women. Obstet. Gynecol. 81:529–535.
Hickey, C.A., S.P. Cliver, S.F. McNeal, H.J. Hoffman, and R.L. Goldenberg. 1995. Prenatal weight gain patterns and spontaneous preterm birth among non obese black and white women. Obstet. Gynecol 85:909–914.

Hogberg, U., S. Wall, and D.E. Wiklund. 1990. Risk determinants of perinatal mortality in a Swedish county, 1980–1984. Acta Obstet. Gynecol. Scand. 69:575–579.

Ikenoue, T., T. Ikeda, S. Ibara, M. Otake, and W.J. Schull. 1993. Effects of environmental factors on perinatal outcome: Neurological development in cases of intrauterine growth retardation and school performance of children perinatally exposed to ionizing radiation. Environ. Health Perspect. 101:53–57.

IOM (Institute of Medicine). 1973. Infant Death: An Analysis By Maternal Risk and Health Care. Report of the Panel on Health Services Research. Washington, D.C.: National Academy Press.

IOM (Institute of Medicine). 1985. Preventing Low Birthweight. Report of the Committee to Study the Prevention of Low Birthweight, Division of Health Promotion and Disease Prevention. Washington, D.C.: National Academy Press.

IOM (Institute of Medicine). 1990. Nutrition During Pregnancy. Part I, Weight Gain; Part II, Nutrient Supplements. Report of the Subcommittee on Nutritional Status and Weight Gain During Pregnancy and Subcommittee on Dietary Intake and Nutrient Supplements During Pregnancy, Committee on Nutritional Status During Pregnancy and Lactation, Food and Nutrition Board. Washington, D.C.: National Academy Press.

IOM (Institute of Medicine). 1991. Nutrition During Lactation. Report of the Subcommittee on Nutrition During Lactation, Committee on Nutritional Status During Pregnancy and Lactation, Food and Nutrition Board. Washington, D.C.: National Academy Press.

IOM (Institute of Medicine). 1992a. Nutrition During Pregnancy and Lactation: An Implementation Guide. Report of the Subcommittee for a Clinical Application Guide, Committee on Nutritional Status during Pregnancy and Lactation, Food and Nutrition Board. Washington, D.C.: National Academy Press.

IOM (Institute of Medicine). 1992b. Nutrition Services in Perinatal Care, 2nd ed. Report of the Committee on Nutritional Status During Pregnancy and Lactation, Food and Nutrition Board. Washington, D.C.: National Academy Press.

Issacs, J.D., E.F. Magann, R.W. Martin, S.P. Chauhan, and J.C. Morrison. 1994. Obstetric challenges of massive obesity complicating pregnancy. J. Perinatol. 14:10–14.

Jacobson, J.L., S.W. Jacobson, R.J. Sokol, S.S. Martier, J.W. Ager, and S. Shankaran. 1994. Effects of alcohol use, smoking, and illicit drug use on fetal growth in black infants. J. Pediatr. 124:731–733.

James, S.A. 1992. Racial and ethnic differences in infant mortality and low birth weight: A psychosocial critique. Ann. Epidemiol. 3:130–136.

Javier-Nieto, F., M. Szklo, and G.W. Comstock. 1992. Childhood weight and growth rate as predictors of adult mortality. Am. J. Epidemiol. 136:201–213.

Johnson, A.A., E.M. Knight, C.H. Edwards, U.J. Oyemade, O.J. Cole, O.E. Westney, H. Laryea, and S. Jones. 1994. Dietary intakes, anthropometric measurements and pregnancy outcomes. J. Nutr. 124:936S–942S.

Johnson, J.W., J.A. Longmate, and B. Frentzen. 1992. Excessive maternal weight and pregnancy outcome. Am. J. Obstet. Gynecol. 167:353–372.

Johnston, E.M. 1991. Weight changes during pregnancy and the postpartum period. Prog. Food Nutr. Sci. 15:117–157.

Jones, D.Y., M.C. Nesheim, and J-P. Habicht. 1985. Influences on child growth associated with poverty in the 1970's: An examination of HANESI and HANESII, cross-sectional U.S. national surveys. Am. J. Clin. Nutr. 42:714–724.

Kanders, B.S. 1995. Pediatric obesity. Pp. 210–233 in Weighing the Options: Criteria for Evaluating Weight-Management Programs, P.R. Thomas, ed. Report of the Committee to Develop Criteria for Evaluating the Outcomes of Approaches to Prevent and Treat Obesity, Food and Nutrition Board, Institute of Medicine. Washington, D.C.: National Academy Press.

Karlberg, J., F. Jalil, B. Lam, L. Low, and C.Y. Yeung. 1994. Linear growth retardation in relation to the three phases of growth. Eur. J. Clin. Nutr. 48:S25–S44.

Kasango Project Team. 1983. Anthropometric assessment of young children's nutritional status as an indicator of subsequent risk of dying. J. Trop. Pediatr. 29:69–75.

Katz, J., K.P. West, Jr., I. Tarwotjo, and A. Sommer. 1989. The importance of age in evaluating anthropometric indices for predicting mortality. Am. J. Epidemiol. 130:1219–1226.

Keen, H., B.J. Thomas, R. J.Jarrett, and J.H. Fuller. 1979. Nutrient intake, adiposity and diabetes. Br. Med. J. 1:655–658.

Keller, W. 1988. The epidemiology of stunting. Pp. 17–29 in Linear Growth Retardation in Less Developed Countries, J.C. Waterlow, ed. New York: Raven Press.

Keppel, K.G., and S.M. Taffel. 1993. Pregnancy-related weight gain and retention: Implications of the 1990 Institute of Medicine guidelines. Am. J. Public Health 83:1100–1103.

Kerr, G.R., E.S. Lee, R.J. Lorimor, W.H. Mueller, and M.M. Lam. 1982. Height distributions of U.S. children: Associations with race, poverty status and parental size. Growth 46:135–149.

Khin-Maung-Naing, T.T.O. 1987. Effect of dietary supplementation on lactation performance of undernourished Burmese mothers. Food Nutr. Bull. 9:59–61.

Khoury, M.J., J.D. Erickson, J.F. Cordero, and B.J. McMarthy. 1988. Congenital malformations and intrauterine growth retardation: A population study. Pediatrics 82:83–90.

Khoury, M.J., C.J. Berg, and E.E. Calle. 1990. The ponderal index in term newborn siblings. Am. J. Epid. 132:576–83.

Kimball, K.J., R.L. Ariagno, D.K. Stevenson, and P. Sunshine. 1982. Growth to age 3 years among very low-birth-weight sequelae-free survivors of modern neonatal intensive care. J. Pediatr. 100:622–624.

Klebanov, P.K., J. Brooks-Gunn, and M.C. McCormick. 1994. Classroom behavior of very low birth weight elementary school children. Pediatrics 94:700–708.

Kleinman, J. 1990. Maternal Weight Gain During Pregnancy: Determinants and Consequences. NCHS Working Paper Series No. 33. Hyattsville, Md.: National Center for Health Statistics.

Klesges, R.C., L.M. Klesges, L.H. Eck, and M.L. Shelton. 1995. A longitudinal analysis of accelerated weight gain in preschool children. Pediatrics. 95:126–130.

Kramer, M.S. 1987a. Determinants of low-birth weight: Methodological assessment and meta-analysis. Bull. WHO 65:663–737.

Kramer, M.S. 1987b. Intrauterine growth and gestational duration determinants. Pediatrics. 80:502–511.

Kramer, M.S. 1993. Effects of energy and protein intakes on pregnancy outcome: An overview of the research evidence from controlled clinical trials. Am. J. Clin. Nutr. 58:627–635.

Kramer, M.S., F.H. McLean, M. Olivier, D.M. Willis, and R.H. Usher. 1989. Body proportionality and head and length 'sparing' in growth-retarded neonates: A critical reappraisal. Pediatrics. 84:717–723.

Kramer, M.S., M. Olivier, F.H. McLean, G.E. Dougherty, D.M. Willis, and R.H. Usher. 1990a. Determinants of fetal growth and body proportionality. Pediatrics 86:18–26.

Kramer, M.S., M. Olivier, F.H. McLean, D.M. Willis, and R.H. Usher. 1990b. Impact of intrauterine growth retardation and body proportionality on fetal and neonatal outcome. Pediatrics 86:707–713.

Kramer, M.S., F.H. McLean, E.L. Eason, and R.H. Usher. 1992. Maternal nutrition and spontaneous preterm birth. Am. J. Epidemiol. 136:574–583.

Krasovec, K., and M.A. Anderson. 1991. Maternal Nutrition and Pregnancy Outcomes: Anthropometric Assessment. Scientific Pub. No. 529. Washington, D.C.: Pan American Health Organization.

Kromhout, D. 1983. Energy and micronutrient intake in lean and obese middle-aged men (the Zutphen study). Am. J. Clin. Nutr. 37:295–299.

Kuczmarski, R.J., K.M. Flegal, S.M. Campbell, and C.L. Johnson. 1994. Increasing prevalence of overweight among U.S. adults. The National Health and Nutrition Examination Surveys, 1960–1991. J. Am. Med. Assoc. 272:205–211.

Kurz, K.M., J-P. Habicht, K.M. Rasmussen, and S.J. Schwager. 1993. Effects of maternal nutritional status and maternal energy supplementation on length of postpartum amenorrhea among Guatemalan women. Am. J. Clin. Nutr. 58:636–642.

Larsen, C.E., M.K. Serdula, and K.M. Sullivan. 1990. Macrosomia: Influence of maternal overweight among a low income population. Am. J. Obstet. Gynecol. 162:490–494.

Larson, B.J. 1991. Relationship of family communication patterns to Eating Disorder Inventory scores in adolescent girls. J. Amer. Diet. Assoc. 91:1065–1067.

Launer, L.J., J-P. Habicht, and S. Kardjati. 1990. Breast feeding protects infants in Indonesia against illness and weight loss due to illness. Am. J. Epidemiol. 131:322–331.

Lawrence, M., T. Yimer, and J.K. O'Dea. 1994. Nutritional status and early warning of mortality in southern Ethiopia, 1988–1991. Eur. J. Clin. Nutr. 48:38–45.

Lechtig, A., and R.E. Klein. 1981. Prenatal nutrition and birth weight: Is there a causal association? Pp. 131–156 in Maternal Nutrition in Pregnancy—Eating for Two? J. Dobbing, ed. London: Academic Press.

Leibel, R.L., M. Rosenbaum, and J. Hirsch. 1995. Changes in energy expenditure resulting from altered body weight. New Engl. J. Med. 332:621–628.

Leiter, E.H. 1993. Obesity genes and diabetes induction in the mouse. Crit. Rev. Food Sci. Nutr. 33:333–338.

Lester, B.M., C. Garcia-Coll, M. Valcarcel, J. Hoffman, and T.B. Brazelton. 1986. Effects of atypical patterns of fetal growth on newborn (NBAS) behavior. Child Dev. 57:11–19.

Leung, A.K., and W.L. Robson. 1990. Childhood obesity. Postgrad. Med. 87:123–130, 133.

Levy, H.L., S.E. Waisbren, D. Lobbregt, E. Allred, A. Schuler, F.K. Trefz., S.M. Schweitzer, I.B. Sardharwalla, J.H. Walter, B.E. Barwell et al. 1994. Maternal mild hyperphenylalaninaemia: An international survey of offspring outcome. Lancet. 344:1589–1594.

Lieberman, E. 1995. Low birth weight—not a black-and-white issue. N. Engl. J. Med. 332:117–118.

Lifshitz, F., and N. Moses. 1989. Growth failure. A complication of dietary treatment of hypercholesterolemia. Am. J. Dis. Child. 143:537–542.

Lifschitz, F., N.M. Finch, and J.Z. Lifschitz, eds. 1991. Failure to thrive. Pp. 253–270 in Children's Nutrition. Boston: Jones and Bartlett Publishers.

Lindtjorn, B., T. Alemu, and B. Bjorvatn. 1993. Nutritional status and risk of infection among Ethiopian children. J. Trop. Pediatr. 39:76–82.

Lindgren, G., G. Aurelius, J. Tanner, and M. Healy. 1994. Standards for height, weight and head circumference of one month to six years based on Stockholm children born in 1980. Acta. Paediatr. 83:360–366.

Listernick, R., K. Christoffel, J. Pace, and J. Chiaramonte. 1985. Severe primary malnutrition in U.S. children. Am. J. Dis. Child. 139:1157–1160.

Little, B.B., and L.M. Snell. 1991. Brain growth among fetuses exposed to cocaine in utero: Asymmetrical growth retardation. Obstet. Gynecol. 77:361–364.

Little, R.E., and C.R. Weinberg. 1993. Risk factors for antepartum and intrapartum stillbirth. Am. J. Epidemiol. 137:1177–1189.

Lubchenco, L.O. 1981. Gestational age, birth weight, and the high-risk infant. Pp. 12–18 in Infants At Risk: Assessment and Intervention, C.C. Brown, ed. Piscataway, N.J.: Johnson & Johnson Baby Products Company.

Lucas, A., R. Morley, T.J. Cole, M.F. Bamford, A. Boon, P. Crowle, J.F. Dossetor, and R. Pearse. 1988. Maternal fatness and viability of preterm infants. Br. Med. J. Clin. Res. Ed. 296:1495–1497.

Luke, B., T. Johnson, and R. Petrie. 1993. Clinical Maternal-Fetal Nutrition. Boston: Little, Brown and Co.

Lutter, C.K., J.O. Mora, J-P. Habicht, K.M. Rasmussen, D.S. Robson, S.G. Sellers, C.M. Super, and M.G. Herrera. 1989. Nutritional supplementation: Effects on child stunting because of diarrhea. Am. J. Clin. Nutr. 50:1–8.

Lutter, C.K., J.O. Mora, J-P. Habicht, K.M. Rasmussen, D.S. Robson, and M.G. Herrera. 1990. Age-specific responsiveness of weight and length to nutritional supplementation. Am J. Clin. Nutr. 51:359–364.

Lutter, C.K., J-P. Habicht, J.A. Rivera, and R. Martorell. 1992. The relationship between energy intake and diarrhoeal disease in their effects on child growth: Biological model, evidence, and implications for public health policy. Food Nutr. Bull. 14:36–42.

Malcolm, L. 1978. Protein energy malnutrition and growth. Pp. 361–371 in Human Growth, 1st ed. Vol. 3: Neurobiology and Nutrition, F. Falkner and J.M. Tanner, eds. New York: Plenum Press.

Malina, R.M., J-P. Habicht, R. Martorell, A. Lechtig, C. Yarbrough, and R.E. Klein. 1975. Head and chest circumferences in rural Guatemalan Ladino children, birth to seven years of age. Am. J. Clin. Nutr. 28:1061–1070.

Mallick, M.J. 1983. Health hazards of obesity and weight control in children: A review of the literature. Am. J. Public Health 73:78–82.

Manser, J.I. 1984. Growth in the high-risk infants. Clin. Perinatol. 2:19–40.
Marchant, K., R. Martorell, and J.D. Haas. 1990. Consequences for maternal nutrition of reproductive stress across consecutive pregnancies. Am. J. Clin. Nutr. 52:616–620.
Martorell, R. 1989. Body size, adaptation, and function. Hum. Org. 48:15–20.
Martorell, R., and J-P. Habicht. 1986. Growth in early childhood in developing countries. Pp. 241–262 in Human Growth: A Comprehensive Treatise, 2nd ed. Vol. 3: Methodology. Ecological, Genetic, and Nutritional Effects on Growth, F. Falkner and J.M. Tanner, eds. New York: Plenum Press.
Martorell, R., and T.J. Ho. 1984. Malnutrition, morbidity, and mortality. Child Survival: Strategies for Research, H. Mosey and L.C. Chen, eds. Pop. Dev. Rev. 10(suppl.):49–68.
Martorell, R., J-P. Habicht, and R.K. Klein. 1982. Anthropometric indicators of changes in nutritional status in malnourished population. Pp. 96–110 in Proceedings, Methodologies for Human Population Studies in Nutrition Related to Health, July 24–25, 1979, B.A. Underwood, ed. NIH Pub. No. 82-2462. Bethesda, Md.: U.S. Department of Health and Human Services.
Martorell, R., J. Rivera, H. Kaplowitz, and E. Pollitt. 1992. Long-term consequences of growth retardation during early childhood. Pp. 143–149 in Human Growth: Basic and Clinical Aspects, M. Hernandez and J. Argente, eds. Amsterdam: Elsevier.
Martorell, R., L.K. Khan, and D.G. Schroeder. 1994. Reversibility of stunting: Epidemiological findings in children from developing countries. Eur. J. Clin. Nutr. 48:S45–S57.
Mascie-Taylor, C.G. 1991. Biosocial influences on stature: A review. J. Biosoc. Sci. 23:113–128.
McCormick, M.C. 1985. The contribution of low birth weight to infant mortality and childhood mortality. N. Engl. J. Med. 312:82–90.
McCormick, M.C., J. Brooks-Gunn, K. Workman-Daniels, J. Turner, and G.J. Peckham. 1992. The health and development status of very low-birth-weight children at school age. J. Am. Med. Assoc. 267:2204–2208.
McCrae, W.M., I.J. Carré, P.W. Brunt, A.P. Mowat, and C.M. Andersen. 1978. Disorders of the alimentary tract. Pp. 438–442 in Textbook of Paediatrics, 2nd ed., vol. 1, J.O. Forfar and G.C. Arneil, eds. Edinburgh and New York: Churchill Livingstone.
Mendelson, R., D. Dollard, P. Hall, S.Y. Zarrabi, and E. Desjardin. 1991. The impact of the healthiest babies possible program on maternal diet and pregnancy outcome in underweight and overweight clients. J. Can. Diet. Assoc. 52:229–234.
Metcoff, J., P. Costiloe, W.M. Crosby, S. Dutta, H.H. Sandstead, D. Milne, C.E. Bodwell, and S.H. Majors. 1985. Effect of food supplementation (WIC) during pregnancy on birth weight. Am. J. Clin. Nutr. 41:933–947.
Meyer, M.B., and G.W. Comstock. 1972. Maternal cigarette smoking and perinatal mortality. Am. J. Epidemiol. 96:1–10.
Michaelson, K.F., P.S. Larsen, B.L. Thomsen, and G. Samuelson. 1994. The Copenhagen Cohort study of infant nutrition and growth: Breast milk intake, human milk macronutrient content, and influencing factors. Am. J. Clin. Nutr. 59:600–611.
Miller, C.A., A. Fine, and S. Adams-Taylor. 1989. Monitoring Children's Health: Key Indicators, 2nd ed. Washington D.C.: American Public Health Association.

Miller, H.C., and T.A. Merritt. 1979. Fetal Growth in Humans. Chicago: Year Book Medical Publishers.

Miller, J.E., and S. Korenman. 1994. Poverty and children's nutritional status in the United States. Am. J. Epidemiol. 140:233–243.

Mitchell, W.G., R.W. Gorrell, and R.A. Greenberg. 1980. Failure to thrive: A study in a primary care setting. Epidemiology and follow-up. Pediatrics 65:971–977.

Mora, J.O., M.G. Herrera, J. Suescun, L. de Navarro, and M. Wagner. 1981. The effects of nutritional supplementation on physical growth of children at risk of malnutrition. Am. J. Clin. Nutr. 34:1885–1892.

Mossberg, H.O. 1989. 40-year follow-up of overweight children. Lancet 2:491–493.

Mumford, P., and J.B. Morgan. 1982. A longitudinal study of nutrition and growth of infants initially on the upper and lower centile of weight and age. Int. J. Obes. 6:335–341.

Naeye, R.L. 1990. Maternal body weight and pregnancy outcome. Am. J. Clin. Nutr. 52:273–279.

Nandi, C., and M.R. Nelson. 1992. Maternal pregravid weight, age and smoking status as risk factors for low birth weight births. Public Heath Rep. 107:658–662.

NIH (National Institutes of Health). 1985. Health Implications of Obesity: National Institutes of Health Consensus Development Conference Statement. Ann. Intern. Med. 103:1073–1077.

NIH (National Institutes of Health) Technology Assessment Conference Panel. 1992. Methods for voluntary weight loss and control. Ann. Intern. Med. 116:942–949.

Niswander, K.R., and M. Gordon. 1972. The Women and Their Pregnancies. The Collaborative Perinatal Study of the National Institute of Neurological Diseases and Stroke. DHEW Pub. No. (NIH) 73–379. Washington, D.C.: U.S. Government Printing Office.

Nommsen, L.A., C.A. Lovelady, M.J. Heinig, B. Lonnerdal, and K.G. Dewey. 1991. Determinants of energy, protein, lipid, and lactose concentrations in human milk during the first 12 months of lactation: The DARLING Study. Am. J. Clin. Nutr. 53:457–465.

NRC (National Research Council). 1989. Diet and Health: Implications for Reducing Chronic Disease Risk. Report of the Commission in Diet and Health, Food and Nutrition Board, Commission on Life Sciences. Washington, D.C.: National Academy Press.

Nulman, I., J. Rovet, D. Altmann, C. Bradley, T. Einarson; and G. Koren. 1994. Neurodevelopment of adopted children exposed in utero to cocaine. Can. Med. Assoc. J. 151:1591–1597.

Oates, R.K., A. Peacock, and D. Forrest. 1985. Long-term effects of nonorganic failure to thrive. Pediatrics. 75:36–40.

Ounsted, M., and C. Ounsted. 1968. Rate of intra-uterine growth. Nature 220:599–600.

Ounsted, M., V.A. Moar, and A. Sott. 1985. Head circumference charts updated. Arch. Dis. Child. 60:936–939.

Owen, G.M., and A.H. Lubin. 1973. Anthropometric differences between black and white preschool children. Am. J. Dis. Child. 126:168–169.

Owen, G.M., K.M. Kram, P.J. Garry, J.E. Lowe, and A.H. Lubin. 1974. A study of nutritional status of preschool children in the United States, 1968–70. Pediatrics 53:597–646.

Palmer, C.G., C. Cronk, S.M. Pueschel, K.E. Wisniewski, R. Laxova, A.C. Crocker, and R.M. Pauli. 1992. Head circumference of children with Down syndrome (0–36 months). Am. J. Med. Genet. 42:61–67.

Parker, J.D. 1994. Postpartum weight change. Clin. Obstet. Gynecol. 37:528–537.

Parker, J.D., and B. Abrams. 1992. Prenatal weight gain advice: An examination of the recent prenatal weight gain recommendations of the Institute of Medicine. Obstet. Gynecol. 79:664–669.

Parker, J.D., and B. Abrams. 1993. Differences in postpartum weight retention between black and white mothers. Obstet. Gynecol. 81:768–774.

Parkinson, C.E., S. Wallis, and D.R. Harvey. 1981. School achievement and behaviour of children who are small-for-dates at birth. Dev. Med. Child. Neurol. 23:41–50.

Paul, A.A., E.A. Ahmed, and R.G. Whitehead. 1986. Head circumference charts updated (letter). Arch. Dis. Child. 61:927–928.

Pelletier, D.L. 1994. The relationship between child anthropometry and mortality in developing countries: Implications for policy, programs and future research. J. Nutr. 124:2047S–2081S.

Pelletier, D.L., E.A. Frongillo, Jr., and J-P. Habicht. 1993. Epidemiologic evidence for a potentiating effect of malnutrition on child mortality. Am. J. Public Health 83:1130–1133.

Perlow, J.H., M.A. Morgan, D. Montgomery, C.V. Towers, and M. Porto. 1992. Perinatal outcome in pregnancy complicated by massive obesity. Am. J. Obstet. Gynecol. 167:958–962.

Petitti, D.B., and C. Coleman. 1990. Cocaine and the risk of low birth weight. Am. J. Public Health 80:25–28.

Petitti, D.B., M.S. Croughan-Minihane, and R.A. Hiatt. 1991. Weight gain by gestational age in both black and white women delivered of normal-birth-weight and low-birth-weight infants. Am J Obstet Gynecol. 164:801–805.

Phillips, D.I., D.J. Barker, C.N. Hales, S. Hirst, and C. Osmond. 1994. Thinness at birth and insulin resistance in adult life. Diabetologia 37:150–154.

Pinstrup-Anderson, P., S. Burger, J-P. Habicht, and K.E. Peterson. 1993. Protein energy malnutrition. Pp. 391–420 in Disease Control Priorities in Developing Countries, D.T. Jamison and W.H. Mostley, eds. London: Oxford University Press.

Pi-Sunyer, F.X. 1993. Metabolic efficiency of macronutrient utilization in humans. Crit. Rev. Food Sci. Nutr. 33:359–361.

Plouin, P.F., G. Breart, Y. Rabarison, C. Rumeau-Rouquette, C. Sureau, and J. Menard. 1983. Fetal growth retardation in gestational hypertension: Relationships with blood pressure levels and the time of onset of hypertension. Eur. J. Obstet. Gynecol. Reprod. Biol. 16:253–262.

Pollitt, E., K.S. Gorman, P.L. Engle, R. Martorell, and J. Rivera. 1993. Early supplementary feeding and cognition: Effects over two decades. Monogr. Soc. Res. Child Dev. 58:1–118.

Prentice, A., and C.J. Bates. 1994. Adequacy of dietary mineral supply for human bone growth and mineralisation. Eur. J. Clin. Nutr. 48(suppl. 1):S161–S177.

Prentice, A.M., R.G. Whitehead, M. Watkinson, W.H. Lamb, and T.J. Cole. 1983. Prenatal dietary supplementation of African women and birth-weight. Lancet 1:489–492.

Price, R.A., A.J. Stunkard, R. Ness, T. Wadden, S. Heshka, B. Kanders, and A. Cormillot. 1990. Childhood onset (age less than 10) obesity has high familial risk. Int. J. Obes. 14:185–195.

Prichard, J.A., P.C. MacDonald, and N.F. Gant. 1985. Williams Obstetrics, 7th ed. Norwalk, Conn.: Appleton-Century-Crofts.

Puffer, R.R., and C.V. Serrano. 1987. Patterns of Birthweights. Washington, D.C.: Pan American Health Organization, Pan American Sanitary Bureau, World Health Organization Regional Office.

Pugliese, M.T., F. Lifshitz, G. Grad, P. Fort, and M. Marks-Katz. 1983. Fear of obesity: A cause for short stature and delayed puberty. N. Engl. J. Med. 309:513–518.

Rahaman, J., G.V. Narayansingh, and S. Roopnarinesingh. 1990. Fetal outcome among obese parturients. Int. J. Gynaecol. Obstet. 31:227–230.

Rao, D.H., and A.N. Naidu. 1977. Nutritional supplementation—whom does it benefit most? Am. J. Clin. Nutr. 30:1612–1616.

Rasmussen, K.M., N.B. Mock, and J-P. Habicht. 1988. The biological meaning of low birthweight and the use of data on low birthweight for nutritional surveillance. Cornell Nutritional Surveillance Program, Working Paper No. 27. Ithaca, N.Y.

Ratcliffe, S.G., N. Masera, and M. McKie. 1994. Head circumference and IQ of children with sex chromosome abnormalities. Dev. Med. Child Neurol. 36:533–544.

Ratner, R.E., L.H. Hamner 3d, and N.B. Isada. 1991. Effects of gestational weight gain in morbidly obese women: 1. Maternal morbidity. Am. J. Perinatol. 8:21–24.

Rawlings, J.S., V.B. Rawlings, and J.A. Read. 1995. Prevalence of low birth weight and preterm delivery in relation to the interval between pregnancies among white and black women. N. Engl. J. Med. 332:69–74.

Read, J.S., J.D. Clemens, and M.A. Klebanoff. 1994. Moderate low birth weight and infectious disease mortality during infancy and childhood. Am. J. Epidemiol. 140:721–733.

Regev, R., and L.M.S. Dubowitz. 1988. Head growth and neurodevelopmental outcome in neonates with intracranial hemorrhage and leukomalacia. Early Human Dev. 16:207–211.

Rimoin, D.L., Z. Borochowitz, and W.A. Horton. 1986. Short stature: Physiology and pathology. West J. Med. 144:710–721.

Rivera, J.A. 1988. Effect of supplementary feeding upon the recovery from mild-to-moderate wasting in children. Ph.D. Dissertation. Cornell University, Ithaca, N.Y.

Rivera, J.A., J-P. Habicht, and D.S. Robson. 1991. Effects of supplementary feeding on recovery from mild to moderate wasting in preschool children. Am. J. Clin. Nutr. 54:62–68.

Roberts, S.B., J. Savage, W.A. Coward, B. Chew, and A. Lucas. 1988. Energy expenditure and intake in infants born to lean and overweight mothers. N. Engl. J. Med. 318:461–466.

Robinson, T.N. 1993. Defining obesity in children and adolescents: Clinical approaches. Crit. Rev. Food Sci. Nutr. 33:313–320.

Roche, A.F., and J.H. Himes. 1980. Incremental growth charts. Am J Clin Nutr. 33:2041–2052.

Rolland-Cachera, M.F., and F. Bellisle. 1986. No correlation between adiposity and food intake: Why are working class children fatter? Am. J. Clin. Nutr. 44:779–787.

Rolland-Cachera, M.F., M. Deheeger, M. Guilloud-Bataille, P. Avons, E. Patois, and M. Sempé. 1987. Tracking the development of adiposity from one month of age to adulthood. Ann. Hum. Biol. 14:219–229.

Rolland-Cachera, M.F., F. Bellisle, and M. Sempé. 1989. The prediction in boys and girls of the weight/height^2 index and various skinfold measurements in adults: A two-decade follow-up study. Int. J. Obes. 13:305–311.

Rosenbaum, M., and R.L. Leibel. 1989. Obesity in children. Pediatr. Rev. 11:43–55.

Rosso, P., E. Donoso, S. Braun, R. Espinoza, and S.P. Salas. 1992. Hemodynamic changes in underweight pregnant women. Obstet. Gynecol. 79:908–912.

Ruel, M.T., J. Rivera, and J-P. Habicht. 1995. Length screens better than weight in stunted populations. J. Nutr. 125:1222–1228.

Rush, D. 1986. The National WIC Evaluation: An Evaluation of the Special Supplemental Food Program for Women, Infants and Children. Research Triangle Park, N.C.: Research Triangle Institute.

Rush, D., J. Leighton, N.L. Sloan, J.M. Alvir, and G.C. Garbowski. 1988a. The National WIC Evaluation: Evaluation of the Special Supplemental Food Program for Women, Infants, and Children. II. Review of past studies of WIC. Am. J. Clin. Nutr. 48 (suppl. 2):394–411.

Rush, D., J. Leighton, N.L. Sloan, J.M. Alvir, D.G. Horvitz, W.B. Seaver, G.C. Garbowski, S.S. Johnson, R.A. Kulka, J.W. Devore, M. Holt, J.T. Lynch, T.G. Virag, M.B. Woodside, and D.S. Shanklin. 1988b. The National WIC Evaluation: Evaluation of the Special Supplemental Food Program for Women, Infants, and Children. VI. Study of infants and children. Am. J. Clin. Nutr. 48 (suppl. 2):484–511.

Rush, D., N.L. Sloan, J. Leighton, J.M. Alvir, D.G. Horvitz, W.B. Seaver, G.C. Garbowsi, S.S. Johnson, R.A. Kulka, M. Holt, J.W. Devore, J.T. Lynch, M.B. Woodside, and D.S. Shanklin. 1988c. The National WIC Evaluation: Evaluation of the Special Supplemental Food program for Women, Infants, and Children. V. Longitudinal study of pregnant women. Am. J. Clin. Nutr. 48 (suppl. 2):439–483.

Rutishauser, I.H., and J.B. Carlin. 1992. Body mass index and duration of breast feeding: A survival analysis during the first six months of life. J. Epidemiol. Community Health 46:559–565.

Sappenfield, W.M., J.W. Buehler, N.J. Binkin, C.J. Hogue, L.T. Strauss, and J.C. Smith. 1987. Differences in neonatal and postneonatal mortality by race, birth weight, and gestational age. Public Health Rep. 102:182–192.

Schelp, F.P., P. Vivatanasept, P. Sitaputra, S. Sornmani, P. Pongpaew, N. Vudhivai, S. Egormaiphol, and D. Bohning. 1990. Relationship of morbidity of under-fives to anthropometric measurements and community health intervention. Trop. Med. Parasitol. 41:121–126.

Scholl, T.O, M.L. Hediger, and I.G. Ances. 1990a. Maternal growth during pregnancy and decreased infant birth weight. Am. J. Clin. Nutr. 51:790–793.

Scholl, T.O., M.L. Hediger, I.G. Ances, D.H. Belsky, and R.W. Salmon. 1990b. Weight gain during pregnancy in adolescence: Predictive ability of early weight gain. Obstet. Gynecol. 75:948–953.

Scholl, T.O., M.L. Hediger, C.S. Khoo, M.F. Healey, and N.L. Rawson. 1991. Maternal weight gain, diet and infant birth weight: Correlations during adolescent pregnancy. J. Clin. Epidemiol. 44:423–428.

Schramm, W.F. 1986. Prenatal participation in WIC related to Medicaid costs for Missouri newborns: 1982 update. Public Health Rep. 101:607–615.
Segel, J.S., and E.R. McAnarney. 1994. Adolescent pregnancy and subsequent obesity in African-American girls. J. Adolesc. Health 15:491–494.
Serdula, M.K., D. Ivery, R.J. Coates, D.S. Freedman, D.F. Williamson, and T. Byers. 1993. Do obese children become obese adults? A review of the literature. Prev. Med. 22:167–177.
Seward, J.F., and M.K. Serdula. 1984. Infant feeding and infant growth. Pediatrics 74:728–762.
Shu, X.O., M.C. Hatch, J. Mills, J. Clemens, and M. Susser. 1995. Maternal smoking, alcohol drinking, caffeine consumption, and fetal growth: Results from a prospective study. Epidemiology 6:115–120.
Sibai, B.M., T. Gordon, E. Thom., S.N. Caritis, M. Klebanoff, D. McNellis, and R.H. Paul. 1995. Risk factors for preeclampsia in healthy nulliparous women: A prospective multicenter study. Am. J. Obstet. Gynecol. 172:642–648.
Siega-Riz, A.M., L.S. Adair, and C.J. Hobel. 1994. Institute of Medicine maternal weight gain recommendations and pregnancy outcome in a predominanty Hispanic population. Obstet. Gynecol. 84:565–573.
Simon, N.P., Brady, N.R., and R.L. Stafford. 1993. Catch-up head growth and motor performance in very-low-birthweight infants. Clin. Pediatr. 32:405–411.
Smedman, L., G. Sterky, L. Mellander, and S. Wall. 1987. Anthropometry and subsequent mortality in groups of children aged 6-59 months in Guinea-Bissau. Am. J. Clin. Nutr. 46:369–373.
Sorensen, T.I., and S. Sonne-Holm. 1988. Risk in childhood of development of severe adult obesity: Retrospective, population-based case-cohort study. Am. J. Epidemiol. 1127:104–113.
Starfield, B., S. Shapiro, M. McCormick, and D. Bross. 1982. Mortality and morbidity in infants with intrauterine growth retardation. J. Pediatr. 101:978–983.
Stark, O., E. Atkins, O.H. Wolff, and J.W.B. Douglas. 1981. Longitudinal study of obesity in the National Survey of Health and Development. Br. Med. J. 283:13–17.
Stein, Z., M. Susser, G. Saenger, and F. Marolla. 1975. Famine and Human Development: The Dutch Hunger Winter of 1944–1945. New York: Oxford University Press.
Stein, Z.A., and M. Susser. 1984. Intrauterine growth retardation: Epidemiological issues and public health significance. Sem. Perinatol. 8:5–14.
Stevens-Simon, C., and E.R. McAnarney. 1992. Determinants of weight gain in pregnant adolescents. J. Am. Diet Assoc. 92:1348–1351.
Stockbauer, J.W. 1987. WIC prenatal participation and its relation to pregnancy outcomes in Missouri: A second look. Am. J. Public Health 77:813–818.
Susser, M. 1991. Maternal weight gain, infant birth weight and diet: Causal sequences. Am. J. Clin. Nutr. 53:1384–1396.
Taffel, S.M. 1986. Maternal Weight Gain and the Outcome of Pregnancy: United States, 1980. National Center for Health Statistics. Vital Health Stat. 21(44).
Taffel, S.M., K.G. Keppel, and G.K. Jones. 1993. Medical advice on maternal weight gain and actual weight gain. Results from the 1988 National Maternal and Infant Health Survey. Ann. N.Y. Acad. Sci. 678:293–305.

Taha, T. el T., R.H. Gray, and A.A. Mohamedani. 1993. Malaria and low birth weight in Central Sudan. Am. J. Epidemiol. 138:318–325.
Taitz, L.S. 1977. Obesity in pediatric practice: Infantile obesity. Pediatr. Clin. North. Am. 24:107–115.
Tanner, J.M. 1981. A History of the Study of Human Growth. Cambridge: Cambridge University Press.
Teberg, A.J., F.J. Walther, and I.C. Pena. 1988. Mortality, morbidity, and outcome of the small-for-gestational age infant. Semin. Perinatol. 12:84–94.
Theron, G.B., and M.L. Thompson. 1993. The usefulness of weight gain in predicting pregnancy complications. J. Trop. Pediatr. 39:269–272.
Tomkins, A. 1981. Nutritional status and severity of diarrhoea among preschool children in rural Nigeria. Lancet 18:860–862.
Tomkins, A., and F. Watson. 1989. Malnutrition and Infection: A Review. ACC/SCN State-of-the-Art Series, Nutrition Policy Discussion Paper No. 5. London: Centre for Human Nutrition, London School of Hygiene and Tropical Medicine.
Torun, B., and F.E. Viteri. 1994. Influence of exercise on linear growth. Eur. J. Clin. Nutr. 48:186–189.
Tsuzaki, S., N. Matsuo, M. Saito, and M. Osano. 1990. The head circumference growth curve for Japanese children between 0–4 years of age: Comparison with Caucasian children and correlation with stature. Ann. Hum. Biol. 17:297–303.
USDA (U.S. Department of Agriculture). 1991. Technical Papers: Review of WIC Nutritional Risk Criteria. Prepared for the Food and Nutrition Service by the Department of Family and Community Medicine, College of Medicine, University of Arizona, Tucson. Washington, D.C.: USDA.
USDA (U.S. Department of Agriculture). 1994. Study of WIC Participant and Program Characteristics, 1992. Background Data. Office of Analysis and Evaluation, Food and Nutrition Service. Washington, D.C.: USDA.
Valdez, R., M.A. Athens, G.H. Thompson, B.S. Bradshaw, and M.P. Stern. 1994. Birthweight and adult outcomes in a biethnic population in the U.S.A. Diabetologia 37:624–631.
Vella, V., A. Tomkins, J. Ndiku, T. Marshal, and I. Cortinovis. 1994. Anthropometry as a predictor for mortality among Ugandan children, allowing for socio-economic variables. Eur. J. Clin. Nutr. 48:189–197.
Verkerk, P.H., F.J. Van Spronsen, G.P. Smit, and R.C. Sengers. 1994. Impaired prenatal and postnatal growth in Dutch patients with phenylketonuria. The National PKU Steering Committee. Arch. Dis. Child. 71:114–118.
Victora, C.G. 1992. The association between wasting and stunting: An international perspective. J. Nutr. 122:1105–1110.
Villar, J., and J. Rivera. 1988. Nutritional supplementation during two consecutive pregnancies and the interim lactation period: Effect on birth weight. Pediatrics. 81:51–57.
Villar, J., V. Smeriglio, R. Martorell, C.H. Brown, and R.E. Klein. 1984. Heterogeneous growth and mental development of intrauterine growth-retarded infants during the first 3 years of life. Pediatrics 74:783–791.
Villar, J., M. Klebanoff, and E. Kestler. 1989. The effect on fetal growth of protozoan and helminthic infection during pregnancy. Obstet Gynecol. 74:915–920.

Villar, J., M. de Onis, E. Kestler, F. Bolanos, R. Cerezo, and H. Bernedes. 1990. The differential neonatal morbidity of the intrauterine growth retardation syndrome. Am. J. Obstet. Gynecol. 163:151–157.

Villar, J., M. Cogswell, E. Kestler, P. Castillo, R. Menendez, and J.T. Repke. 1992. Effect of fat and fat-free mass deposition during pregnancy on birth weight. Am. J. Obstet. Gynecol. 167:1344–1352.

Vobecky, J.S., J. Vobecky, D. Shapcott, and P.P. Demers. 1983. Nutrient intake patterns and nutritional status with regard to relative weight in early infancy. Am. J. Clin. Nutr. 38:730–738.

Wadden, T.A., G.D. Foster, K.D. Brownell, and E. Finley. 1984. Self-concept in obese and normal weight children. J. Consul. Clin. Psychol. 52:1104–1105.

Walker, S.P., C.A. Powell, M. Grantham-MaGregor, J.H. Himes, and S.M. Chang. 1991. Nutritional supplementation, psychosocial stimulation, and growth of stunted children: The Jamaican study. Am. J. Clin. Nutr. 54:642–648.

Waller, D.K., J.L. Mills, J.L. Simpson, G.C. Cunningham, M.R. Conley, M.R. Lassman, and G.G. Rhoads. 1994. Are obese women at higher risk for producing malformed offspring? Am. J. Obstet. Gynecol. 170:541–548.

Wang, X., B. Guyer, and D.M. Paige. 1994. Differences in gestational age-specific birthweight among Chinese, Japanese and white Americans. Int. J. Epidemiol. 23:119–128.

Waterlow, J.C. 1978. Observations on the assessment of protein-energy malnutrition with special reference to stunting. Courrier. 28:455–460.

Waterlow, J.C. 1994a. Relationship of gain in height to gain in weight. Eur. J. Clin. Nutr. 48:S72–S74.

Waterlow, J.C. 1994b. Causes and mechanisms of linear growth retardation (stunting). Eur. J. Clin. Nutr. 48:S1–S4.

Wen, S.W., R.L. Goldenberg, G.R. Cutter, H.J. Hoffman, and S.P. Cliver. 1990. Intrauterine growth retardation and preterm delivery: Prenatal risk factors in an indigent population. Am. J. Obstet. Gynecol. 162:213–218.

West, K.P., E. Djunaedi, A. Pandji, Kusdiono, I. Tarwotjo, A. Sommer, and the Aceh Study Group. 1988. Vitamin A supplementation and growth: A randomized community trial. Am. J. Clin. Nutr. 48:1257–1264.

WHO (World Health Organization). 1988. Breast-feeding and Child Spacing: What Health Workers Need to Know. Geneva: WHO.

WHO (World Health Organization). 1991. Indicators for Assessing Breast-feeding Practices: A Report of an Informal Meeting, 11–12 June, 1991. WHO/CDD/SER 91.4. Geneva: WHO.

WHO (World Health Organization). 1995. Physical Status: The Use and Interpretation of Anthropometry. WHO Technical Report Series 854. Geneva: WHO.

Wilcox, L.S., and J.S. Marks, eds. 1995. From Data to Action: CDC's Public Health Surveillance for Women, Infants and Children. Atlanta: Centers for Disease Control.

Williams, R.L., R.K. Creasy, G.C. Cunningham, W.E. Hawes, F.D. Norris, and M. Tashiro. 1982. Fetal growth and perinatal viability in California. Obstet. Gynecol. 59:624–632.

Winick, M. 1969. Malnutrition and brain development. J. Pediatr. 74:667–679.

Winick, M., and P. Rosso. 1969. Head circumference and cellular growth of the brain in normal and marasmic children. J. Pediatr. 74:774–778.

Witter, F.R., L.E. Caulfield, and R.J. Stolzfus. 1995. Influence of maternal anthropometric status and birth weight on the risk of cesarean delivery. Obstet. Gynecol. 85:947–951.

Wolke, D., D. Skuse, and B. Mathisen. 1990. Behavioral style in failure-to-thrive infants: A preliminary communication. J. Pediatr. Psychol. 2:237–254.

Wright, C.M., A. Aynsley-Green, P. Tomlinson, L. Ahmed, and J.A. MacFarlane. 1992. A comparison of height, weight and head circumference of primary school children living in deprived and non-deprived circumstances. Early Hum. Dev. 31:157–162.

Yip, R. 1993. Expanded usage of anthropometry z-scores for assessing population nutrition status and data quality (abstract). P. 279 in Proceedings of the 15th International Congress of Nutrition, Adelaide.

Yip, R., and T.W. Sharp. 1993. Acute malnutrition and high childhood mortality related to diarrhea: Lessons from the 1991 Kurdish refugee crisis. J. Am. Med. Assoc. 270:587–590.

Yip, R., N.J. Binkin, and F.L. Trowbridge. 1988. Altitude and child growth. J. Pediatr. 113:486–489.

Yip, R., I. Parvanta, K. Scanlon, E.W. Borland, C.M. Russell, and F.L. Trowbridge. 1992a. Pediatric nutrition surveillance system—United States, 1980–1991. Morbid. Mortal. Weekly Rep. 41(SS-7):1–24.

Yip, R., K. Scanlon, and F. Trowbridge. 1992b. Improving growth status of Asian refugee children in the United States. J. Am. Med. Assoc. 267:937–940.

Yip, R., K. Scanlon, and F. Trowbridge. 1993. Trends and patterns in height and weight status of low-income U.S. children. Crit. Rev. Food Sci. Nutr. 33:409–421.

Zhang, Y., R. Proenca, M. Maffei, M. Barone, L. Leopold, and J.M. Friedman. 1994. Positional cloning of the mouse obese gene and its human homologue. Nature 372:425–432.

5

Biochemical and Other Medical Risk Criteria

Biochemical and other medical risk criteria are used during the certification process for the WIC program (Special Supplemental Nutrition Program for Women, Infants, and Children) to establish eligibility for participation in the program and as a basis for either preventive or curative nutrition or health interventions. WIC program regulations define this group of nutrition risks in two categories:

- those determined by biochemical measures such as hemoglobin as a measure of anemia, and
- other documented nutritionally related medical conditions, such as clinical signs of nutrition deficiencies, metabolic disorders, preeclampsia in pregnant women, failure to thrive in an infant, chronic infections in any person, alcohol or drug abuse or mental retardation in women, lead poisoning, history of high-risk pregnancies or factors associated with high-risk pregnancies (such as smoking; conception before 16 months postpartum; history of low birth weight, premature births, or neonatal loss; adolescent pregnancy; or current multiple pregnancy) in pregnant women, or congenital malformations in infants or children or infants born to women with alcohol or drug abuse histories or mental retardation (7 CFR Subpart C, Section 246.7(e)(2)(i and ii); *Federal Register* 60(75):19,487–19, 491).

Currently, biochemical risk or documented nutrition-based medical conditions fall under Priority I for pregnant women, breastfeeding women, and infants; Priority III for children; and Priority VI for nonbreastfeeding postpartum women. Biochemical and other medical risk criteria are used to certify applicants for participation in the WIC program within the same priority as anthropometric risk criteria. These criteria are assigned a higher priority for participation than dietary or predisposing risk criteria (e.g., homelessness or migrancy) (see Chapter 3, Table 3-2). In the WIC program's certification process, medical risk is based on an assessment by a competent professional authority on the staff of the WIC agency or is based on referral data submitted by a competent professional authority not on the staff of the WIC agency (7 CFR Subpart C, Section 246.7(d)).

This chapter covers the medical nutrition risk criteria related to nutrient deficiencies, medical conditions applicable to the entire WIC population, conditions related to intake of specific foods, conditions specific to pregnancy, conditions specific to infants, and potentially toxic substances. These groupings are somewhat different from those used by the WIC program to reduce overlap in content. A list of medical risk criteria that are used by state WIC programs appears in Table 5-1. A summary of the criteria as predictors of risk and benefit appears in Table 5-2.

TABLE 5-1 Summary of Biochemical and Other Medical Risk Criteria in the WIC Program and Use by States

Risk Criterion	States Using		
	Women	Infants	Children
Criteria Related to Nutrient Deficiencies			
Anemia	54	54	54
Nutrient deficiencies including failure to thrive			
Malnutrition	—	8	8
Nutrition related illness	—	25	27
Failure to thrive	—	30	27
Medical Conditions Applicable to the Entire WIC Population			
Gastrointestinal disorders	13	30	24
Nausea and vomiting of pregnancy	26	—	—
Chronic diarrhea	—	16	15
Chronic vomiting	—	15	7
Crohn's disease	—	7	—
Liver disease	—	15	14
Hepatitis	—	18	14
Intestinal diseases	—	6	7
Cystic fibrosis	—	30	32
Endocrine disorders	—	—	6
Diabetes mellitus (Types I and II)	54	35	41
Hypo- or hyperthyroidism	6	6	—

Continued

TABLE 5-1 *Continued*

Risk Criterion	States Using		
	Women	Infants	Children
Medical Conditions Applicable to the Entire WIC Population *(Continued)*			
Chronic hypertension	54	19	25
Renal disease	54	35	35
Cancer	20	26	30
Central nervous system disorders	—	12	10
Epilepsy	5	6	6
Cerebral palsy	—	36	37
Spina bifida	—	12	13
Myelomeningocele	—	—	6
Genetic and congenital disorders	21	—	38
Cleft lip or palate	—	41	39
Down syndrome	—	16	10
Pyloric stenosis	—	7	—
Thalassemia	14	6	7
Sickle cell anemia	16	20	21
History of an infant with congenital disorder	32	—	—
History of a genetic disorder in infant	17	—	—
Nutritionally significant genetic disease	8	—	—
Congenital disorder	—	37	—
Genetic disorder	—	8	—
Inborn errors of metabolism			
Phenylketonuria	—	29	28
Maple syrup urine disease	—	13	12
Galactosemia	—	19	15
Metabolic disorder	32	24	26
Tyrosinemia and homocystinuria	—	7	6
Other inborn errors of metabolism	—	19	20
Chronic infections	52	21	10
Recurrent infections	25	—	11
Infectious disorder	28	—	—
Nutrition-related infectious disease	14	9	—
Respiratory infections	—	12	19
Tuberculosis	—	25	25
Pneumonia	—	19	18
Bronchitis	—	7	12
Otitis media	—	21	19
Meningitis	—	14	15
HIV infection and AIDS	20	22	20
Recent surgery or trauma	18	28	27
Burns	10	24	24
Severe acute infections	28	—	—
Other medical conditions			
Juvenile rheumatoid arthritis	—	—	—
Arthritis	2	—	—

Continued

TABLE 5-1 *Continued*

Risk Criterion	States Using Women	States Using Infants	States Using Children
Medical Conditions Applicable to the Entire WIC Population *(Continued)*			
Lupus erythematosus	6	—	—
Cardiorespiratory disorders	17	37	38
Conditions Related to the Intake of Specific Foods			
Food allergies	27	29	34
Celiac disease or intolerance	—	24	24
Food intolerances			
Lactose intolerance	—	20	16
Asthma	—	6	8
Conditions Specific to Pregnancy			
Pregnancy at a young age	52	—	—
Pregnancy age older than 35	43	—	—
Closely spaced pregnancies	52	—	—
High parity	43	—	—
History of preterm delivery	42	—	—
History of postterm delivery	8	—	—
History of low birth weight	49	—	—
History of neonatal loss	43	—	—
History of previous birth of an infant with a congenital or birth defect	32	—	—
Lack of prenatal care	18	—	—
Multifetal gestation	51	—	—
Fetal growth restriction	17	—	—
Preeclampsia and eclampsia	54	—	—
Placental abnormalities	15	—	—
Conditions Specific to Infants and/or Children			
Prematurity	—	39	6
Hypoglycemia	12	—	—
Fetal alcohol syndrome	—	12	9
Potentially Toxic Substances			
Drug-nutrient interactions	9	—	—
Inappropriate use of medication	—	23	23
Maternal smoking	51	—	—
Alcohol and illegal drug use			
Alcohol use	51	36	23
Illegal drug use	50	36	23
Lead poisoning	19	24	24

NOTE: Dashes indicate risk is not applicable or not reported for that population.

TABLE 5-2 Summary of Broad Categories of Biochemical and Other Medical Risk Criteria as Predictive of Risk or Benefit Among Women, Infants, and Children

Risk Criterion[a]	Women Risk	Women Benefit	Infants Risk	Infants Benefit	Children Risk	Children Benefit
Women, Infants, and Children						
Anemia	✓	✓	✓	✓	✓	✓
Nutrition deficiencies	✓	✓	✓	✓	✓	✓
Gastrointestinal disorders	✓	✓	✓	✓	✓	✓
Endocrine disorders	✓	✓	✓	✓	✓	✓
Hypertension	✓	✓	✓	✓	✓	✓
Renal disease	✓	✓	✓	✓	✓	✓
Cancer	✓	✓	✓	✓	✓	✓
Central nervous system disorders	✓	✓	✓	✓	✓	✓
Genetic and congenital disorders	✓	✓	✓	✓	✓	✓
Inborn errors of metabolism	✓	✓	✓	✓	✓	✓
HIV infection and AIDS	✓	✓	✓	✓	✓	✓
Recent major surgery or trauma, burns, and severe acute infections	✓	✓	✓	✓	✓	✓
Food allergies	✓	✓	✓	✓	✓	✓
Lead poisoning	✓	✓	✓	✓	✓	✓
Women During Pregnancy						
Nausea and vomiting	✓	✓				
Diabetes mellitus	✓	✓				
Pregnancy at low age	✓	✓				
Pregnancy age older than 35	✓	0				
Closely spaced pregnancies	✓	✓				
High parity	?	0				
History of preterm delivery	✓	✓				
History of postterm delivery	?	0				
Lack of prenatal care	✓	✓				
Multifetal gestation	✓	✓				
Fetal growth restriction	✓	✓				
Preeclampsia and eclampsia	✓	0				
Placental abnormalities	✓	0				
Maternal smoking	✓	?				
Alcohol and illegal drug use	✓	✓				

Continued

TABLE 5-2 *Continued*

Risk Criterion[a]	Women Risk	Women Benefit	Infants Risk	Infants Benefit	Children Risk	Children Benefit
Infants and Children						
Prematurity			✓	✓	?	?

NOTE: ✓ = predictive of risk or benefit; ? = evidence unclear; 0 = no evidence, or evidence but no effect; blank = not applicable to that group.

[a] Within the broad category *chronic or recurring infections*, there is evidence for nutrition risk and benefit for some specific criteria, such as tuberculosis, but not for other specific criteria, such as upper respiratory infections, bronchitis, and otitis media. The same is true within the broad categories *drug-nutrient interactions* and *food intolerances*.

CRITERIA RELATED TO NUTRIENT DEFICIENCIES

Anemia

Anemia is defined as a reduction of the red blood cell (erythrocyte) volume or hemoglobin concentration greater than two standard deviations below the mean (i.e., below the 2.5th percentile) occurring in healthy persons of the same age, gender, or, for women, stage of pregnancy (IOM, 1990, 1993). Anemias are generally classified into two groups—those resulting primarily from decreased production of red blood cells or hemoglobin, or those in which increased destruction or loss of red blood cells is the predominant mechanism. Megaloblastic anemia is associated with deficiencies of folate and vitamin B_6 and/or vitamin B_{12}. Microcytic anemia is associated with thalassemia trait, iron deficiency, and/or copper deficiency. The most common nutrition-related anemia is iron deficiency, which may be caused by diets low in iron, the insufficient assimilation of iron from the diet, the utilization of iron for rapid growth or pregnancy, or blood loss.

Prevalence of and Factors Associated with Anemia

Information on the prevalence of iron deficiency anemia in the United States comes from the National Health and Nutrition Examination Surveys (NHANES), conducted by the National Center for Health Statistics; the Pregnancy (PNSS) or Pediatric Nutrition Surveillance System (PedNSS), conducted by the Centers for Disease Control and Prevention (CDC); the U.S. Department of Agriculture's (USDA) WIC Eligibility Study; and the National WIC Evaluation. Between 1980 and 1991, the prevalence of anemia among United States infants and children through 5 years of age declined dramatically, from 7 to

3 percent, according to most recent data from the PedNSS, a low-income sample that includes many WIC program participants (Yip et al., 1992). However, there has been negligible decrease in anemia among black and Hispanic infants and children less than 2 years of age (Figure 17, p. 20, Yip et al., 1992).

In 1990, the PNSS reported prevalences of iron deficiency anemia of 10, 14, and 33 percent in the first, second, and third trimesters of pregnancy, respectively, for low-income pregnant women of all races (Kim et al., 1992). Black women exhibited a significantly higher prevalence of iron deficiency anemia than did women of other races. PNSS data show that the prevalence of iron deficiency anemia among low-income pregnant women has remained stable since 1979.

Estimates of the prevalence of iron deficiency anemia among the population potentially eligible for participation in the WIC program were reported in the 1985 WIC Eligibility Study (USDA, 1987) and were based on data from the NHANES II survey. These prevalence estimates were 2.3 percent for women 12 through 49 years of age, 14.3 percent for infants 6 to 11 months of age, 13.5 percent for children 12 to 23 months of age, 14.8 percent for children 2 to 3 years of age, 8.6 percent for children 3 to 4 years of age, and 8.4 percent for children 4 to 5 years of age.

Factors associated with anemia in women include poverty, low education, high parity, and black and Hispanic ethnicity (IOM, 1990; LSRO, 1991), with pregnancy imposing increased iron needs for the growth of the fetus and for expansion of the maternal blood volume (IOM, 1993). Factors associated with anemia in infants and children include poverty, inadequate dietary intake, malabsorption, and moderate to severe malnutrition (Behrman, 1992; IOM, 1993). Low-birth-weight (LBW) infants are at increased risk of developing anemia because of low neonatal iron stores (IOM, 1993).

Anemia as an Indicator of Nutrition and Health Risk

Anemia can impair energy metabolism, temperature regulation, immune function, and work performance (IOM, 1993). Anemia during pregnancy may increase the risk of prematurity, poor maternal weight gain, LBW, and infant mortality (IOM, 1990). CDC recently confirmed earlier associations between anemia during pregnancy, hemoglobin concentrations of less than 10 g/dl in the first trimester, and delivery of LBW infants (Kim et al., 1992). Other studies (Ulmer and Goepel; 1988; Scholl et al., 1992) report that maternal iron deficiency is associated with both LBW and poor gestational weight gain.

Data from the National WIC Evaluation (Rush et al., 1988b) showed a significant negative relationship between the woman's initial hemoglobin concentration and birth weight. There was no evidence of a relationship between a hemoglobin concentration of less than 10 g/dl or greater than 14 g/dl and adverse perinatal outcomes among white women. Among a small group of black WIC participants, however, a high hemoglobin concentration (> 14 g/dl) at entry in either the first or second trimester was associated with LBW, and low hemoglobin concentration (< 10 g/dl) in the first trimester was associated with LBW. There was no association of low hemoglobin concentration at entry in the second trimester with LBW.

In infants and children, the greatest risk from iron deficiency anemia (even if mild) is a delay in mental and motor development. Consistently, the mental and motor development scores of iron deficient anemic infants and toddlers fall behind those of children of the same age with replete iron stores (Idjradinata and Pollitt, 1993; Lozoff et al., 1982; Walter et al., 1989). Among preschool and school age children, iron deficiency anemia is associated with comparatively poor scores in tests of intelligence, school achievement, and specific cognitive processes (Pollitt et al., 1989; Seshadri and Gopaldas, 1989; Soewondo et al., 1989).

Anemia as an Indicator of Nutrition and Health Benefit

Because low-income women (and to a lesser extent infants and children) are at increased risk for iron deficiency anemia, their potential to benefit through participation in the WIC program is clear. Iron is one of the nutrients targeted in the WIC program food package through the provision of iron-fortified cereals and infant formula. The WIC program food package also supplies sources of folate and vitamin B_{12}, which can assist in the prevention of other nutritional anemias. Additionally, the WIC program encourages mothers to breastfeed their infants, which normally ensures adequate iron status for the first 4 to 6 months in infants born at term.

Studies have shown that the provision of supplemental iron (through food or supplements, or both) can reduce the prevalence of iron deficiency anemia in women, infants, and children (IOM, 1990, 1993; Rush et al., 1988a, b; Yip et al., 1992). The large decline in the prevalence of anemia since 1980 is principally attributed to participation in the WIC program. Studies show that prevention or treatment of anemia during pregnancy improves pregnancy outcomes (primarily LBW) (Kim et al., 1992; Rush et al., 1988b).

Studies in infants and children have revealed mixed results in the reversal of cognitive delays and behavioral changes through the delivery of supplemental iron (Lozoff et al., 1991; Pollitt, 1993). Some studies have shown that impaired cognitive function is still present at the time when formerly anemic children enter school, whereas others have shown strong evidence of complete recovery in response to iron treatment. Among infants, the administration of iron-fortified infant formula contributed to the prevention of anemia and of the motor delays observed among iron deficient anemic infants who received non-iron-fortified formula (Moffat et al., 1994). Similarly, in a randomized trial, the administration of ferrous sulfate led to the saturation of iron stores among previously anemic infants and toddlers and was accompanied by a full reversal of the developmental delays in these children (Idjradinata and Pollitt, 1993). Such developmental improvement was not observed among those anemic children who received a placebo. In other studies, iron treatment failed to improve performance on the Bayley Mental Development Scale (Pollitt, 1994). Various experimental and quasi-experimental studies have shown that iron repletion therapy among anemic preschool and school children improves cognitive test performance and school achievement (Watkins and Pollitt, in press).

Use of Anemia as a Nutrition Risk Criterion in the WIC Setting

Measurement of either hemoglobin or hematocrit concentration is used to detect the presence of anemia or putative iron deficiency because both are easy to use and inexpensive. These measurements are the methods most frequently used to identify the presence of anemia among participants in the WIC program. Among women and children, hemoglobin and hematocrit values vary by age, stage of pregnancy, smoking status, and altitude (see Table 5-3). During pregnancy, hemoglobin values gradually fall to a low point near the end of the second trimester, largely because of expanded blood volume. From this point until term, the concentration of hemoglobin rises again.

Serum ferritin concentration, erythrocyte protoporphyrin, mean corpuscular volume, serum iron concentration and iron-binding capacity, and serum transferrin receptor concentration are other biochemical tests used to define anemia. However, they are more expensive and less practical for use in the WIC program.

In the WIC program, anemia is the most frequently cited nutrition risk among participants in all categories. (The WIC program's priority system gives individuals with hematologic- and anthropometric-based nutrition risks priority for participation in the WIC program.) According to 1992 state WIC agency plans, all states use hematocrit or hemoglobin concentration measurements to evaluate the risk of anemia (see Table 5-1) (USDA, 1994).

The recommended cutoff values for anemia from the CDC (1989) and the Institute of Medicine (IOM, 1993) are found in Table 5-3. The cutoff points for anemia currently in use vary substantially among states and by participant category.

TABLE 5-3 Cutoff Points for Anemia Used in the WIC Program and Recommended Cutoff Points from the Centers for Disease Control and Prevention and the Institute of Medicine for Women, Infants, and Children

	Cutoff Point		
Population	WIC Programs	CDC[a]	IOM[a,b]
Pregnant Women			
First trimester	10.0–12.6 g/dl Hgb 30–38% Hct	11.0 g/dl Hgb 33% Hct	11.0 g/dl Hgb, with ferritin <20 µg/l
Second trimester	10.0–12.0 g/dl Hgb 30–37% Hct	10.5 g/dl Hgb 32% Hct	10.5 g/dl Hgb, and 20 µg/l ferritin
Third trimester	10.0–12.6 g/dl Hgb 30–37% Hct	11.5 g/dl Hgb 34% Hct	11.0 g/dl Hgb, and no ferritin collected
Lactating Women	12.0 g/dl Hgb 36% Hct	12.0 g/dl Hgb 36% Hct	12.0 g/dl Hgb 36% Hct
Postpartum, Nonlactating Women	12.0 g/dl Hgb 36% Hct	12.0 g/dl Hgb 36% Hct	12.0 g/dl Hgb 36% Hct
Infants			
(birth to 6 mo)	9.9–15 g/dl Hgb 30.9–44% Hct	N/A N/A	11.0 g/dl Hgb 33% Hct
Children			
(> 6 mo to 23 mo)	9.9–13 g/dl Hgb 30.9–39% Hct	11.0 g/dl Hgb 33% Hct	11.0 g/dl Hgb 33% Hct
(2 to 5 yr)	10.0–12.7 g/dl Hgb 31–38% Hct	11.0 g/dl Hgb 33% Hct	11.0 g/dl Hgb 33% Hct

NOTE: Hgb = hemoglobin; Hct = hematocrit.

[a] Adjustments for altitude (> 5,000 feet, add 0.5 g/dl hemoglobin or 1.5 percent hematocrit) or smoking (add 0.3 to 0.5 g/dl hemoglobin or 1 to 1.5 percent hematocrit, depending on the number of cigarettes smoked per day) should be added to the cutoff points for pregnant, breastfeeding, and nonlactating postpartum women.

[b] The IOM recommendations listed here for lactating and nonlactating postpartum women correspond to the IOM recommendations for women of childbearing age.

SOURCE: WIC program cutoff values reported in 1992 state plans (USDA, 1994); CDC guidelines for pregnant women (CDC, 1989); Report of the Committee on the Prevention, Management, and Treatment of Iron Deficiency Anemia Among U.S. Infants, Children, and Women of Childbearing Age (IOM, 1993).

Recommendation for Anemia

The risk of *anemia* is well documented for women, infants, and children; anemia can be identified by measures of hemoglobin or hematocrit concentration. There is empirical evidence and a theoretical basis for benefit from participation in the WIC program. Therefore, the committee recommends use of *anemia* as a nutrition risk criterion for women, infants, and children in the WIC program, using cutoff values from the CDC (1989) or the IOM (1993) (see Table 5-3). Use of higher cutoff values is not recommended because the yield of risk will be very low for both anemia and iron deficiency. The committee's recommendations for biochemical and other medical risk criteria are summarized in Table 5-4.

Failure to Thrive and Other Nutrient Deficiency Diseases

Failure to thrive (FTT) is ordinarily a mild form of protein-energy malnutrition (PEM) that is manifested by a reduction in the rate of somatic growth. Severe PEM presents as marasmus or kwashiorkor. Marasmus (less than 60 percent median weight for age) is characterized by severe loss of muscle and fat. Kwashiorkor is characterized by edema and hypoproteinemia, but loss of lean body mass and fat is less severe than in marasmus. Examples of micronutrient deficiencies include scurvy (vitamin C deficiency) and vitamin D deficiency rickets.

Prevalence of and Factors Associated with Failure to Thrive and Other Nutrient Deficiency Diseases

Although clinically obvious undernutrition is relatively uncommon in the United States, it does occur; FTT is the form most commonly encountered among infants and young children. On occasion, severe forms of protein-energy malnutrition (PEM) or micronutrient deficiency diseases are encountered. PEM results from a combination of social, economic, biologic, and environmental factors (Torun and Chew, 1994). Impaired family dynamics, lack of knowledge on the part of the caregiver for the infant or child, and, in some instances, organic diseases are all major factors contributing to failure to thrive in infants and young children in this country. Whatever the primary factor, however, malnutrition is the final common pathway.

Inappropriately low weight for the stature of the infant or child provides a clear indication of recent malnutrition. Impaired linear growth, with weight appropriate for stature, is also a frequent end result of malnutrition, although other causes, e.g., endocrinopathies, need to be excluded. Approximately 1 to 5 percent of all pediatric hospital admissions are for FTT (Bithoney et al., 1991; Phelps, 1991). A large number of infants and children with FTT are managed as outpatients by physicians throughout the United States (Mitchell et al., 1980). FTT without an apparent medical cause accounts for a majority of cases of FTT

TABLE 5-4 Summary of Medical Risk Criteria and Committee Recommendations for the Specific WIC Population

Risk Criterion	Committee Recommendation	Pregnant Women	Postpartum Women Lactating	Postpartum Women Nonlactating	Infants	Children
Criteria Related to Nutrient Deficiencies						
Anemia	Use with CDC or IOM cutoffs	✓	✓	✓	✓	✓
Failure to thrive	Use[a]				✓	✓
Nutrient deficiency diseases	Use[a]	✓	✓	✓	✓	✓
Medical Conditions Applicable to the Entire WIC Population[b]						
Gastrointestinal disorders	Use	✓	✓	✓	✓	✓
Nausea and vomiting during pregnancy	Use only if serious and prolonged	✓				
Diabetes mellitus	Use	✓	✓	✓	✓	✓
Gestational diabetes	Use	✓	✓	✓		
Thyroid disorders	Use	✓	✓	✓	✓	✓
Chronic hypertension	Use	✓	✓	✓	✓	✓
Renal disease	Use, but not for chronic urinary tract infections	✓	✓	✓	✓	✓
Cancer	Use	✓	✓	✓	✓	✓
Central nervous system disorders	Use	✓	✓	✓	✓	✓
Genetic and congenital disorders	Use	✓			✓	✓
Pyloric stenosis	Do not use					
Inborn errors of metabolism	Use[a]	✓			✓	✓
Chronic or recurrent infections	Use, with exceptions	✓			✓	✓
Upper respiratory infections	Do not use					
Bronchitis	Do not use					
Otitis media	Do not use					
Urinary tract infections	Do not use					
HIV infections and AIDS	Use	✓	✓	✓	✓	✓

Recent major surgery, trauma, burns, or severe acute infections	Use		✓		✓
Other medical conditions (juvenile rheumatoid arthritis, lupus erythematosus, and cardiorespiratory disorders)	Use		✓		✓
Conditions Related to the Intake of Specific Foods					
Food allergies	Use		✓	✓	✓
Celiac disease	Use		✓	✓	✓
Lactose intolerance	Use		✓	✓	✓
Other food intolerance	Do not use				
Asthma	Do not use				
Conditions Specific to Pregnancy					
Pregnancy at a young age	Use with cutoff value of 2 years postmenarche	✓			
Pregnancy age older than 35 years	Do not use				
Closely spaced pregnancies	Use with an interconceptional interval of 6 months (9 months if concurrently lactating)	✓			
High parity	Do not use				
History of preterm delivery	Use	✓			
History of postterm delivery	Do not use				
History of low birth weight	Use	✓			
History of neonatal loss	Do not use				
History of birth with congenital or birth defect	Use	✓			

Continued

TABLE 5-4 Continued

Risk Criterion	Committee Recommendation	Pregnant Women	Postpartum Women Lactating	Postpartum Women Nonlactating	Infants	Children
Conditions Specific to Pregnancy *(Continued)*						
Lack of prenatal care	Use with cutoff value of care beginning after 1st trimester or long intervals between visits[c]	✓				
Multifetal gestation	Use	✓				
Fetal growth restriction	Use	✓				
Preeclampsia and eclampsia	Do not use			✓		
Placental abnormalities	Do not use					
Conditions Specific to Infants and/or Children						
Prematurity	Use with cutoff value of ≤37 weeks' gestation; do not use for children				✓	✓
Hypoglycemia	Use				✓	
Potentially Toxic Substances						
Long-term drug-nutrient interactions	Use for selected drugs	✓	✓			
Maternal smoking	Use, with cutoff of any smoking[c,d]	✓	✓		✓	
Alcohol and illegal drug use	Use with cutoff of any use[c,e]	✓	✓	✓		
Lead poisoning	Use with cutoff value of >10 µg/dl				✓	✓

NOTE: ✓ = subgroup to which the recommendation applies.

[a] This criterion merits higher priority among children.
[b] Diagnosis of the condition is the cutoff point used.
[c] This criterion merits lower priority.
[d] Two committee members (Barbara Abrams and Barbara Devaney) preferred to (1) set a higher cutoff point that would more clearly identify women whose cigarette use places them at higher risk of poor outcomes and (2) maintain this criterion at high priority.
[e] Three committee members (Barbara Abrams, Barbara Devaney, and Roy Pitkin) preferred to (1) set a higher cutoff point that would more clearly identify women whose alcohol use places them at higher risk of poor outcomes and (2) maintain these criteria at high priority.

(Powell, 1988). As discussed in Chapter 4, weight change is the anthropometric measurement that is most indicative of recent malnutrition, especially in infants and young children. No data were available to the committee on the prevalence of failure to thrive in the WIC population.

Clinically evident deficiencies of micronutrients other than iron are generally uncommon in otherwise healthy infants and children in the United States. Increased rates of breastfeeding and supplementation of infant formulas with vitamins and trace elements have undoubtedly reduced the risk of micronutrient deficiencies. However, overdilution of formula or substitution of sugar-based beverages for formula can lead to general malnutrition. Breastfed infants are at risk for deficiency of vitamin D if they do not receive adequate exposure to sunlight but are otherwise at very low risk of nutrient deficiencies. There is evidence to suggest that zinc deficiency may occur after 3 months of age in some breastfed infants (Krebs et al., in press; Walravens et al., 1992). Deficiencies of other micronutrients may occur in the breastfed infant if there is a serious maternal deficiency of that nutrient. Causes of maternal deficiencies include very low intake of fruits and vegetables (folate), vegan diets (vitamins B_{12} and D), and alcoholism (thiamin). Osteopenia secondary to calcium deficiency may occur in premature infants, and decreased bone density attributable to inadequate calcium intake has been documented during the reproductive cycle in adolescents.

Although the incidence of neural tube defects (spina bifida and anencephaly) can be reduced by approximately 50 percent by ensuring a folate intake of at least 400 µg/day in the periconceptional period (CDC, 1992), women are ordinarily not eligible for participation in the WIC program during this period.

Many disease states increase the risk of clinically significant micronutrient deficiencies. For example, fat soluble vitamin deficiencies, including vitamin E deficiency, may occur in individuals who malabsorb nutrients because of cystic fibrosis or liver disease. Data on the prevalence of other nutrient deficiency diseases among the general and WIC populations were not available to the committee.

Failure to Thrive and Other Nutrient Deficiency Diseases as Indicators of Nutrition and Health Risk

The presence of clinical signs and symptoms of PEM or of specific micronutrient deficiencies indicates current nutrition and health risks. Persistent malnutrition may lead to elevated morbidity and mortality rates. Infants and children with FTT may remain developmentally delayed, despite weight gain (Drotar and Sturm, 1992; Wolke et al., 1990). Important functional disturbances may occur as a result of single or multiple nutrient deficiencies. Examples in-

BIOCHEMICAL AND OTHER MEDICAL RISK CRITERIA

clude impaired cognitive function, impaired function of the immune system, and impaired function of skeletal muscle.

Failure to Thrive and Other Nutrient Deficiency Diseases as Indicators of Nutrition and Health Benefit

Participation in the WIC program provides key nutrients and education to help restore nutrition status and promote full rehabilitation of those with an overt nutrient deficiency. Infants and children with FTT can definitely benefit from nutrition and health interventions to improve weight gain. The benefit is so clear that a formal diagnosis of nonorganic FTT (FTT without a medical basis) must be based on a positive response of weight gain to nutrition rehabilitation (Lifshitz et al., 1991). Intervention promotes compensatory catch-up growth in weight and other dimensions of growth (Casey and Arnold, 1985); developmental delays may be less responsive to complete recovery (Frank and Zeisel, 1988).

When clinically evident undernutrition is first identified in the WIC program setting, immediate referral for nutrition and health intervention is required.

The supplemental food provided by the WIC program, as well as nutrition education and referrals for other health and social services, can benefit those at risk of nutrient deficiencies. Data on the benefit of participation in the WIC program for those identified as being at risk of nutrient deficiency diseases were not available to the committee.

Use of Failure to Thrive and Other Nutrient Deficiency Diseases as Nutrition Risk Criteria in the WIC Setting

The diagnosis of most nutrient deficiency diseases, including failure to thrive, is based on clinical evidence (including laboratory or radiological findings), performed by a health care provider, and reported to WIC program staff. See Table 5-1 for risk criteria used by states.

Recommendations for Failure to Thrive and Other Nutrient Deficiency Diseases

The risk of *failure to thrive* is well documented in infants and children, and the risk of *other nutrient deficiency diseases* is well documented in women as well. These diseases can be diagnosed clinically. There is a strong theoretical and empirical basis for benefit from participation in the WIC program. Therefore, the committee recommends use of *nutrient deficiency diseases* as a nutrition risk criterion for women, infants, and children in the WIC program and it recommends use of diagnosis of *failure to thrive* as a nutrition risk criterion for infants and children. The committee believes that these nutrition risk criteria deserve high priority for children because of the yield of benefit.

MEDICAL CONDITIONS APPLICABLE TO THE ENTIRE WIC POPULATION

Gastrointestinal Disorders

For growth, development, or maintenance of normal nutrition status, food must be ingested, digested, and absorbed. Conditions associated with protracted vomiting, parasitic and bacterial infections of the gastrointestinal tract, malabsorption, and diarrhea interfere with those processes. Quality of the water supply, sanitation systems, and household food preparation habits are environmental factors associated with gastrointestinal disorders (Lutter et al., 1992).

Prevalence of and Risks Associated with Specific Gastrointestinal Disorders

Nausea and vomiting of pregnancy. Some degree of nausea is extremely common in early gestation, and at least half of normal pregnant women experience vomiting (Klebanoff et al., 1985). Vomiting severe enough to warrant a diagnosis of hyperemesis gravidarum is much less frequent.

Inflammatory bowel disease. Inflammatory bowel disease occurs in two forms, ulcerative colitis and Crohn's disease. Pregnancy does not exert any consistent effect on the course of inflammatory bowel disease, but active disease at conception increases the risk of poor pregnancy outcome. Crohn's disease usually appears during the second and third decade of life; however, approximately 20 percent of cases occur during childhood or adolescence (Ekvall, 1993).

It is estimated that there are approximately 800,000 individuals with inflammatory bowel disease in the United States. Women are more likely than men to develop Crohn's (Eisen and Sandler, 1994). The inflammatory process in Crohn's disease causes symptoms of diarrhea, blood and protein loss in the gastrointestinal tract, abdominal pain, weight loss, fever, anemia, and growth failure (Rosenberg and Mason, 1994). The cause of the growth failure is multifactorial and includes enteric losses, malabsorption of fat and carbohydrates, and increased nutrient needs due to inflammatory processes. The major cause of poor growth is inadequate energy intake.

Short bowel syndrome. Short bowel syndrome is most often seen as a result of surgical resections due to conditions such as necrotizing enterocolitis and

Crohn's disease. Loss of absorptive surface is the primary problem in short bowel syndrome, and the nutrition risk depends in large part on the extent and site of the resection. Motility disturbances, bile acid deficiency, and bacterial overgrowth are additional complications seen with this syndrome.

Liver disease. Most liver diseases have a significant cholestatic component (Balistreri, 1985). Bile flow is obstructed from the hepatocyte into the biliary system and hence the intestine; there is a marked decrease in concentration of intraluminal bile acids, often below the concentration necessary for micelle formation and fat absorption. Growth failure is a frequent complication of liver disease.

Vital hepatitis. Viral hepatitis exists in at least five forms, is highly infectious, can progress from acute to chronic disease, and can be transferred from mother to fetus.

Cystic fibrosis. Cystic fibrosis is an inherited disorder in which there is a generalized dysfunction of the exocrine glands. This results in the production of abnormally thick, sticky mucus, and involves the lungs, pancreas, liver, and intestines (Ekvall, 1993). The most severe presentation of this disease is failure to thrive combined with respiratory distress and malabsorptive syndrome in infants. Cystic fibrosis occurs more in whites (1 in about 1,800 live births) than in blacks (1 in 17,000 live births), and is rare in Asians. Cystic fibrosis affected over 19,000 individuals in 1994, and 43 percent of cases were among females (Cystic Fibrosis Foundation, 1995).

Data on the prevalence of specific gastrointestinal disorders among the WIC population were not available to the committee.

Gastrointestinal Disorders as Indicators of Nutrition and Health Risk

Gastrointestinal disorders increase nutrition risk through any of a variety of mechanisms: impaired food intake, abnormal deglutition, impaired digestion of food in the intestinal lumen, generalized or specific nutrient malabsorption, or excessive gastrointestinal losses of endogenous fluids and nutrients. Nutrient intake may need to be increased to correct existing deficiencies or to counterbalance excessive losses of nutrients or fluid.

Because of frequent loss of nutrients through vomiting, diarrhea, malabsorption, or infections, individuals experiencing chronic symptoms are often malnourished. Chronic vomiting and diarrhea can lead to a rapid breakdown in body functions with such consequences as dehydration and malnutrition, resulting in lowered resistance to disease.

Pregnant women with severe vomiting during pregnancy are at risk of weight loss, dehydration, and metabolic imbalances—particularly in severe cases of vomiting (hyperemesis gravidarum). Risk from mild forms of nausea and vomiting during pregnancy is low; the condition generally responds to small frequent feedings, usually of simple carbohydrates, and avoidance of any foods that cause nausea. More severe cases of vomiting require medical management to prevent serious complications. In rare cases, total parenteral nutrition may be necessary (Godsey and Newman, 1991).

Gastrointestinal Disorders as Indicators of Nutrition and Health Benefit

The goal of nutritional management of gastrointestinal disorders is to restore or preserve nutrition status. Treatment of any gastrointestinal disorder requires an appropriate source of nutrients. The WIC program provides nutritious supplemental foods or special dietary formulas, general nutrition education, and support for the initiation and maintenance of breastfeeding (which provides antimicrobial benefits as well as nutrients for infants (IOM, 1991; Lutter, 1992). The WIC program helps keep the family linked with health and social services.

Ekvall (1993), Boyle (1995), and others discuss nutritional management of gastrointestinal disorders to restore or improve nutrition and health—a vital part of the medical management of the individual.

Use of Gastrointestinal Disorders as Risk Criteria in the WIC Setting

Diagnosis of gastrointestinal disorders or diseases by a health care provider is reported to the WIC agency staff. WIC program regulations allow for the provision of special dietary formulas indicated for many gastrointestinal disorders as part of the supplemental food package. Table 5-1 summarizes the extent to which various gastrointestinal disorders (including the category nausea and vomiting of pregnancy) are used as nutrition risk criteria by state WIC agencies.

Recommendations for Gastrointestinal Disorders

The risk of chronic *gastrointestinal disorders* is well documented among women, infants, and children, and clinical methods are available to identify these risk criteria. There is a theoretical basis for benefit from participation in the WIC program and empirical evidence of the importance of nutritious foods in restoring or maintaining satisfactory nutrition and health. Therefore, the committee recommends use of *gastrointestinal disorders* as nutrition risk criteria for women, infants, and children by the WIC agencies and with high priority.

The committee cautions, however, that nutrition risk criteria for conditions such as vomiting and diarrhea be defined by state WIC agencies as chronic conditions, not single episodes.

Diabetes Mellitus

Diabetes mellitus results from an absolute insulin deficiency (Type I) or a functional insulin deficiency (Type II). Genetic and environmental factors are involved. Type I diabetes mellitus is associated with histocompatibility antigen, autoimmunity, and/or islet cell antibodies. Peak ages for presentation of absolute insulin deficiency are between 5 and 7 years of age and at puberty. There is a seasonal variability in onset and association with mumps, rubella, and cytomegalo viruses. Diabetes mellitus is the most common endocrine disorder to complicate pregnancy. *Gestational diabetes* refers to diabetes mellitus that is diagnosed during pregnancy; in most cases it is non-insulin-dependent.

Prevalence of and Factors Associated with Diabetes Mellitus

More than 13 million persons in the United States have diabetes mellitus, and 60 percent of newly diagnosed cases occur in women (Tinker, 1994). Estimates of the prevalence of diabetes mellitus during pregnancy depend on the diagnostic criteria employed; a rate of 2 to 3 percent is a reasonable conservative estimate. The occurrence of diabetes mellitus is more prevalent among overweight women (Colditz et al., 1995) and in certain American-Indian and Latino populations (Baxter et al., 1993; Valway et al., 1993). No information on the prevalence of diabetes mellitus or gestational diabetes among the WIC population was available to the committee.

Diabetes Mellitus as an Indicator of Nutrition and Health Risk

Insulin deficiency results in major disturbances of carbohydrate, protein, and lipid metabolism. With inadequate insulin, lipid metabolism increases. Insulin and growth hormone work synergistically to promote the movement of amino acids from the extracellular to the intracellular space, increase protein synthesis, and decrease protein degradation.

Individuals with Type I diabetes mellitus nearly always require insulin and are at risk for developing ketoacidosis, hypoglycemic reactions, and such long-term serious complications as cardiovascular disease, renal disease, and loss of vision (Crofford, 1995; Shaughnessy and Slawson, 1994). Type I diabetes mellitus during pregnancy is associated with increased risk of preeclampsia, fetal malformation, macrosomia, fetal and neonatal death, and other complications.

Women with gestational diabetes are at increased risk of developing Type II diabetes mellitus later in life (Coustan et al., 1993). Their infants are at increased risk of macrosomia. Breastfeeding women with diabetes mellitus are at risk for delayed lactogenesis, mastitis, and lower plasma glucose levels (Ferris et al., 1988; Neubauer et al., 1993).

Diabetes Mellitus as an Indicator of Nutrition and Health Benefit

The WIC program provides supplemental food, nutrition education, and access to health services that can benefit individuals with diabetes mellitus and women with gestational diabetes. Foods in the WIC package can help individuals to follow their diet plan. Individuals with diabetes mellitus benefit from referral for nutrition management (American Diabetes Association and American Dietetic Association, 1994, 1995; Bourgeosis and Duffer, 1990; Jovanovic-Peterson and Peterson, 1990).

Dietary management and attention to exercise play a key role in maintaining euglycemia. There is ample evidence that normalization of maternal blood glucose diminishes the risk of virtually all complications in the mother, fetus, and newborn (Cunningham et al., 1993).

Use of Diabetes Mellitus as a Nutrition Risk Criterion in the WIC Setting

A health care provider reports the diagnosis of diabetes mellitus to WIC program staff. Table 5-1 lists the use of this nutrition risk criterion by state WIC programs.

Recommendation for Diabetes Mellitus

The risk of *diabetes mellitus* is well documented for women, infants, and children, and this condition can be diagnosed clinically. There is a theoretical basis for benefit from participation in the WIC program and empirical evidence that appropriate diet is a key to maintenance of euglycemia. Therefore, the committee recommends use of *diabetes mellitus* as a nutrition risk criterion for women, infants, and children and *gestational diabetes* for pregnant women in the WIC program.

Thyroid Disorders

Hypothyroidism results from deficient levels of production of thyroid hormone, or a defect in its receptor; *hyperthyroidism* results from excessive levels

BIOCHEMICAL AND OTHER MEDICAL RISK CRITERIA

of secretion of thyroid hormone (Behrman, 1992; Clugson and Hetzel, 1994). Hypothyroidism and hyperthyroidism may be associated with the autoimmune process. The drug thiourea has been associated with hypothyroidism and should be used with caution during pregnancy (ACOG, 1995).

Prevalence of and Factors Associated with Thyroid Disorders

Data on the prevalence of hypo- or hyperthyroidism among women, infants, or children in the United States or in WIC program participants were not available to the committee. Hyperthyroidism can occur in infants and children born to mothers with a history of hyperthyroidism.

Thyroid Disorders as Indicators of Nutrition and Health Risk

Congenital or neonatal hypothyroidism results in severe mental and physical retardation. Hyperthyroidism in infants may result in failure to thrive, cardiac failure, and a variety of other clinical abnormalities.

The hypermetabolic state in individuals with hyperthyroidism is accompanied by increased caloric needs, and those affected may have a voracious appetite. On the other hand, hypothyroidism is accompanied by decreased metabolism and decreased caloric needs.

Thyroid Disorders as Indicators of Nutrition and Health Benefit

As part of the medical management of hypothyroidism, attention must be directed to anthropometric status. Nutrition education may help promote normal growth and development and avoidance of excessive weight gain. A low-fat version of the WIC food package would assist with weight management in hypothyroidism. The management of hyperthyroidism requires a diet high in energy, carbohydrates, and vitamins and minerals to maintain or achieve desirable weight, growth, and development. The WIC program provides supplemental food that helps achieve improved nutrient intake. Nutrition education and referrals to health care and social services may also assist individuals in managing their condition.

Use of Thyroid Disorders as a Risk Criterion in the WIC Setting

The diagnosis of hypo- or hyperthyroidism is performed by a health care provider, and the diagnosis is reported to WIC program staff.

Recommendation for Thyroid Disorders

The risk of *hypo- and hyperthyroidism* is well documented in women, infants, and children, and these conditions can be diagnosed clinically. There is a theoretical basis for benefit from participation in the WIC program. Therefore, the committee recommends that the WIC program use *hypo- and hyperthyroidism* as nutrition risk criteria for women, infants, and children in the WIC program.

Chronic Hypertension

Hypertension is defined as elevated arterial blood pressure measured indirectly by an inflatable cuff and pressure manometer (NRC, 1989). The health risk of hypertension increases steadily with blood pressure level (either systolic or diastolic). Diastolic blood pressure is generally the value used to diagnose hypertension. Normotension in adults is defined as systolic blood pressure less than or equal to 140 mm Hg and diastolic blood pressure less than or equal to 90 mm Hg (in infants 80/60, and in children approximately 100/65 mm Hg) (WHO, 1978).

Factors associated with hypertension include excessive body weight; intake of salt, fat, and perhaps other dietary components (e.g., potassium and calcium may be protective); alcohol consumption; race; and age (Kotchen et al., 1991; NRC, 1989). In children there is a strong correlation between obesity and blood pressure, and a direct association between changes in body weight and blood pressure (Kotchen et al., 1989).

Prevalence of and Factors Associated with Chronic Hypertension

Approximately 30 percent of adult Americans have definitive hypertension using criteria of the Joint National Committee on Detection, Evaluation, and Treatment of High Blood Pressure (NRC, 1989); and about 22 percent of women have hypertension (Burt et al., 1995). Using 1984 program data, USDA (1987) estimated that approximately 9 percent of women who are income-eligible for participation in the WIC program would present with hypertension as a nutrition risk. Hypertension is far less prevalent among infants and children and generally accompanies other chronic diseases (Pruitt, 1992). Data on the prevalence of hypertension among infants and children participating in the WIC program were not available to the committee.

Chronic Hypertension as an Indicator of Nutrition and Health Risk

Hypertension diagnosed through elevated diastolic blood pressure is a major risk factor for stroke, hypertensive heart disease, coronary heart disease, and kidney disease (Kotchen and Kotchen, 1994; NRC, 1989). Individuals with mild hypertension have twice the risk of cardiovascular disease than normotensive persons.

Women with hypertension antedating pregnancy are at increased risk for several types of adverse pregnancy outcomes (IOM, 1990). Fetal growth restriction, presumably reflecting impairment of uteroplacental perfusion from vascular disease, is relatively common. Abruptio placentae occurs with increased frequency in women with chronic hypertension. There is also a tendency for women with chronic hypertension to experience an acute worsening of the condition, termed "superimposed preeclampsia," or pregnancy-aggravated hypertension. These conditions account for a substantial proportion of perinatal morbidity and mortality in populations with a high baseline incidence of chronic hypertension.

Chronic Hypertension as an Indicator of Nutrition and Health Benefit

Evidence for the prevention and control of hypertension through altered dietary intake comes from many studies in adults and longitudinal studies that have followed blood pressures in children over time (NRC, 1989; Pruitt, 1992). Management of hypertension—either pharmacologic or nonpharmacologic—can reduce the development of serious conditions. Nonpharmacologic treatment for postpartum women includes a combined intervention of weight loss, sodium restriction, moderate alcohol restriction, and moderate isotonic physical activity. The WIC food package provides compatible foods. Nutrition education provided in the WIC setting can address topics pertinent to the prevention and management of hypertension in general and during pregnancy, the postpartum period, infancy, and childhood.

Use of Chronic Hypertension as a Risk Criterion in the WIC Setting

Diagnosis of hypertension can be reported to WIC program staff by health care providers. Trained health care staff can obtain blood pressure measurements in the WIC setting and refer for a confirming diagnosis and medical management. See Table 5-1 for the use of hypertension as a nutrition risk criterion in the WIC program.

Recommendation for Chronic Hypertension

The risk of *chronic hypertension* is well documented for women, infants, and children, and this condition can be diagnosed clinically. There is a theoretical and empirical basis for benefit from participation in the WIC program. Therefore, the committee recommends the use of *chronic hypertension* as a nutrition risk criterion for women, infants, and children in the WIC program.

Renal Disease

Either acute or chronic *renal disease* may complicate pregnancy. Urinary tract infections are the most common acute infection during pregnancy. However, most urinary tract infections involve the bladder; infection of the renal parenchyma (i.e., pyelonephritis) is less frequent. Nonetheless, acute pyelonephritis is the most common serious medical complication of pregnancy.

Even though renal disease among infants and children has many etiologies (acute, chronic, or congenital), the rate of deterioration of nutrition status is fastest among infants and children with glomerulonephritis, followed by hereditary nephropathies and renal dysplasia, and then by urinary tract malformation (Gonzalez, 1992; Bergstein, 1992).

Prevalence of and Factors Associated with Renal Disease

Based on 1984 WIC program data, the expected frequency of renal disease (including chronic urinary tract infections) among women in the WIC program was estimated to be 19 percent (USDA, 1987). Estimates were not made for infants or children. Data on the prevalence of specific renal diseases or disorders among U.S. women, infants, and children were not available to the committee.

Renal Disease as an Indicator of Nutrition and Health Risk

With chronic renal disease in pregnant women, fetal growth is often restricted and there is a high likelihood of developing a preeclampsia-like syndrome superimposed on underlying vascular disease. The woman with chronic renal disease often has proteinuria, but is also at the risk of azotemia if she increases her dietary protein intake.

Growth failure in children with renal disease can result from PEM, chronic acidosis, osteodystrophy, uremic conditions, and endocrine dysfunction (Bergstein, 1992). Uremia has a broad spectrum of neurologic, gastrointestinal, metabolic, hematologic, cardiovascular, and immunologic effects. Metabolic changes in amino acid transport change peripheral insulin resistance and the process of glucose utilization. In renal insufficiency, a significant deficit in height is usually observed in infants and children.

Renal Disease as an Indicator of Nutrition and Health Benefit

The WIC program can benefit the nutrition and health of affected individuals by providing modified food packages, sometimes including special dietary formulas, and referrals to medical care that will include dietary counseling and management. Dietary management in renal disease helps to preserve renal function, treat symptoms, prevent states of nutrient deficiency or excess, and promote positive pregnancy outcomes and growth and development in infants and children.

Use of Renal Disease as a Risk Criterion in the WIC Setting

Renal disease is diagnosed by a medical care provider and reported to WIC agency staff. See Table 5-1 for the use of renal disease as a nutrition risk criterion in the WIC program.

Recommendations for Renal Disease

The risk of *renal disease* is well documented in women, infants, and children, and this condition can be diagnosed clinically. There is a theoretical and empirical basis for benefit from participation in the WIC program. Therefore, the committee recommends use of *renal disease* (including chronic pyelonephritis with persistent proteinuria) as a nutrition risk criterion in the WIC program for women, infants, and children. However, the committee recommends that diagnosis of other chronic urinary tract infections not be used as a nutrition risk criterion.

Cancer

An individual's nutrition status at the time of diagnosis of *cancer* (populations of cells that have acquired the ability to multiply and spread without the usual biologic restraints; NRC, 1982) is associated with the outcome of treatment (Shils et al., 1994). The type of cancer and stage of disease progression determines the type of medical treatment, and, if indicated, nutrition management.

Prevalence of and Factors Associated with Cancer

The incidence of cancer in 1995 was estimated to be 575,000 new cases among women, and 8,000 new cases among children (American Cancer Society, 1995). Data on the prevalence of cancer among the WIC population were not available to the committee.

Cancer as an Indicator of Nutrition and Health Risk

Individuals with a diagnosis of cancer are at significant health risk and under specific circumstances may be at increased nutrition risk, depending upon the stage of disease progression or type of ongoing cancer treatment.

The most common nutritional risk for individuals with cancer is PEM and wasting (Shils et al., 1994). Energy and protein needs are often increased as a result of the disease or its therapy. Cancer treatment interventions that promote the development of PEM are irradiation to the head, neck, esophagus, abdomen, or pelvis, or intense or frequent use of corticosteroid therapy. PEM is associated with impaired immune competence, increased susceptibility to infections, major organ dysfunction, and increased morbidity and mortality. Hematopoietic, gastrointestinal, and immunologic systems are most affected by PEM. Some chemotherapy drugs (e.g., cytosine arabinoside) are toxic to the gastrointestinal tract and, thus, pose additional nutrition risks.

Cancer as an Indicator of Nutrition and Health Benefit

Individuals with cancer should maintain adequate nutrition status to promote normal growth patterns in infants and children and to maintain weight in women. The food package, in conjunction with nutrition education and referrals, may help prevent the development of nutrition problems that are secondary to the disease or its therapy.

Use of Cancer as a Risk Criterion in the WIC Setting

A diagnosis of cancer is made by a health care provider and reported to WIC agency staff. See Table 5-1 for use of this criterion by state WIC programs.

Recommendation for Cancer

The risk of *cancer* is well documented for women, infants, and children, and a clinical method is available to identify this condition. There is a theoretical basis for benefit from participation in the WIC program. Therefore, the committee recommends the use of *cancer* or *ongoing chemotherapy* as a nutrition risk criterion in the WIC program for women, infants, and children.

Central Nervous System Disorders

Central nervous system (CNS) *disorders* can be categorized as conditions that alter nutrition status metabolically, mechanically, or both. CNS disorders such as cerebral palsy (CP) and neural tube defects (NTD; e.g., spina bifida or myelomeningocele) affect energy requirements and may affect the individual's ability to feed himself.

Prevalence of and Factors Associated with Central Nervous System Disorders

Epilepsy is a symptom of brain dysfunction characterized by excessive fluctuations in electromechanical balance that may be expressed in spontaneous recurring seizures (Ekvall, 1993). Epilepsy affects 2.5 million individuals in the Unites States, with 30 percent of cases in children under 18 years of age (approximately 5 per 1,000) (Epilepsy Foundation of America, 1993). Data on the prevalence of epilepsy among the WIC population were not available to the committee.

Cerebral palsy in infants and children is a group of chronic, nonprogressive disorders of the brain that produce abnormalities of posture, muscle tone, and motor coordination (Ekvall, 1993). The prevalence of cerebral palsy is approximately 2 per 1,000 live births, with cases occurring more than twice as often in whites as in blacks. Factors associated with CP are LBW and birth asphyxia.

NTDs account for most congenital anomalies of the CNS; they are estimated to occur in approximately 5 in 10,000 live births (approximately 2,500 to 3,000/yr), with cases occurring more than twice as often in whites as in blacks. NTDs result from the failure of the neural tube to close between the third and fourth week of gestation. Maternal intake of at least 400 µg of folic acid daily (4 mg daily by women who have had an affected infant previously) in the periconceptional period is believed to greatly reduce the risk of having an infant with NTD (MMWR, 1992; MRC Vitamin Study Research Group, 1991). Infants born with an NTD exhibit high infant mortality; but over the past several decades, survival has dramatically increased with prompt correction of the tube defect and multidisciplinary management of the infant's condition.

Data on the prevalence of CNS disorders among the WIC population were not available to the committee.

Central Nervous System Disorders as an Indicator of Nutrition and Health Risk

Individuals with epilepsy are at risk of physical injury resulting from seizures, inadequate growth, and alteration in nutrient status from prolonged anticonvulsant therapy (e.g., hydantoins alter folate metabolism) (Ekvall, 1993). Infants and children with cerebral palsy often grow poorly and have decreased energy and nutrient intake, primarily because of poor motor skills. Infants with NTDs may be at increased risk of abnormal growth and development because of limited mobility or paralysis, hydrocephalus, limited feeding skills, and genitourinary problems. Because of immobility, reduced respiratory capacity, or other physical problems, women with cerebral palsy, or neural tube defects who become pregnant may find it very difficult to meet their increased nutrient requirements.

Central Nervous System Disorders as an Indicator of Nutrition and Health Benefit

Individuals with CNS disorders need adequate nutrients and sometimes feeding assistance for proper growth and development (Ekvall, 1993). Women, infants, and children with epilepsy, cerebral palsy, or NTDs can benefit from participation in the WIC program by the provision of nutritious supplemental food, nutrition education, and referrals to health care and social services.

Use of Central Nervous System Disorders as a Risk Criterion in the WIC Setting

CNS disorders are diagnosed by a health care provider and reported to WIC agency staff. Table 5-1 summarizes how many states use these risk indicators in the WIC setting.

Recommendation for Central Nervous System Disorders

The risk of *central nervous system disorders* is well documented in women, infants, and children, and clinical methods are available to identify these risks. There is a theoretical basis for benefit from participation in the WIC program. Therefore, the committee recommends use of *central nervous system disorders* as nutrition risk criteria for women, infants, and children in the WIC program. This includes diagnosis of epilepsy, cerebral palsy, and neural tube defects (spina bifida or myelomeningocele).

Genetic and Congenital Disorders

Genetic abnormalities and *congenital malformations* are common causes of disease, disability, or death among infants, and their complications can persist throughout life (Holmes, 1992). Many genetic alterations are associated with congenital heart or kidney disease (see the section on renal disease).

Prevalence of and Factors Associated with Genetic and Congenital Disorders

Approximately 0.5 to 1 percent of infants have a hereditary malformation at birth that causes no physical or metabolic abnormality. Approximately 2 percent of newborns have a major congenital malformation. Genetic and congenital disorders affect nutrition if they cause problems with self-feeding, digestion, absorption or utilization of nutrients, and/or hypoxia.

Cleft lip or palate reflects a failure of the palate shelves to meet and fuse. The prevalence of cleft lip or palate in the general population ranges from 0.03 to 0.2 percent (Behrman, 1992). Populations at greater risk for cleft lip or palate are white, Asian, some tribes of American Indians, or infants delivered postterm. The condition occurs more in males than in females, and more frequently in children born subsequent to a previous child with cleft lip or palate.

Down syndrome results from the presence of an extra 21st chromosome, and is the most common chromosomal abnormality associated with mental retardation (Ekvall, 1993). Down syndrome occurs in approximately 1 in 800 live births, and occurrence increases with advancing maternal age. Over 50 percent of individuals with Down syndrome have congenital heart disease. Children with Down syndrome also have an increased incidence of duodenal atresia and imperforate anus.

Pyloric stenosis and other gastrointestinal obstructive processes have multifactorial inheritance (Shandling, 1992). Pyloric stenosis is more prevalent in first-born male infants (1:150 live male births compared to 1:750 live female births) and males born to mothers who had pyloric stenosis. The condition is generally corrected surgically within the first month of life.

Thalassemia major is a severe, progressive hemolytic anemia usually presenting during the infant's second 6 months (Holmes, 1992). Higher prevalence of thalassemia major occurs in ethnic groups from Mediterranean countries, Africa, the Middle East, and India. In the United States, Berini and Kahn (1987) reported that blacks have a higher incidence of the thalassemia gene than the general population.

Sickle cell anemia is an inherited disorder in which the sickle gene is obtained from each parent (Hb SS) (Ekvall, 1993). Sickle cell anemia occurs in approximately 1 in 625 U.S. blacks (1 in 12 are carriers [Hb AS]), but it is also observed in individuals of Italian, Sicilian, Egyptian, Turkish, Arabic, and Asian ancestry.

Data on the prevalence of specific genetic and congenital disorders among women, infants, and children participating in the WIC program were not available to the committee.

Genetic and Congenital Disorders as Indicators of Nutrition and Health Risk

Genetic and congenital disorders often adversely affect the metabolism of nutrients or normal physiological processes, or cause mechanical barriers to adequate nutrition—resulting in severe health or nutrition problems. Even though the nutritional needs of infants and children with cleft lip or palate are the same as those of other children, mechanical difficulties in feeding may exist. Infants may have insufficient suction when sucking, swallowing problems, and slow weight gain during their first few months. Bowers (1987) found that those with unilateral clefts and isolated clefts of the lip and palates were significantly shorter that their unaffected peers and boys were thinner.

Infants and children with Down syndrome often have feeding problems, growth retardation, dental problems, and changes in nutrient metabolism (Ekvall, 1993). Additional physical factors contributing to nutrient inadequacies include increased mucus production, late appearance of the chewing reflex and of teeth, other dental problems, storage of food in the high-arched palate, and/or thrusting of food out of the mouth with the tongue.

Children with congenital heart disease often experience delayed growth and developmental delay. Hypoxia retards cell growth and multiplication. Impaired energy intake and hypermetabolism may both contribute to malnutrition.

Individuals with thalassemia major have severe anemia, spleen and liver enlargement, impaired growth, and endocrine and cardiac problems (Holmes, 1992). Virtually every organ in the body can be affected by the two primary manifestations of sickle cell anemia: severe hemolytic anemia and vaso-occlusion and infarction of organs and tissues.

Genetic and Congenital Disorders as Indicators of Nutrition and Health Benefit

For infants and children with these disorders, special attention to nutrition may be essential to achieve adequate growth and development and to maintain their health. The WIC program can provide supplemental food, special formula as appropriate, general nutrition and health education, and improved linkages with health care and social services. It does not provide counseling about therapeutic diets. Affected infants, children, and women need dietary management as part of the overall medical management of their conditions.

BIOCHEMICAL AND OTHER MEDICAL RISK CRITERIA

Use of Genetic and Congenital Disorders as Nutrition Risk Criteria in the WIC Setting

Genetic and congenital disorders are diagnosed by a medical care provider and reported to WIC program staff. Table 5-1 summarizes the use of various types of genetic or congenital disorders as nutrition risk criteria by state WIC agencies.

Recommendations for Genetic and Congenital Disorders

The risk of *genetic or congenital disorders* is well documented in women, infants, and children, and clinical methods are available to identify these disorders. There is a theoretical and empirical basis for benefit from participation in the WIC program. Therefore, the committee recommends use of *genetic or congenital disorders* as nutrition risk criteria for women, infants, and children in the WIC program. This includes the use of specific disorders discussed in this section, except for *pyloric stenosis*. Pyloric stenosis is usually repaired within the first month of life. After the infant has recovered from the surgery, gastrointestinal function returns to normal and health and nutrition risk is eliminated.

Inborn Errors of Metabolism

Inborn errors of metabolism include phenylketonuria (PKU), maple syrup urine disease, galactosemia, hyperlipoproteinuria, homocystinuria, tyrosinemia, histidinemia, urea cycle disorders, glutaric aciduria, methylmalonic acidemia, glycogen storage disease, galactokinase deficiency, fructoaldolase deficiency, propionic acidemia, and hypermethioninemia. These and the many other inborn errors of metabolism are either gene mutations or gene deletions that translate into altered metabolism in the body. They can be identified through metabolic assessment performed prenatally or at birth.

Prevalence of and Factors Associated with Inborn Errors of Metabolism

The occurrence of many inborn errors of metabolism is concentrated among individuals of specific ethnic origins (e.g., tyrosinemia type I is seen most often in persons having a French-Canadian ancestry, and glutaric aciduria is most prevalent among Swedish and Pennsylvania Amish populations). The prevalence of inborn errors of metabolism ranges from extremely rare (1 in more than 200,000 live births) to approximately 1 in 10,000 live births (USDA, Report on Ad Hoc Task I.3. Estimated Demand and Cost of WIC Food Package III, USDA, Food and Nutrition Service, Washington, D.C., unpublished information). No prevalence estimates on the number of WIC participants with inborn errors of metabolism were available to the committee.

Inborn Errors of Metabolism as Indicators of Nutrition and Health Risk

Untreated pregnant women with certain inborn errors of metabolism have a higher risk of spontaneous abortion or other health or nutrition risks. Infants born to mothers with untreated PKU may show fetal growth restriction, microcephaly, LBW, and congenital heart disease (Barness, 1993; Rohr et al., 1985).

If inborn errors of metabolism are not detected and treated soon after birth, infants accumulate abnormal metabolites in their blood, resulting in a spectrum of clinical presentations such as mental retardation, seizures, microcephaly, eczema, growth retardation, speech defects, developmental delay, and abnormal eye and bone formation.

Inborn Errors of Metabolism as Indicators of Nutrition and Health Benefit

For many inborn errors of metabolism, appropriate dietary management, which includes the use of special formulas, can minimize the medical risk to affected individuals (COG-AAP, 1991). The benefit of nutrition and medical intervention is illustrated through the example of PKU, which is the most prevalent inborn error in the United States for which dietary management has been provided over an extended period (since the mid-1960s). Such dietary management is not provided by the WIC program, but the special formulas may be.

Individuals with PKU lack the enzyme to convert phenylalanine to tyrosine, and high levels of phenylalanine and its metabolites are toxic to the developing central nervous system. Therefore, restricting intake of phenylalanine reduces the risk of damage to the fetus or the newborn. Early results from a large collaborative study indicate that a phenylalanine-restricted diet, if instituted early in gestation, can result in apparently normal outcome (Platt et al., 1992).

Recently, it has been shown that children with PKU who receive early and continuous dietary treatment with a phenylalanine-free amino acid mixture have only mildly elevated levels of phenylalanine and reduced levels of tyrosine. Children whose phenylalanine levels were three to five times normal (6–10 mg/dl) showed signs of poor performance in tests of object retrieval, attention control, and motor tapping but no signs of deficits in other functions. The nature of the selective deficits observed indicated an impairment in the dorsolateral prefrontal cortex (Diamond, 1995).

Infants with PKU would receive excessive phenylalanine if breastfed exclusively. Therefore, all mothers, whether breastfeeding or not, should be re-

BIOCHEMICAL AND OTHER MEDICAL RISK CRITERIA

ferred for dietary treatment of the infant, which includes use of low phenylalanine or phenylalanine-free formula. Such special formulas may be provided by the WIC program. A phenylalanine-restricted diet during infancy and early childhood normalizes blood phenylalanine levels, permitting normal mental development. Similar dietary management is indicated for individuals with other inborn errors of metabolism.

Use of Inborn Errors of Metabolism as Risk Criteria in the WIC Setting

Inborn errors of metabolism are reported to WIC programs from diagnosis by a medical care provider. Table 5-1 summarizes how many states use these risk criteria in the WIC setting.

Recommendations for Inborn Errors of Metabolism

The risks of *PKU and other inborn errors of metabolism* are well documented in women, infants, and children, and these risks can be identified clinically. The benefit of use of special formulas is well established. Therefore, the committee recommends use of *PKU* and other *inborn errors of metabolism* as nutrition risk criteria for women, infants, and children in the WIC program.

Chronic or Recurrent Infections

The relationship between nutrition and infection has been appreciated for centuries: tuberculosis was known as "consumption," and HIV/AIDS was categorized as "slim disease" when first discovered in East Africa (Keusch, 1994). Individuals with chronic or recurrent infections such as tuberculosis, pneumonia, bronchitis, upper respiratory infections, otitis media, meningitis, and hepatitis may have increased nutrition needs. Nutrition deficits can impair the host's ability to sustain cellular proliferation and other defense mechanisms. HIV/AIDS is covered separately in the next section.

Prevalence of and Factors Associated with Chronic or Recurrent Infections

Data on prevalence of chronic or recurrent infections among the U.S. or the WIC population were not available to the committee. In the United States, the probability of children developing acute otitis media is understood to be very high (Infante-Rivard and Fernandez, 1993).

Chronic or Recurrent Infections as Indicators of Nutrition and Health Risk

Catabolic responses to infection increase energy and nutrient requirements and may exacerbate medical conditions associated with infection (Keusch, 1994). Iron, zinc, vitamin A, and other nutrients are associated with the host's ability to fight infection, and deficiencies of these nutrients are associated with negative health outcomes with chronic or recurrent infections. Hepatitis increases risk for nutrient imbalances, anorexia, and emesis (Brunell, 1992).

Infants and children with otitis media in the first year of life have an increased risk of recurrent acute or chronic disease (Bluestone and Nozza, 1992).

The committee did not find any research studies indicating nutrition risk resulting from upper respiratory infections, bronchitis, or otitis media.

Chronic or Recurrent Infections as Indicators of Nutrition and Health Benefit

The relationship between nutrition, the immune system, and health is very complex. The supplemental food provided through the WIC program provides nutrients that may be needed to maintain an individual's ability to fight chronic or recurrent infections. The WIC program's role in referring participants to health services provides additional benefits. The committee found no studies that indicated that supplemental food or nutrition education would improve the health of women, infants, or children with chronic or recurrent upper respiratory infections, bronchitis, or otitis media.

Use of Chronic or Recurrent Infections as Risk Criteria in the WIC Setting

Diagnosis of chronic or recurrent infections is made by a medical care provider and reported to WIC program staff. State WIC agency plans generally define "chronic" as a persistent condition present at the time of certification for the program, and "recurrent" as a condition that must have occurred more than 2 times over the past 12 months (USDA, 1994). Table 5-1 summarizes use of this risk indicator by state WIC agencies.

Recommendations for Chronic or Recurrent Infections

The risk of certain *chronic or recurrent infections* has been well documented for women, infants, and children. There is a theoretical and empirical basis for benefit from participation in the WIC program for individuals with serious infections such as tuberculosis. The committee recommends use of selected *chronic or recurrent infections* as a nutrition risk criterion for women, infants, and children in the WIC program. However, the committee cautions that state WIC agency program plans should clearly define *chronic* or *recurrent* with each condition in its listing of nutrition risk criteria. The committee recommends discontinuation of *chronic upper respiratory infections, bronchitis, otitis media,* and *chronic urinary tract infection* (see earlier section) as nutrition risk criteria in the WIC program because of lack of scientific evidence to support nutrition benefit.

HIV Infection and AIDS

Prevalence of and Factors Associated with HIV Infection and AIDS

The growing prevalence of human immunodeficiency virus (HIV) infection and acquired immunodeficiency syndrome (AIDS) among women (CDC, 1995b) has been accompanied by an increase in the number of children who have been infected perinatally. Mother-to-infant transmission cumulatively accounts for about 90 percent of all pediatric cases (CDC, 1994a). The CDC estimates that 1.6 to 1.7 of every 1,000 women tested in 1992 were HIV seropositive (CDC, 1994b). The prevalence of seropositive infants is much lower.

Women made up 18 percent of adults and adolescents with AIDS reported in 1994. In 1994, CDC estimated that black women made up more than half of all reported cases of HIV/AIDS among women older than 13 years of age, and Hispanic women were also heavily overrepresented. The racial/ethnic distribution was similar for infants and children (CDC, 1994b). No data on the prevalence of HIV/AIDS in the WIC program population were available to the committee.

The strikingly higher rates of HIV/AIDS in blacks and Hispanics are closely linked to poverty; and the ethnic distribution of Americans living in poverty closely resembles the distribution of AIDS cases (National Commission on AIDS, 1992). Populations living in poverty tend to have unequal access to preventive and medical care, lower standards of living, higher levels of unemployment, and higher rates of drug use and alcoholism. A study in Seattle, Washington, found that after controlling for other demographic and behavioral risk, income level was independently associated with HIV infection (Krueger et al., 1990).

Risk indicators for HIV/AIDS include unprotected maternal or paternal sexual activity, maternal or paternal injection of illegal drugs, sexual abuse, bisexuality, exposure to HIV-contaminated blood or blood products, and consumption of HIV-contaminated breast milk (infants only).

HIV/AIDS as an Indicator of Nutrition and Health Risk

As a member of the retrovirus family, HIV enters the cell and causes cell dysfunction or death. Since this virus primarily affects cells of the immune system, immunodeficiency results. HIV can replicate in T cells, B cells, monocytes, and macrophages. Recent evidence suggests that monocytes and macrophages may be the most important target cells and indicates that HIV can infect bone marrow stem cells.

The leading indicators of AIDS are HIV-related immunosuppression (81 percent) and *Pneumocystis carinii* pneumonia (12 percent) in adults, and bacterial infections (19 percent) and *P. carinii* pneumonia (18 percent) in infants and children (CDC, 1994b). HIV wasting syndrome accounted for 10 percent of all conditions that are indicators of AIDS for adults and 17 percent for infants and children. Other major clinical findings associated with HIV infection (Chachoua et al., 1989) are failure to thrive, poor growth (McKinney and Robertson, 1993; Saavedra et al., 1995), oral candidiasis, parotitis, chronic or recurrent diarrhea, malabsorption, lymphoid interstitial pneumonitis, bacterial and viral infections, opportunistic infections, hepatomegaly, splenomegaly, encephalopathy, developmental delay, loss of developmental milestones, cardiomyopathy, and nephropathy. In addition to all the clinical findings presented above, other clinical symptoms associated with HIV infection in adults include such conditions as Kaposi's sarcoma, B-cell lymphoma, and lymphopenia (Chachoua et al., 1989).

HIV infection is associated with the risk of malnutrition at all stages of infection. In the early stages, malnutrition may result from lifestyle factors such as drug abuse. As the disease process progresses, anorexia, intestinal malabsorption, diarrhea, drug-nutrient interactions, fever, secondary infection, and increased cytokine production may all contribute to PEM, the wasting syndrome, and to specific micronutrient deficiencies (Baum et al., 1994). PEM and specific micronutrient deficiencies have adverse effects on the immune system, pregnancy outcome, growth and development of infants and young children, organ (e.g., cardiac) function, and tolerance to treatment.

HIV has been reported in human milk and has been documented to be passed from mother to infant by breastfeeding (Newell and Peckham, 1994; Ruff, 1994). A separate study by Semba et al. (1994) reported an increased risk of mother-to-child transmission of HIV among vitamin A deficient mothers.

HIV/AIDS as an Indicator of Nutrition and Health Benefit

Some prospective, observational evidence, mainly obtained from studies on homosexual men, indicates that optimizing nutrition among individuals with

HIV infection may retard disease progression (Abrams et al., 1993; LSRO/FASEB, 1990; Semba et al., 1995; Tang et al., 1993). The observational study by Semba et al. (1994) indicates that optimal vitamin A status may have a protective effect on mother-to-child transmission of HIV, but this finding needs to be tested in an intervention study. A recent study of 118 vitamin A supplemented children of HIV-infected women in Durban, South Africa, found that these children had lower overall morbidity than the control group and that morbidity associated with diarrhea was significantly reduced in the supplemented infected children (Coutsoudis et al., 1995).

HIV-infected women in the United States need to be advised against breast-feeding because of the risk of the vertical transmission of maternal virus to the infant (IOM, 1991), and their infants are likely to benefit from the formula WIC provides. Special interventions (e.g., special infant or enteral formula) may be necessary in infants and children with clinical evidence of HIV/AIDS. The potential benefits of ensuring optimal nutrition for HIV-infected women (during pregnancy and the postpartum period), infants, and children include improved maternal nutrition and health, improved infant and child growth and development, and, possibly, a slowing of disease progression. At present, there is a paucity of studies to demonstrate clear benefits of WIC program interventions for those with HIV/AIDS. However, the American and Canadian Dietetic Associations have taken the position that therapeutic and educational nutrition interventions should be components of care provided to HIV-infected individuals (American Dietetic Association, 1994). WIC program-related referrals to health care and social services may benefit those with HIV/AIDS and uninfected infants of infected mothers.

Use of HIV/AIDS as a Nutrition Risk Criterion in the WIC Setting

Health care providers report diagnoses of HIV infection or AIDS to WIC program staff. Table 5-1 lists the numbers of states using this diagnosis as a nutrition risk criterion.

Recommendation for HIV/AIDS

The risk of *HIV/AIDS* is well documented in women, infants, and children, and can be identified by clinical diagnosis. There is a theoretical basis for benefit from participation in the WIC program. Therefore, the committee recommends use of *HIV/AIDS* as a nutrition risk criterion for women, infants, and children in the WIC program.

Recent Major Surgery, Trauma, Burns, or Severe Acute Infections

Most patients having major surgery do not experience serious malnutrition. However, the disease process or metabolic response to *recent major surgery, trauma, burns,* or *severe acute infection* can increase the risk of malnutrition and affect subsequent nutrient requirements for rehabilitation and recovery (Souba and Wilmore, 1994). The variability in the metabolic and physiologic responses to major surgery, trauma, burns, and severe acute infections is related in part to the patient's age, previous state of health, preexisting disease, previous stress, and specific pathogens.

Prevalence of and Factors Associated with Recent Major Surgery, Trauma, Burns, or Severe Acute Infections

Data on the prevalence of recent major surgery, trauma, burns, or severe acute infections among women, infants, and children in the U.S. population or participating in the WIC program were not available to the committee. Chronic and recurrent infections and HIV infection are discussed in previous sections of this chapter.

Recent Major Surgery, Trauma, Burns, or Severe Acute Infections as Indicators of Nutrition or Health Risk

The catabolic response to surgery occurs as a result of the traumatic insult of surgery and other complications of both preexisting disease and gastrointestinal function that diminish food intake (Souba and Wilmore, 1994). Persons experiencing severe trauma such as automobile accidents or burns exhibit a hypermetabolic state that may reach twice the basal levels and persist for 2 months or longer (Wilmore, 1977). Alterations in the metabolism of glucose, protein, and fat occur following injury. There is a marked rise in the regulatory hormones (glucagon, glucocorticoids, and catecholamines) in all phases of injury or after severe burn.

The gut functions as a central organ of amino acid metabolism, a role that becomes more pronounced during a critical illness. Disuse of the gastrointestinal tract during major illnesses may lead to numerous physiologic derangements, changes in the microflora, impaired immune function in the gut, and disruption of the integrity of the mucosal barrier.

Severe infections are characterized by prolonged fever, hypermetabolism, diminished protein economy, altered glucose dynamics, and accelerated lipolysis. Anorexia associated with severe infections contributes to the loss of lean body mass. Multiorgan and system involvement surrounding surgery, trauma, or

BIOCHEMICAL AND OTHER MEDICAL RISK CRITERIA

burns compound these metabolic effects and often affect function of the gastrointestinal tract, liver, heart, and lungs. Women who conceive during recovery from recent surgery, trauma, or burns may be at increased nutrition risk because the special nutritional needs of pregnancy are superimposed on those related to the metabolic response to trauma.

Recent Major Surgery, Trauma, Burns, or Severe Acute Infections as Indicators of Nutrition or Health Benefit

In part because of technologic and scientific advances in nutritional support, individuals who would have died in the past are now surviving complex surgical procedures, major trauma, burns, and sepsis (Souba and Wilmore, 1994). After discharge, there may be a continued need for high nutrient intake to promote completion of healing and to return to optimal weight and nutrition status. Supplemental food supplied by the WIC program is a source of key nutrients.

Use of Recent Major Surger, Trauma, Burns, or Severe Acute Infections as Nutrition Risk Criteria in the WIC Setting

Recent major surgery, trauma, burns, or severe acute infections are diagnosed by a health care provider and reported to WIC program staff or are self-reported during the certification process for participation in the WIC program, or at follow-up visits. See Table 5-1 for a summary of use of these specific nutrition risk criteria by WIC state agencies. In many cases, the recency of the condition is not specified.

Recommendation for Recent Major Surgery, Trauma, Burns, or Severe Acute Infections

The risk of *recent major surgery, trauma, burns,* or *severe acute infections* is well documented for women, infants, and children, and these conditions are identified easily. There is a theoretical and empirical basis for benefit from participation in the WIC program. Therefore, the committee recommends the use of *recent major surgery, trauma, burns,* or *severe acute infections* as nutrition risk criteria by the WIC program for women, infants, and children. If self-report is used as the basis for certification, a cutoff point of 2 months (Wilmore, 1977) is recommended.

Other Medical Conditions

There are other medical conditions with nutrition implications that are used as nutrition risk indicators in the WIC program that do not fit into the categories previously discussed in this chapter. This section covers the conditions of *juvenile rheumatoid arthritis, lupus erythematosus,* and *cardiorespiratory disorders.*

Prevalence of and Factors Associated with Other Medical Conditions

Juvenile rheumatoid arthritis. Juvenile rheumatoid arthritis (JRA) is the most common pediatric rheumatic disease and is the most common cause of chronic arthritis among children, occurring in approximately 0.01 percent of infants and children (Ekvall, 1993). JRA is thought to result from infection with unidentified microorganisms or an autoimmune reaction (Schaller, 1992). The disease persists throughout life.

Individuals with JRA are at risk of joint stiffness, fever, anorexia, weight loss, failure to grow, and fatigue (Ekvall, 1993). Approximately 36 percent of these individuals experience PEM and have lower than recommended intakes of energy, vitamin E, calcium, and iron. Serum vitamin C is often low among patients who receive high dosages of aspirin.

Lupus erythematosus. Lupus erythematosus is also an autoimmune disorder—one that affects multiple organ systems. Lupus erythematosus is more common in dark-skinned ethnic groups including blacks, Hispanics, Asians, and some American-Indian tribes, and is estimated to occur in 1 in 700 women between 15 and 65 years of age (Ferris and Reece, 1994).

Lupus erythematosus increases risk of infections, malaise, anorexia, and weight loss (Schaller, 1992). Pregnant women with lupus erythematosus are at increased risk of late pregnancy losses (after 28 weeks gestation) secondary to hypertension and renal failure, of cardiac defects or heart block in the fetus, and spontaneous abortion (Ferris and Reece, 1994). Little is known about nutrient metabolism or requirements of pregnant or breastfeeding women with lupus erythematosus.

Cardiorespiratory diseases. Cardiorespiratory diseases interfere with the normal physiological process. Congestive heart failure in infants and children is often accompanied by failure to thrive and malnutrition. Prevalence estimates on cardiorespiratory diseases in the U.S. population were not available to the committee.

Growth failure can be present in individuals with cardiorespiratory disease and can be aggravated because of increased metabolic requirements and difficulty in sucking and swallowing (Ekvall, 1993). Salt intake must be limited for persons having congestive heart failure. Low calorie intake and hypermetabolism are both postulated as causes of malnutrition among individuals with cardiorespiratory diseases.

Data on the prevalence of the above disorders among women, infants, and children participating in the WIC program were not available to the committee.

Other Medical Risks as Indicators of Nutrition and Health Benefit

The WIC program can benefit individuals with medical risks through the provision of supplemental food, special dietary formulas as indicated, and referrals for health care services. WIC provides general nutrition and health education that focuses on maintaining dietary intake to meet the Recommended Dietary Allowance for age and the promotion of optimal growth or the prevention of obesity (Ekvall, 1993). Nutrition-related interventions as a part of medical management help correct growth and weight problems in children with JRA and lupus erythematosus (Schaller, 1992).

Use of Other Medical Risks as Risk Indicators in the WIC Setting

Other medical risks are diagnosed by a health care provider and reported to WIC staff. See Table 5-1 for a summary of use of these specific nutrition risk indicators by WIC state agencies. Note that JRA has not been used as a nutrition risk criterion in the WIC by state WIC agencies for infants or children (USDA, 1994).

Recommendations for Other Medical Conditions

The risks of *juvenile rheumatoid arthritis, lupus erythematosus,* and *cardiorespiratory disorders* are documented in women, infants, and children, and they can be identified by a clinical diagnosis. There is a theoretical and empirical basis for benefit from participation in the WIC program. Therefore, the committee recommends the use of *juvenile rheumatoid arthritis, lupus erythematosus,* and *cardiorespiratory disorders* as nutrition risk criteria for women, infants, and children in the WIC program. The committee recommends deletion of general diagnosis of *arthritis* as a nutrition risk criterion in the WIC program for women.

CONDITIONS RELATED TO THE INTAKE OF SPECIFIC FOODS

Food Allergies

Food represents the largest antigenic challenge confronting the human immune system. *Food allergies* are illnesses that affect only part of the population. True food allergies involve abnormal immunologic responses to food-borne substances. With true food allergy, even minute amounts of the offending food can cause potentially life-threatening reactions.

Two types of true food allergies occur: antibody-mediated and cell-mediated (Sampson, 1994). Allergens are typically naturally occurring proteins from the implicated food. Those proteins that are resistant to digestion can elicit the formation of antibodies, but only the formation of allergen-specific immunoglobulin E (IgE) elicits allergic sensitization.

The antibody-mediated allergies (also known as atopy or immediate hypersensitivity) occur immediately after consumption of the offending food. The foods most commonly involved in IgE-mediated food allergies are peanuts, cow milk, eggs, soybeans, nuts from trees, wheat, and seafood.

The sole known example of a cell-mediated food allergy is celiac disease, also known as gluten-sensitive enteropathy. This is a delayed hypersensitivity reaction because the onset time between ingestion of the offending food and development of symptoms can be from 24 to 72 hours later. Signs and symptoms of celiac disease result from the ingestion of the gluten protein fraction of wheat, rye, barley, triticale, and oats.

Prevalence of and Factors Associated with Food Allergies

The prevalence of IgE-mediated food allergies in the population is estimated to be between 4 and 8 percent of young infants, 1 and 2 percent of children, and less than 1 percent of adults (Sloan and Powers, 1986). The prevalence of celiac disease has been estimated at 1 in every 3,000 individuals in the United States (Ekvall, 1993). The prevalence of food allergies among the WIC population was not available to the committee.

Food Allergies as Indicators of Nutrition and Health Risk

Atopic diseases such as asthma, allergic rhinitis, and atopic dermatitis can all be precipitated by antigenic foods. Both upper and lower respiratory symptoms have been demonstrated as a result of food allergy; however, the role of nutrition apart from avoidance of the allergenic food could not be documented.

Infants are more susceptible to the development of food allergies than are adults: their digestive system may not yet be fully functional and the intestinal mucosa may be more permeable to proteins. Infants born to parents with histories of IgE-mediated allergies are most at risk for the development of food allergies. Many infants outgrow allergies to milk within a few months or years, but some food allergies, such as peanut allergy, may be more intransigent.

Individuals with IgE-mediated food allergies are at risk of gastrointestinal disorders (e.g., nausea, vomiting, diarrhea, colic), atopic dermatitis, urticaria, angioedema, rhinitis, and the potentially life-threatening conditions anaphylactic shock and asthma.

Celiac disease is a malabsorption syndrome that primarily affects the absorptive functions of the small intestine. The primary symptoms are body wasting, diarrhea, anemia, and bone pain.

Food Allergies as Indicators of Nutrition and Health Benefit

The avoidance of the offending food is the primary method of treatment for food allergies. Referral for dietary management is indicated for those with true food allergy.

Exclusive breastfeeding for several months appears to reduce severe allergic disease in high-risk infants, but debate continues over whether restricting the mother's diet during lactation to avoid the common antigens (cow milk, seafood, soy, nuts, and eggs) confers additional benefit (Harrison, 1994). A prospective, randomized, controlled study of food allergen avoidance in infancy by Zeiger and Heller (1995) confirms benefit of nutrition intervention to reduce risk of severe food allergy but reports no benefit from third trimester food restrictions. Breastfeeding for 1 year may delay the onset of food allergies, but it does not decrease the likelihood of their development by 7 years of age. For allergic infants who are formula fed, WIC may provide special milk-free formula.

A modified food package may be needed for maximum benefit.

Use of Risk of Food Allergies as Nutrition Risk Criteria in the WIC Setting

Food allergies are diagnosed by a physician and reported to the WIC program. Table 5-1 lists the use of food allergies as a nutrition risk criterion by state WIC agencies.

Recommendation for Food Allergies

The risk of *food allergies* is well documented for women, infants, and children, and this condition can be identified clinically. There is a theoretical basis for benefit from participation in the WIC program. Therefore, the committee recommends use of *food allergy* and *celiac disease* as nutrition risk criteria for women, infants, and children in the WIC program.

Food Intolerances

Food intolerances occur through many different mechanisms. The primary categories of food intolerance include enzyme deficiencies, pharmacologic reactions, and idiosyncratic reactions with unknown mechanisms. These illnesses are of lesser importance than allergy because of finite tolerance levels for the offending foods among affected individuals. Also, the link between specific foods or food additives and food intolerances has not been proven in many cases. The best examples of food intolerances are lactose intolerance and sulfite-induced asthma.

Lactose intolerance is a disorder in which a deficiency of ß-galactosidase in the small intestine results in reduced ability to digest and absorb lactose. Sulfite-induced asthma is an idiosyncratic illness—the mechanism of this reaction is not known.

Prevalence of and Factors Associated with Food Intolerances

The prevalence of lactose intolerance varies from 6 to 12 percent in northern European Caucasians to 60 to 80 percent in most other ethnic groups (Rohr et al., 1985). The prevalence of noticeable lactose intolerance increases with advancing age; it is rare in otherwise healthy young infants but is a frequent occurrence following infectious diarrhea. In these individuals, recovery can be anticipated within a few weeks.

Sulfites are a comparatively minor cause of asthma, affecting perhaps 1 to 2 percent of all asthmatic individuals. The prevalence of food intolerances among the WIC population was not available to the committee.

Food Intolerances as Indicators of Nutrition and Health Risk

The symptoms of lactose intolerance include abdominal cramps, flatulence, and frothy diarrhea. However, many individuals with lactose intolerance can tolerate the ingestion of small amounts of dairy products at any one time and a number of small servings over the course of a day. Asthma is the only well-documented adverse effect of sulfite ingestion.

Food Intolerances as Indicators of Nutrition and Health Benefit

The committee found no empirical evidence of direct benefit of the WIC program for individuals with food intolerances other than lactose intolerance. Participation in the WIC program can provide special formula for affected infants; cheese, which is low in lactose, for women and children; and education about food sources of lactose and foods that can be substituted for milk to maintain a nutritionally balanced diet.

Use of Food Intolerances as Nutrition Risk Criteria in the WIC Setting

Diagnosis of food intolerance is reported to the WIC agency by a health care provider. Table 5-1 lists use of food intolerance as a nutrition risk criterion by WIC state agencies.

Recommendations for Food Intolerances

The risk of *food intolerances* other than lactose intolerance is not well documented in women, infants, and children. For *lactose intolerance*, there is a theoretical and empirical basis for benefit from participation in the WIC program, especially when lactose-reduced milk products are part of the food package. Therefore, the committee recommends use of well-documented symptomatic *lactose intolerance* as a risk criterion for women, infants, and children. However, the committee recommends discontinuation of nonspecific and poorly identified *food intolerances*. Given the lack of evidence to support the role of nutrition as an indicator of benefit for *asthma*, the committee recommends discontinuation of use of diagnosis of *asthma* as a nutrition risk criterion for women, infants, and children in the WIC program.

CONDITIONS SPECIFIC TO PREGNANCY

Pregnancy at a Young Age

Pregnancy at young ages (i.e., before growth is complete) carries particular nutritional risk because of the potential for competition for nutrients between the needs for pregnancy and those for the woman's own growth. Adolescent pregnancy is generally regarded as conception before the 18th birthday, but postmenarchal age may be more important than chronologic age in quantifying risk, with the first 2 years after menarche the most critical time (Zlatnik and Burmeister, 1977).

Prevalence of and Factors Associated with Pregnancy at a Young Age

The rate of births to teens ages 15 to 19 increased 24 percent between 1986 and 1991, from 50 to 62 births per 1,000 females (IOM, 1995). Low income, minority status, and disadvantaged backgrounds are common scenarios among pregnant teenagers.

Pregnancy at a Young Age as an Indicator of Nutrition and Health Risk

Weight gain during pregnancy is more likely to be low in very young mothers, and adolescents often follow dietary practices that lead to low intakes of a variety of nutrients (IOM, 1990). Maternal age less than 15 years has been identified as a risk factor for LBW (IOM, 1995).

Pregnancy at a Young Age as an Indicator of Nutrition and Health Benefit

In one study of pregnant teens who participated in the WIC program, mean birth weight appeared to be increased, and the percentage of mothers delivering LBW infants decreased (Kennedy and Kotelchuck, 1984), but confirmation of these findings is needed. Since pregnant adolescents are likely to have many risk factors, they have substantial potential to benefit from the food package, nutrition education, and referral to health and social services.

Use of Pregnancy at a Young Age as a Risk Criterion in the WIC Setting

Table 5-1 lists the use of pregnancy at a young age as a nutrition risk criterion by state WIC programs. Cutoff points in use include conception at a specified number of years postmenarche and specific actual ages at conception.

Recommendation for Pregnancy at a Young Age

The risk of *pregnancy at a young age* is well documented in women, and it is easy to identify this condition. There is empirical evidence and a theoretical basis for benefit from participation in the WIC program. Therefore, the committee recommends use of *pregnancy at a young age* as a nutrition risk for women in all state WIC programs, with a cutoff value of 2 years postmenarche.

Pregnancy Age Older than 35 Years

Prevalence of and Factors Associated with Pregnancy Age Older than 35 Years

In the United States, the prevalence of women delaying childbearing continues to increase; from 1976 to 1986 the rate of first births among women 40 years of age or older doubled (NCHS and Ventura, 1989). Data on the prevalence of pregnancy above 35 years of age among the WIC population were not available to the committee.

Pregnancy Age Older than 35 Years as an Indicator of Nutrition and Health Risk

With advancing age, especially after age 35, risks associated with pregnancy increase. Most or all of this is due to the increasing likelihood of medical illnesses in the mother and congenital defects (i.e., chromosomal abnormalities) in the fetus (Berkowitz et al., 1990; Cefalo and Moos, 1988; Fretts et al., 1995). The extent of risk attributable specifically to nutrition in older mothers is highly questionable.

Pregnancy Age Older than 35 Years as an Indicator of Nutrition and Health Benefit

Although medical complications of pregnancy increase with increased age, and yield of risk would be high, there is little evidence of nutrition benefit from WIC participation and the services offered by the program.

Recommendation for Pregnancy Age Older than 35 Years

The risk of *pregnancy age older than 35 years* is well documented in women, and this condition can be identified easily. However, there is no theoretical or empirical basis for benefit from participation in the WIC program. Therefore, the committee recommends discontinuation of use of *pregnancy age older than 35 years* as a nutrition risk criterion for women in the WIC program.

Closely Spaced Pregnancies

Closely spaced pregnancies are commonly defined using either of two indicators: short interpregnancy interval (birth to conception interval), or short birth interval (the interval between the previous and sampled births). The interpregnancy interval is not affected by the length of gestation of the second pregnancy.

Prevalence of and Factors Associated with Closely Spaced Pregnancies

In 1991, 14 percent of all second- and higher-order U.S. births occurred within 18 months of the mother's previous birth, 28 percent within 2 years, and 52 percent within 3 years (CDC/NCHS, 1993). Black women are more likely than white women to have closely spaced pregnancies, regardless of the definition used (CDC/NCHS, 1993; Kalmuss and Namerow, 1994; Rawlings et al., 1995). For WIC program participants, over 30 percent had an interpregnancy interval of 23 months or less (Gordon and Nelson, 1995); only about 3 percent had intervals of 11 months or less. No data were found for the prevalence of shorter interpregnancy intervals.

In a study of adolescent mothers, Kalmuss and Namerow (1994) reported that approximately 25 percent of adolescent mothers have a second child within 24 months of their first birth. The percentage is even higher (31 percent) for those age 17 years or less at the time of the first birth. Poverty is associated with closely spaced births among adolescents, while higher educational level of the parents is associated with longer intervals between births.

Closely Spaced Pregnancies as an Indicator of Nutrition and Health Risk

Mothers with closely spaced pregnancies have little time to recover from the physiologic and nutrition demands of the previous pregnancy. If such women are also breastfeeding, any negative effects of lactation on maternal nutritional status may further increase the risks of adverse outcomes of pregnancy, such as prematurity or fetal growth restriction (Cleland and Sathar, 1984; Hobcraft et al., 1985). This may occur because both the last portion of pregnancy and full lactation are periods of potential nutritional depletion for the mother (Winkvist et al., 1992). Becoming pregnant soon after the end of this period of depletion allows the mother little or no time for nutritional repletion.

Prematurity leading to shorter birth intervals has also been suggested as an explanation for the relationship of closely spaced pregnancies with prematurity and fetal growth restriction. Where investigated (DaVanzo, 1984), both maternal depletion and prematurity seemed to play an equally important role.

Studies of lactating women indicate that their nutrient or energy stores may be depleted if nutrient and energy intake are marginal, while milk tends to remain adequate in nutrient content (IOM, 1991). Although overlapping of lactation with pregnancy is uncommon in the United States, when it does occur, it can increase the risk of nutrient depletion. Using data from Guatemala, Merchant and colleagues (1990) found evidence of depletion of maternal nutrient stores caused by substantial overlapping of pregnancy and lactation.

In studies using multivariate analysis, an interpregnancy interval of 3 months (or a comparable birth interval of 12 months) is reported to increase the risk of delivering an infant born preterm and with low birth weight (Rawlings et al., 1995), delivering an infant small for gestational age (SGA) (Miller, 1989), and neonatal death (Miller, 1989). None of these studies focused on low-income populations. In a study by Lang and co-workers (1990), the risk of preterm labor was increased twofold but was not statistically significant. In the Rawlings et al. (1995) study of 1,922 U.S. military families who have health care available without charge, the increased risk of delivering a preterm, low-birth-weight infant was seen for whites only for interpregnancy intervals of less than 3 months, while for blacks the cutoff was less than 9 months.

Lieberman and colleagues (1989), in a study of nearly 4,500 women in Boston, found that women with interpregnancy intervals of 18 months or fewer were at twice the risk of giving birth to a full-term SGA infant when compared with women with interpregnancy intervals of 24 to 36 months. These results were obtained after adjusting for multiple confounding factors. The risk was lowest (2.4 percent) at interpregnancy intervals of 24 to 36 months. In contrast, for more than 2,000 low-income women with a birth interval of 2 years or less (which approximates a 15-month interpregnancy interval), multivariate analyses indicated an increased risk of spontaneous preterm delivery (Abrams et al., 1989) but not SGA (Abrams et al., 1991).

In a much smaller study of healthy, nonsmoking women from private obstetric practices in Chicago, differences in interpregnancy interval were not associated with higher postpartum weight, subsequent pregravid weight, birth weight, or length of gestation (Farahati et al., 1993). A number of U.S. studies showed that closely spaced pregnancies increase the risk of the low birth weight (e.g., Brody and Bracken, 1987; Eisner et al., 1979; Spiers and Wang, 1976) without differentiating whether the low birth weight was a result of preterm birth or intrauterine growth retardation.

In a multivariate analysis that used data from Hungary, Sweden, and the United States, Miller (1989) reported that maternal depletion did not explain the association of closely spaced pregnancies with SGA because the risk did not decrease with increasing length of the birth interval in the under-18-months range; however, in the Lieberman (1989) study, it did.

Closely Spaced Pregnancies as an Indicator of Nutrition and Health Benefit

The shorter the time between pregnancies, the shorter the time for repletion of nutrient stores. As reported in Chapter 4, women who received postpartum WIC program benefits for 5 to 7 months delivered infants with higher mean birth weights and birth lengths and a lower risk of low birth weight (Caan et al., 1987) than did women who received supplements for 2 months or less. Moreover, the women who were supplemented longer had higher mean hemoglobin values and lower risk of maternal obesity at the beginning of their subsequent pregnancies. These results suggest that more repletion occurred in the women who received WIC program benefits for the longer period and suggests that WIC program participation may be beneficial to postpartum women with closely spaced pregnancies.

Use of Closely Spaced Pregnancies in the WIC Setting

Interpregnancy interval is the most practical and informative definition of closely spaced pregnancies to use in the WIC setting. Health care providers in the WIC setting can obtain the date of the previous delivery from self-report and the estimated date of conception from the patient's record. Table 5-1 shows that 52 states use closely spaced pregnancies as a risk criterion for pregnant women. The cutoff point varies widely, from three births in 24 months to intervals of ≤ 25 months, and two states do not give a cutoff point.

Recommendations for Closely Spaced Pregnancies

Health risks of closely spaced pregnancies are reasonably well documented for pregnancy outcomes, especially those of women who have low incomes and for interpregnancy intervals of 3 months or less. There is a theoretical basis for nutrition risk during the subsequent pregnancy and period of lactation, but information linking nutrition to the health risks is equivocal. Closely spaced pregnancies can be identified using information easily available through self-report and the patient's record.

The committee recommends use of closely spaced pregnancies as a nutrition risk criterion for pregnant women, using a 6-month *interpregnancy* interval as the usual cutoff point, but increasing the cutoff point to a 9-month interpregnancy interval for women who are concurrently pregnant and lactating. The committee assumes that a postpartum woman with a previous short interpregnancy interval will qualify under another risk criterion.

The committee recommends research on the associations of short interpregnancy intervals and such nutritional risk factors as prepregnancy weight, weight gain, and diet.

High Parity

Parity refers to the number of a woman's completed pregnancies that have reached the stage of viability. The cutoff values defining different parity groups are usually first-order births or first pregnancy, first- and second-order births, and births of higher orders. Often, studies examine very high parity births, defined variously as four, five, or more previous pregnancies. High parity is closely related to other risk criteria, especially prior miscarriages and abortions, closely spaced pregnancies, and high age at conception.

Prevalence of and Factors Associated with High Parity

Estimates of the prevalence of high parity vary because of differences in the definition of high parity and the data source used. Population-based data generally use natality data from birth certificates for live-born U.S. infants and refer to the number of previous births since the number of previous viable pregnancies is not available. In 1993, 11 percent of all live births were fourth- and high-order births (Ventura et al., 1995). Black women giving birth are more likely than white women to be at higher parity; 16 percent of all births to black women were fourth- or higher-order births compared with 10 percent of all births to white women (Ventura et al., 1995; Cogswell and Yip, 1995). Among women of Hispanic origin, 15 percent of all live births in 1993 were fourth- or higher-order births, and among American-Indian women, 22 percent of all births were fourth- or higher-order births.

Data from the 1988 National Maternal and Infant Health Survey (NMIHS) indicate that 16 percent of low-income pregnant women who were income-eligible for the WIC program had four or more previous pregnancies and 32 percent had three or more previous pregnancies (Gordon and Nelson, 1995). The percentage of prenatal WIC participants with three or more pregnancies was higher than this percentage among income-eligible nonparticipants (34 percent versus 29 percent).

High Parity as an Indicator of Nutrition and Health Risk

Empirical evidence points to two main risks of high parity: (1) poor pregnancy outcomes and infant growth and (2) long-term health risks to women. The rationale typically offered for expecting poorer pregnancy outcomes for women of high parity is maternal depletion (Merchant and Martorell, 1988). High parity implies frequent, and often closely-spaced, pregnancies, which could result in a deterioration in maternal nutrition status and increased risks of intrauterine growth retardation, low birth weight, and poor lactation performance. However, the relationship between maternal depletion and parity may be more complicated. Women of high parity may be those who are most fecund. If a woman's nutritional status deteriorates, her fecundity may decrease, resulting in lower parity (Winkvist et al., 1992).

In a comprehensive review of numerous studies of the determinants of low birth weight, Kramer (1987) concluded that, although lower mean birth weight is frequently observed for women of very high parity, few studies have adequately controlled for important confounding factors such as age, socioeconomic status, cigarette and alcohol use, genital infection, and interpregnancy intervals. Moreover, the few studies with adequate controls found either no significant effects of parity on mean birth weight or negative effects that only occurred at parity 14 or 15 (Kramer, 1987). Some recent studies also find no significant effects of high parity on the risk of intrauterine growth retardation (Miller, 1989; Springer et al., 1992).

In contrast, an analysis of trends in low birth weight in the United States from 1975 through 1985 reported that, within each age group, the rates of low birth weight were higher for third- and higher-order births than for second-order births (Taffel, 1989). A study of the effects of maternal age and parity on birth weight in New York City reported significant increases in mean birth weight from parity 1 to parity 3, but marked declines in mean birth weight among higher parity groups (MacLeod and Kiely, 1988). Neither of these studies had adequate controls for socioeconomic status. An analysis of the determinants of infant and child mortality also found that higher-order births were at higher risk of poor birth outcomes, although the authors hypothesized that this increased risk could reflect the risks of advanced maternal age and close birth spacing (Hobcraft et al., 1985).

Many studies find interaction effects of parity and age and parity and short interpregnancy birth interval on birth weight. In particular, multiparity increases the risk of low birth weight for women under age 20, although the independent effects of parity and short interpregnancy intervals for young women are difficult to disentangle (Kramer, 1987; MacLeod and Kiely, 1988). Kramer (1987) concluded that multiparity increases the risk of low birth weight for women under age 20, has little effect for women ages 20 to 34 years, and decreases the risk for women over age 35.

High parity is also thought to be related to the long-term health status of women. Studies of the long-term effects of childbearing found that parous women had lower mortality from breast, ovarian, and endometrial cancer than did nulliparous women but a higher mortality from diabetes mellitus, gallbladder disease, cancer of the uterine cervix, nephritis and nephrosis, hypertension, ischemic and degenerative heart disease, cerebrovascular disease, and all causes of death (Beral, 1985).

Focusing on specific health problems, high parity is associated with significantly increased risks of both non-insulin-dependent diabetes mellitus and impaired glucose tolerance, after controlling for age, obesity, and family history (Kritz-Silverstein et al., 1989). High parity has also been found to be associated with increased risks of obesity and excessive weight gain, which in turn are risk factors for cardiovascular disease (Brown et al., 1992; Williamson et al., 1994).

The weight gain associated with increased parity is generally thought to be modest. A prospective study of childbearing and 10-year weight gain in U.S. white women found an average weight gain of 1.7 kg associated with having one additional live birth after age 25. Nonetheless, the modest effect of each additional birth on weight gain shows potentially strong effects of very high parity on the risk of excessive weight gain and obesity. Specifically, the risk of gaining more than 13 kg and of becoming overweight was increased by 60 to 110 percent in women having live births during the 10-year study period (Williamson et al., 1994). Moreover, multivariate analysis of the participants in the 1988 NIMHS who began pregnancy with normal body mass index suggests that high multiparity[1] was significantly associated with excessive maternal postpartum weight retention (> 20 lb) in black but not white mothers (Parker and Abrams, 1993).

Overall, studies of the nutrition and health risks of high parity report mixed findings and often suffer from incomplete controls for potential confounding factors.

High Parity as an Indicator of Nutrition and Health Benefit

The equivocal evidence on the risks associated with high parity suggests that high parity is likely to be a poor indicator of nutrition and health benefit. Since the effects of high parity on mean birth weight and the risk of low birth weight are modest, at best, prenatal WIC participation by women at high parity is unlikely to influence birth outcomes. Finally, although there are some important long-term effects of high parity on women's health status, WIC participation is only likely to modify these effects through nutrition education and, perhaps, health care referrals. The WIC food package for women at high parity would not be expected to influence these long-term health impacts. No studies were identified that examined the effects of WIC participation for women at high parity.

Use of High Parity in the WIC Setting

State WIC agencies typically define high parity on the basis of the number of previous pregnancies and rely on self-report. Table 5-1 indicates the extent to which state WIC agencies use high parity as a risk criterion. In 1992, the cutoff

---

[1] High multiparity was defined as more than three births if older than 25 years or more than two births if younger than 25 years; the reference group was other multiparous women.

for high parity ranged from more than three to more than five pregnancies, and one state that used high parity as a risk indicator did not indicate a cutoff value.

Recommendations for High Parity

Studies of the nutrition and health risks of *high parity* are inconclusive and suggest few significant effects on birth outcomes that can be attributed specifically to high parity. While there is some evidence of long-term health risks of high parity, WIC participation is not likely to modify these long-term effects. Therefore, the committee recommends that *high parity* be discontinued as a nutrition risk criterion.

Empirical evidence on the interactions of high parity with both age and short interpregnancy interval does suggest significant risks associated with high parity at young ages and high parity with short interpregnancy intervals. The committee recommends that consideration be given to the development of a nutrition risk criterion that reflects the combination of high parity and other nutrition risk criteria, such as age and interpregnancy interval.

In addition, during the review of high parity as a risk criterion, it became clear that the highest parity-related risk is for first-order births. Specifically, first-borns have lower mean birth weight and a higher risk of low birth weight than subsequent births (Kramer, 1987; Cogswell and Yip, 1995; Macleod and Kiely, 1988; Miller, 1989; IOM, 1985; Taffel, 1989). An obstetrical risk screening system developed and used in a community-based setting in Massachusetts weighted the risks of parity 0 and parity 5+ equally, while parity 1–5 was considered to be the lowest risk (Kennedy, 1986). Current WIC nutrition risk criteria do not include a criterion for parity 0 (nulliparous women). While parity 0 is likely to be closely related to young age at conception, it is not perfectly correlated, and adverse outcomes have been documented for nulliparous women at older ages. Parity 0 may also be a marker for several important perinatal risk factors: a low level of knowledge about nutrition and the importance of health care, inadequate social support, and a lack of knowledge about eligibility for public assistance. The committee recommends that further research be conducted on the nutrition and health risks of parity 0 and on the effects of WIC participation on birth outcomes for women pregnant for the first time.

History of Preterm Delivery

Prevalence of and Factors Associated with History of Preterm Delivery

Preterm birth (delivery before 37 completed weeks of gestation) is generally acknowledged to represent the predominant problem in obstetrics, in both

BIOCHEMICAL AND OTHER MEDICAL RISK CRITERIA 205

industrialized and developing societies. In 1991, approximately 11 percent of pregnancies in the United States ended early (Paneth, 1995); this was about 15 percent higher than in 1981. The prevalence of history of preterm delivery in the WIC program was not known to the committee. Maternal factors associated with history of preterm delivery or shortened gestational duration are low income, ethnic background (blacks at higher risk), young age, smoking, poor nutrition, and low educational attainment (IOM, 1990; Paneth, 1995).

History of Preterm Delivery as an Indicator of Nutrition and Health Risk

Preterm delivery itself is the largest contributor to neonatal, infant, and perinatal mortality in the United States (IOM, 1990). History of preterm delivery is a major risk factor for preterm delivery in industrialized countries (Shoino and Behrman, 1995).

History of Preterm Delivery as an Indicator of Nutrition and Health Benefit

Nutrition interventions play a role in the prevention of preterm delivery by minimizing preventable factors such as anemia and inappropriate weight gain. While there are few published reports on nutrition intervention and gestational duration, low weight gain during pregnancy may increase risk of reduced gestational duration (see Chapter 4). Through the provision of supplemental foods, nutrition education, and referrals for health and social services the WIC program supports desirable weight gain during pregnancy and thus the potential to improve gestational duration. WIC program evaluations reported longer duration of gestation for WIC participants than for nonparticipants (Edozien et al., 1979; Rush et al., 1988b), although with uncertain statistical significance.

Use of History of Preterm Delivery as a Nutrition Risk Criterion in the WIC Setting

Table 5-1 lists the use of history of preterm delivery by state WIC programs.

Recommendation for History of Preterm Delivery

The risk of *history of preterm delivery* is well documented in women, and it can be identified from medical records or self-report. There is a theoretical basis for benefit from participation in the WIC program. The committee recommends use of *history of preterm delivery* as a nutrition risk criterion for women in the

WIC program, using the IOM (1990) cutoff value of 37 weeks' gestation for the previous occurrence.

History of Postterm Delivery

Prevalence of and Factors Associated with Postterm Delivery

Postterm delivery (typically defined as pregnancy extending beyond 42 weeks from the onset of the last menstruation) is a fairly frequent occurrence. The prevalence of history of postterm delivery is difficult to ascertain because of uncertainties that typically surround estimation of gestational age. The prevalence of history of postterm delivery among WIC participants was not available to the committee.

History of Postterm Delivery as an Indicator of Nutrition and Health Risk

History of postterm delivery is associated with increased risks for the fetus, such as hypoxia, meconium aspiration, and macrosomia (ACOG, 1989).

History of Postterm Delivery as an Indicator of Nutrition and Health Benefit

The committee finds no evidence of benefit to support retaining history of postterm delivery as a nutrition risk criterion in the WIC program.

Recommendation for History of Postterm Delivery

The risk of *history of postterm delivery* is not well documented in women, and it is difficult to identify this because of uncertainties that typically surround estimation of gestation age. There is no theoretical or empirical basis for benefit from participation in the WIC program. Therefore, the committee recommends discontinuation of use of *history of postterm delivery* as a nutrition risk criterion for women by state WIC programs.

History of Low Birth Weight

Low birth weight (see section "Low Birth Weight" in Chapter 4) occurs because of either preterm birth or fetal growth restriction. As discussed above, women who have delivered early are at increased risk of repeat preterm birth in a subsequent pregnancy, and those who have delivered an infant who is small for gestational age are also at increased risk to repeat, especially if fetal growth was restricted because of a persistent condition such as maternal hypertensive disease. Thus, a history of LBW identifies a cohort of women at increased risk of delivering another LBW infant.

There is some basis for anticipating benefit from nutritional intervention in case of preterm birth and fetal growth restriction. Since a history of LBW identifies women at increased risk for either of these two conditions, the committee recommends use of *a history of LBW* as a nutrition risk criterion.

History of Neonatal Loss

Neonatal loss is a vague term that encompasses death of the neonate from any cause. As such, it is not a useful nutritional risk criterion for the WIC program. History of LBW already encompasses a major contributing factor to neonatal death.

History of Previous Birth of an Infant with a Congenital or Birth Defect

Prevalence of and Factors Associated with a History of Previous Birth of an Infant with a Congenital or Birth Defect

See the section "Genetic and Congenital Disorders" for information.

History of Previous Birth of an Infant with a Congenital or Birth Defect as an Indicator of Nutrition and Health Risk

Women who have previously had an infant affected by a neural tube defect are at increased risk of a recurrence (MRC Vitamin Study Research Group, 1991). Recent studies suggest that intake of folic acid may also be inversely related to the occurrence of cleft lip or cleft palate (Shaw et al., 1995).

History of Previous Birth of an Infant with a Congenital or Birth Defect as an Indicator of Nutrition and Health Benefit

For improved nutrition to reduce risk of recurrence of birth defects, the woman's increased nutrient intake needs to occur prior to and in the early weeks of pregnancy. Except in the case of closely spaced pregnancies, this is not ordinarily a period when women are served by the WIC program. It is not known if improved nutrient intake will lead to other improvements in pregnancy outcome.

Use of History of Previous Birth of an Infant with a Congenital or Birth Defect in the WIC Setting

In 1992, at least 32 states used this criterion (Table 5-1).

Recommendation for History of Previous Birth of an Infant with a Congenital or Birth Defect

The risk of *history of previous birth of an infant with a congenital or birth defect* is well documented. The potential to benefit from WIC program participation is uncertain. The committee recommends use of *history of a previous birth of an infant with a congenital or birth defect*, particularly a neural tube defect, as a nutrition risk criterion for pregnant women.

Lack of Prenatal Care

Prenatal care is defined in *Standards for Obstetric-Gynecologic Services* (ACOG, 1985) and *Guidelines for Perinatal Care* (AAP-ACOG, 1992). Prenatal care serves as a means to monitor the progress of the mother and the developing fetus. The components of prenatal care include pregnancy dating, establishing goals, risk assessment, education, and clinical and laboratory tests. As risks are identified, referrals should be made to appropriate medical and social services, including referrals to the WIC program (IOM, 1985).

Prevalence of and Factors Associated with Lack of Prenatal Care

Lack of or inadequate prenatal care is defined as lack of entry into prenatal care by a specified number of weeks' gestation or fewer than a specified number of prenatal care visits for stage of gestation as recognized by the American College of Obstetricians and Gynecologists (ACOG) (Witwer, 1990). Although recent surveys report that 98 percent of American women receive some form of prenatal care, in 1992, 22 percent of all women did not begin prenatal care during the first trimester (Shiono and Behrman, 1995). A study by the U.S. General Accounting Office (1987) reported 71 percent of low-income women experienced problems obtaining prenatal care because of inadequate financial resources and barriers to transportation and health care services. Data on the lack of prenatal care among WIC participants were not available to the committee.

Documented risk factors for lack of or inadequate prenatal care include young maternal age, nonwhite ethnic background, and low maternal education

BIOCHEMICAL AND OTHER MEDICAL RISK CRITERIA

(Curry, 1990). In addition, poverty, unemployment, other socioeconomic factors, and single marital status have been reported as risk factors (IOM, 1990).

Lack of Prenatal Care as an Indicator of Nutrition and Health Risk

Women who do not receive early and adequate prenatal care are more likely to deliver premature, growth-retarded, or low-birth-weight infants and to gain too little weight during pregnancy (Alexander and Korenbrot, 1995; IOM, 1990; USDA, 1991a).

Lack of Prenatal Care as an Indicator of Nutrition and Health Benefit

Several studies have reported significant nutrition and health benefits for pregnant women through early enrollment in the WIC program (Rush et al., 1988b). Other studies have reported improved birth outcomes and associated savings in health care expenditures in pregnant women enrolled early in the WIC program (Buescher et al., 1993; Devaney et al., 1990). However, there were not any studies available to the committee to evaluate definitively the effects of timing of prenatal care in relation to WIC services on pregnancy outcome, and most studies treated prenatal care as the presence or absence of care, not number of visits or timing of care (USDA, 1991a). Many studies predict improved birth outcomes through participation in the WIC program, but the results cannot be considered conclusive because of methodological problems (Rush et al., 1988a). However, Alexander and Korenbrot (1995) report that the interventions of most benefit to the mother and fetus include nutrition (to improve prepregnancy weight or gestational weight gain and reduce risk of low-birth-weight infants), smoking cessation (to prevent low-birth-weight infants), and medical care (to improve general morbidity). The review concludes that access to and utilization of prenatal care services reduces risk factors for poor pregnancy outcomes and must be part of a broad, unified approach to public health that includes nutrition interventions.

Use of Lack of Prenatal Care as a Nutrition Risk Criterion in the WIC Setting

According to 1992 state plans, lack of prenatal care or inadequate prenatal care is used as a risk criterion in 18 state WIC agencies (USDA, 1994). Cutoffs for establishing the presence of this risk criterion in the WIC program are generally based on the interval between conception and initiation of prenatal care or less than a specified number of prenatal care visits at a stated length of gestation.

Recommendations for Lack of Prenatal Care

The nutritional risk of *lack of prenatal care* is documented in women, and this can be identified readily. There is empirical evidence and a theoretical basis for benefit from WIC program participation. Therefore, the committee recommends use of *lack of prenatal care* or *inadequate prenatal care* as a nutrition risk criterion for women in the WIC program, with a cutoff value of care beginning after the first trimester or long intervals between additional visits (see AAP-ACOG, 1992). In addition, the committee recommends that its relative priority be reduced to priority level VII.

Multifetal Gestation

Prevalence of and Factors Associated with Multifetal Gestation

The prevalence of *multifetal gestation* is considerably higher than the traditional estimate of one in 75 conceptions. Part of this increase reflects improved methods of early diagnosis with sonography, and part reflects the use of ovulation-inducing agents in assisted reproductive technologies. Older maternal age, black race, and previous family history are also associated with increased prevalence of multifetal gestation. Although less than 2 percent of all births are twin births, twins accounted for 16 percent of LBW infants (IOM, 1990). Data on the prevalence of multifetal gestation in the WIC program are not available.

Multifetal Gestation as an Indicator of Nutrition and Health Risk

The woman carrying more than one fetus presents a high-risk situation, with increased risk of preterm labor, impaired fetal growth, placental and cord accidents, and preeclampsia. The risk increases markedly as the number of fetuses increases, but even with twins the incidence of complications is substantial. There is considerable reason to believe that nutrition is involved. Based on a review of evidence regarding weight gain in women carrying twins, the IOM (1990) concluded that a total gain of 16 to 20.5 kg (35–45 lb) is consistent with a favorable outcome in a full-term twin pregnancy. This range, which represents the first weight gain recommendation for twins, translates to a weekly gain of about 750 g during the second and third trimesters. Women pregnant or breastfeeding with twins have greater requirements for all nutrients than those with only one infant.

Multifetal Gestation as an Indicator of Nutrition and Health Benefit

The need for increased weight gain associated with multifetal gestation and the increased nutrient needs mentioned above suggest that this nutrition risk criterion is a good predictor of benefit from the supplemental food, nutrition education, and health and social service referrals provided by the WIC program. No empirical evidence of this relationship was available to the committee.

Use of Multifetal Gestation in the WIC Setting

Multifetal gestation is generally determined via sonography and reported to WIC by the health care provider. Multifetal gestation is used as a nutrition risk criterion in the WIC by 51 state WIC agencies (USDA, 1994).

Recommendation for Multifetal Gestation

The risk of *multifetal gestation* is well documented in women, and this condition can be identified by a clinical diagnosis. There is a theoretical basis for benefit from participation in the WIC program. Therefore, the committee recommends use of *multifetal gestation* as a nutrition risk criterion for pregnant, breastfeeding, and postpartum women in the WIC program.

Fetal Growth Restriction

Physical examination of the pregnant woman by a health care provider may allow diagnosis of *fetal growth restriction*. The many causes of fetal growth restriction (this term replaces intrauterine growth retardation) can be conveniently grouped as intrinsic or extrinsic to the fetus. Intrinsic causes include fetal infections and chromosomal and other congenital anomalies; extrinsic causes include maternal dietary inadequacy, vascular disease, and placental and cord abnormalities. Whenever fetal growth restriction is suspected, a careful dietary assessment of the mother is advised (Luke et al., 1993). Although inadequate maternal nutrition is but one cause of fetal growth restriction, it is one of the few causes that are responsive to remedial therapy.

Prevalence of and Factors Associated with Fetal Growth Restriction

Data on the prevalence of fetal growth restriction among WIC participants or in the U.S. population were not available to the committee. Restricted fetal growth usually results in an infant who is small for gestational age, discussed in Chapter 4.

Fetal Growth Restriction as an Indicator of Nutrition and Health Risk

Infant size at birth is a critical determinant of long-term child health outcomes (see review by McCormick, 1985). Newborn infants whose growth was restricted during gestation are at risk of respiratory distress, hypoglycemia, hypocalcemia, polycythemia, birth asphyxia, intracranial hemorrhage, and long-term cognitive delays (IOM, 1990).

Fetal Growth Restriction as an Indicator of Nutrition and Health Benefit

Decreased cigarette smoking, improved diets, and improved utilization of early prenatal care during the 1970s may have contributed to the observed improvement in birth weights. Energy supplementation during pregnancy may decrease the incidence of fetal growth restriction with or without concurrent increases in gestational weight gain (IOM, 1990). Studies have shown that food supplementation during pregnancy to improve weight gain reduces the risk of fetal growth restriction (IOM, 1990). The WIC program holds potential to reduce fetal growth restriction by providing supplemental foods and nutrition education to improve weight gain.

Use of Fetal Growth Restriction as a Risk Criterion in the WIC Setting

Fetal growth restriction is a diagnosis reported to WIC programs by a health care provider. An abnormally slow rate of intrauterine growth may be detected by careful serial measurements of uterine fundal height and abdominal girth and confirmed by ultrasonography. Fetal growth restriction is usually defined as a fetal weight below the 10th percentile for gestational age. Fetal growth restriction is used as a risk indicator for pregnant women in 17 state WIC agencies (USDA, 1994).

Recommendation for Fetal Growth Restriction

The risk of *fetal growth restriction* is well documented in women, and a suitable method for identifying this condition is available. There is a theoretical and empirical basis for benefit from participation in the WIC program. Therefore, the committee recommends use of *fetal growth restriction* as a nutrition risk criterion for pregnant women in the WIC program.

Preeclampsia and Eclampsia

Preeclampsia is diagnosed when a previously normal gravida develops hypertension and proteinuria in late gestation, and *eclampsia* refers to preeclampsia plus either convulsions or coma. Both conditions are limited largely to women in their first pregnancy, and they are strongly associated with low income, low educational attainment, and poor nutrition (Henderson and Little, 1990).

Prevalence of and Factors Associated with Preeclampsia and Eclampsia

Preeclampsia occurs in approximately 6 to 8 percent of all pregnancies. Data on the prevalence of preeclampsia or eclampsia among the WIC population were not available to the committee.

Preeclampsia and Eclampsia as Indicators of Nutrition and Health Risk

Preeclampsia is strongly associated with an increased risk of LBW in infants (Henderson and Little, 1990). It is also associated with fetal growth restriction resulting from decreased delivery of nutrients or oxygen through the uteroplacental circulation (Henderson and Little, 1990), and with preterm delivery (IOM, 1985).

Preeclampsia and Eclampsia as Indicators of Nutrition and Health Benefit

Although high calcium intake may reduce the risk of developing preeclampsia (IOM, 1990; Ito et al., 1994; Repke, 1994; van den Elzen et al., 1995), the committee could find no theoretical or empirical basis for expecting those with a diagnosis of preeclampsia or eclampsia to benefit from participation in the WIC Program.

Use of Preeclampsia and Eclampsia as Risk Criteria in the WIC Setting

Preeclampsia or eclampsia are diagnosed by a health care provider. As a risk criterion for pregnant women in the WIC program, preeclampsia or eclampsia is used by all state WIC agencies (USDA, 1994).

Recommendation for Preeclampsia and Eclampsia

The risk of *preeclampsia* or *eclampsia* is well documented in pregnant women, and this condition can be identified by a clinical diagnosis. There is no theoretical basis or scientific evidence for nutrition benefit from participation in the WIC program. Therefore, the committee recommends discontinuation of use of *preeclampsia* or *eclampsia* as a nutrition risk criterion for pregnant women in the WIC program.

Placental Abnormalities

Prevalence of and Factors Associated with Placental Abnormalities

The placenta normally implants in the uterine fundus and remains attached until after delivery of the infant. Occasionally, the placenta may be found in the lower portion of the uterus, near or over the cervix, where the normal prelabor changes of late gestation can lead to premature separation of a portion. This condition is called placenta previa. In addition, the normally implanted placenta can separate prematurely, a condition known as abruptio placentae or abruption.

Placental Abnormalities as an Indicator of Nutrition and Health Risk

Extreme and acute placental separation interferes with fetal oxygenation and can lead to fetal death, but small and gradual separation may be tolerated reasonably well. If continued over long periods, such a case of chronic separation can lead to blood loss anemia in the pregnant woman. Medical care and monitoring is indicated in the case of placental separation. The committee found no evidence of nutrition-related risks in placental abnormalities, except for the occasional case of anemia due to chronic blood loss.

Placental Abnormalities as an Indicator of Nutrition and Health Benefit

No theoretical base or studies were identified by the committee related to the benefits of nutrition intervention for pregnant women with placental abnormalities or with a history of placental abnormalities.

Use of Placental Abnormalities in the WIC Setting

Presence of placental abnormalities are diagnosed and reported by a health care provider. According to 1992 state WIC plans, diagnosis of a placental abnormality (abruptio placentae) is used as a nutrition risk criterion by 15 state WIC agencies (USDA, 1994) (see Table 5-1).

Recommendation for Placental Abnormalities

The risk of *placental abnormalities* is well documented in women, and this condition can be identified by a clinical diagnosis. There is no theoretical basis for benefit from participation in the WIC program. Therefore, the committee recommends discontinuation of use of *placental abnormalities* as a nutrition risk criterion for women in the WIC program.

CONDITIONS SPECIFIC TO INFANTS AND/OR CHILDREN

Prematurity

Causes of *prematurity* include preterm spontaneous labor, antepartum hemorrhage, premature rupture of membranes, and maternal hypertension (IOM, 1990). Other associated conditions are low maternal age, low maternal weight, poor socioeconomic status, diabetes mellitus, nephritis, anemia, fetal anomalies, and multiple pregnancies (IOM, 1985; IOM, 1990).

Incidence of and Factors Associated with Prematurity

The incidence of prematurity ranges from approximately 8 percent for white infants to 18 percent for black infants. No estimate of the prevalence of prematurity among the WIC population was available to the committee.

Prematurity as an Indicator of Nutrition and Health Risk

Most premature infants have low birth weights (< 2,500 g); some have very low birth weights (VLBW, < 1,500 g). Other problems of prematurity that may have nutritional implications include immature sucking and swallowing; immature digestion and absorption of carbohydrates and lipids; immature excretory capacity; patent ductus arteriosus; poorly developing nutrient stores of vitamin E and iron; need for high mineral accretion rate (calcium and phosphorus); necrotizing enterocolitis; and small gastric capacity (Paneth, 1995).

Prematurity as an Indicator of Nutrition and Health Benefit

Despite their increased caloric and nutrient needs for rapid growth, premature infants grow well on breast milk and may benefit from some of its unique nonnutritional components. Thus, encouragement to express milk until the newborn can feed orally and other forms of breastfeeding promotion may promote infant health. However, the mother's milk may need to be supplemented (from 20 kcal/oz to 24 to 30 kcal/oz). When used, formulas may need to be somewhat concentrated to optimize growth. A choice of feeding method—parenteral, enteral, gavage, bottle, or breast—is determined after evaluation of the infant's suck-swallow mechanism, gut maturity, and general clinical condition. After a preterm infant is large enough to leave the hospital, macro- and micronutrient needs continue to be higher than for term infants, especially during the first few months. The WIC program provides education about infant feeding and either an expanded breastfeeding supplemental food package (see Chapter 1) for mothers, to help cover the increased energy and nutrient demands of breastfeeding, or infant formula.

Most premature infants catch up to normal growth and development indices by the second year of life. There is no indication of benefit of nutrition services to children who were premature at birth but who meet no other risk criteria (see earlier sections of this chapter on health problems associated with prematurity and Chapter 4 on growth delay).

Use of Prematurity as a Risk Criterion in the WIC Setting

Prematurity is reported to WIC program staff either by the mother or a health care provider. Table 5-1 lists the use of prematurity as a risk criterion by state WIC programs for infants and children. The cutoff point used by state WIC programs is 37 or 38 weeks.

Recommendations for Prematurity

The risk of *prematurity* is well documented in infants, and a suitable method is available to identify this condition. There is a theoretical and empirical basis for benefit from participation in the WIC program. Therefore, the committee recommends the use of *prematurity* as a nutrition risk criterion for infants, with a cutoff value of 37 weeks; but it recommends discontinuation of *prematurity* as a nutrition risk criterion for children.

Hypoglycemia

Hypoglycemia is defined as a blood glucose concentration less than 40 mg/dl (Sperling, 1992). Symptomatic hypoglycemia is a risk observed in a substantial proportion of newborns who are small for gestational age (SGA), but it is uncommon and of shorter duration in newborns who are of the appropriate size for gestational age (IOM, 1990). In newborns, the symptoms may consist of jitters, tremors, lethargy, and apneic spells. Significant risk factors for hypoglycemia in infants include black race for males (Cole and Peevy, 1994), preterm birth, small for gestational age infant, and maternal diabetes mellitus (Singhal et al., 1992).

Prevalence of and Factors Associated with Hypoglycemia

Data on the prevalence of hypoglycemia among infants or children in the United States or among WIC program participants were not available to the committee.

Hypoglycemia as an Indicator of Nutrition and Health Risk

For SGA newborns, there may be a defect in the gluconeogenesis pathway and an imbalance among glycogen stores, fatty acid oxidation, and endocrine controls. All infants with fetal growth restriction must be considered at high risk for hypoglycemia during their first few days.

Hypoglycemia as an Indicator of Nutrition and Health Benefit

Nutrition management for infants and children with hypoglycemia must concentrate on frequent feedings and the provision of adequate glucose and nutrients to prevent deficiencies and to support adequate growth.

Use of Hypoglycemia as a Risk Criterion in the WIC Setting

Table 5-1 lists the number of states that use hypoglycemia as a nutrition risk criterion in the WIC.

Recommendation for Hypoglycemia

The risk of *hypoglycemia* is well documented among infants, and this condition can be diagnosed clinically. There is a theoretical basis for benefit from participation in the WIC program. Therefore, the committee recommends use of *hypoglycemia* as a nutrition risk criterion for infants and children in the WIC program.

POTENTIALLY TOXIC SUBSTANCES

Long-Term Drug-Nutrient Interactions or Misuse of Medications

This section covers interactions between prescription and over-the-counter medications and nutrients. Illegal drug use is discussed in the section "Alcohol and Illegal Drug Use."

Interactions between drugs and nutrients can be physicochemical, physiologic, or patho-physiologic (Roe, 1994). Physicochemical interactions result in reduced absorption of the drug, one or more nutrients, or both. Physiologic interactions are those that either slow or accelerate the uptake of drugs. Pathophysiologic interactions include those in which drugs, through their toxicologic effect, cause cellular damage so that nutrients cannot be activated within, used by, stored in, or removed from the body.

Prevalence and Factors Associated with Drug-Nutrient Interactions or Misuse of Medications

Prescription or over-the-counter drugs are widely used, and are sometimes misused. All drugs provided to or taken by pregnant women can be considered potentially harmful to the fetus because of cross-placental transfer and teratogenicity (Roe, 1994). Data on the prevalence of the use of prescription or over-the-counter drugs or drug-nutrient interactions in the WIC program were not available to the committee.

Drug-Nutrient Interactions or Misuse of Medications as Indicators of Nutrition and Health Risk

Predicting the risk of drug-nutrient interactions requires consideration of multiple factors. In addition to pharmaceutical preparations, some vitamins and their analogs may have both pharmacologic and nutrient properties.

Absorption of most drugs occurs by diffusion through any portion of the mucosa of the gastrointestinal tract. Food components affect drug absorption and bioavailability (Welling, 1977), but effects differ for different drugs. Three general mechanisms explain these effects: gastric emptying time, interactions with the gut, and competitive inhibition. High-protein diets enhance metabolism of some drugs, and protein-deficient diets tend to slow drug metabolism (Anderson et al., 1979; Kato et al., 1968). The level and type of dietary fat may affect drug absorption and metabolism.

Drugs may affect appetite by their central and peripheral effects. Any drug that induces nausea, impairs the sense of taste, or has adverse effects on the gastrointestinal tract is likely to reduce food intake and hence to contribute to weight loss. Drugs used for cancer chemotherapy are the most important group of drugs that reduce appetite. Drugs such as phenothiazine, lithium, and benzodiazepine increase appetite. Certain drugs can deplete stores of such nutrients as vitamin K, calcium, and vitamin D. The mechanisms responsible for drug-induced maldigestion and malabsorption include the interactions of the drug and nutrients in the gastrointestinal tract, drug-induced changes in gastrointestinal function, and drug-induced enteropathy causing damage to the brush border of the intestinal villi, which results in interference with active transport mechanisms for nutrients (Roe, 1994).

The risk of adverse side effects of drugs depends on the toxicity of the drug and secondary effects on appetite, and it increases with the number of drugs taken at the same time and with the duration of exposure.

Misuse of certain drugs during early pregnancy can result in fetal malformations. Recently intake of more than 10,000 I.U. of vitamin A (retinol) daily from supplements was associated with increased risk of cranial-neural-crest origin birth defects (Rothman et al., 1995).

Use of some prescription or over-the-counter drugs is not advisable when breastfeeding because of health risks to the infant, as covered in detail by the Committee on Drugs of the American Academy of Pediatrics (COD-AAP, 1994).

Drug-Nutrient Interactions or Misuse of Medications as Indicators of Nutrition and Health Benefit

Adverse effects of drug-nutrient interactions can be minimized through adequate nutrient intake and education about meeting dietary needs and timing of drug intake in relation to meals or breastfeeding.

Participation in the WIC program may provide health and nutrition benefit through basic health education, particularly during pregnancy, supplemental foods that help maintain nutrient stores, and referrals to health care services for those in need of additional counseling or medical management because of adverse effects of drug-nutrient interactions.

Use of Drug-Nutrient Interactions or Misuse of Medications as Risk Indicators in the WIC Setting

No cutoff point for prescription or over-the-counter drug use or drug-nutrient interactions has been identified beyond the actual existence of documented drug-nutrient interactions or occurrences of misuse. Table 5-1 summarizes use of the risk indicator by state WIC agencies.

Recommendations for Drug-Nutrient Interactions or Misuse of Medications

The risk of specific *drug-nutrient interactions* or *misuse of medications* is documented in pregnant and lactating women, and the use of prescription and over-the-counter medications can be identified by the health care provider. There is a theoretical basis for benefit from participation in the WIC program. However, the potential to benefit is divided between those drugs for which a clear nutrient interaction is present, and those for which the interaction is weak or unclear. Therefore, the committee recommends use of *drug-nutrient interactions* or *misuse of medications* as a nutrition risk criterion for pregnant and lactating women in the WIC program, but only for a predetermined listing of pharmaceutical agents that have a known direct effect on nutrition. The committee encourages that such a listing be developed and made available to state WIC agency staff to ensure adequate assessments and referrals.

Maternal Smoking

Cigarette smoking continues to be a major public health threat in the United States, particularly among families who meet the WIC criteria for eligibility. Smoking generally refers to the active use of cigarettes and the recurring inhalation of tobacco smoke. In the present context, exposure to tobacco smoke is defined by: (1) fetal exposure to the components of tobacco that cross the placenta and enter fetal circulation, and (2) exposure after birth to tobacco-smoke-contaminated air either at home or in other environmental contexts (Samet et al., 1994). This section covers fetal exposure to maternal smoking. Exposure to tobacco smoke among infants and children after birth is discussed in Chapter 7.

Prevalence and Factors Associated with Maternal Smoking

The prevalence of tobacco use has decreased dramatically since the first report issued by the Surgeon General's Advisory Committee on Smoking and Health in 1964. This decline resulted from widespread educational efforts to discourage tobacco and a substantial increase in the cessation of smoking among older adults. In 1991, 22 percent of women 18 to 24 years of age smoked, as did 28 percent of women 25 through 44 years of age (U.S. Department of Commerce, 1993). Of concern to WIC is that young females with low levels of education have shown the least reduction in smoking. The change in prevalence of smoking among white adolescents was negligible from 1980 to 1992 (DHHS, 1994). Prevalence of smoking is comparatively high among blacks, blue collar workers, and workers with lower levels of education (DHHS, 1989). According to WIC program data, in 1986, approximately 12 percent of pregnant women participating in the WIC program were certified using smoking as a nutrition risk criterion in the WIC program (USDA, 1987), and 16 percent were certified on the same basis in 1988 (USDA, 1994).

Maternal Smoking as an Indicator of Health and Nutrition Risk

Maternal cigarette smoking during pregnancy is associated with high rates of spontaneous abortions, stillbirths, bleeding during pregnancy, placental complications (abruptio placentae, placenta previa), complications of labor (preterm labor, prolonged and premature rupture of the membranes), fetal growth restriction (measured as decreased total body weight, decreased lean body weight, decreased length and head circumference), increased rates of small size for gestational age (SGA), and perinatal mortality. (For recent reviews, see Abel 1980; Berkowitz 1988; DHHS, 1989; Fredricsson and Giljam, 1992; Garn, 1985; Gilstrap and Little, 1992; Lincoln, 1986; Luke et al., 1993; and Naeye, 1992). Many reviewers concluded that adverse effects of maternal smoking on prematurity (Kramer, 1987; Shiono et al., 1986a) and certain types of neonatal mortality (e.g., respiratory distress syndrome and sudden infant death syndrome) are firmly established, and that they increase with maternal age (Luke et al., 1993).

A number of studies conclude that there is no association between maternal smoking and congenital malformations (de Haas, 1975; Malloy et al., 1989; Seidman et al., 1990; Shiono et al., 1986b); however, one study indicated there may be an increased risk for specific malformations, including microcephalus, cleft defects, and club foot (Van den Eeden et al., 1990). There is ongoing debate about the exact nature of the mechanisms associated with smoking in the prenatal environment (e.g., Backe 1993; Cliver et al. 1992; English and Eskenazi 1992; Goldstein 1977; Hebel et al. 1988; Kleinman et al. 1988; Kline et al. 1977; Macarthur and Knox, 1988; Naeye, 1978; Shiono et al., 1986a; Wen et al., 1990; Yerushalmy, 1971).

Several large prospective studies (the National Child Development Study of Great Britain; the U.S. National Collaborative Perinatal Project (NCPP); the Seattle, Washington, Longitudinal Study; and the Ottawa Prenatal Prospective

Study) and a few smaller studies have revealed consistent deficits in stature and other anthropometric measures among infants of smokers (reviewed by Rush and Callaghan, 1989). Heavy maternal smoking causes up to 10 percent deficits in birth weight, 5 percent deficits in birth length, and 2 percent deficits in head circumference. These deficits are proportional to the level of smoking and the duration of smoking while pregnant and are not rapidly countered by postnatal catch-up growth (Elwood et al., 1987).

In most smokers the cumulative effects of smoking combined with alcohol or caffeine consumption must be considered. In a prospective study in Denmark (Olsen et al., 1991), higher levels of alcohol consumption were associated with a reduction in average birth weight of about 40 g, which increased to 200 g when the mother also smoked. Mean birth weights were more than 500 g higher for nonsmoking abstainers than for heavy smokers and drinkers.

A Canadian study involving heavy smokers (15+ cigarettes per day) found a reduction in birth weight of more than 200 g when the mother consumed 300 mg or more of caffeine per day (Beaulac-Baillargeon and Desrosiers, 1987). Similarly, in London (Brooke et al., 1989; Peacock et al., 1991), consumption of caffeine and alcohol was found to be directly related to birth weights that were 10 to 18 percent lower for babies of smokers, independent of smoking levels (actual birth weights not reported). These effects were strongest when consumption was early in the pregnancy.

Longitudinal data on postnatal growth and development from studies in Pittsburgh (Day et al., 1992), Ottawa (Fried and O'Connell, 1987), and Michigan (Jacobson et al., 1994) suggest that the interaction of alcohol consumption and smoking during pregnancy may have significant adverse effects on postnatal growth and development.

Evidence is equivocal that maternal smoking during pregnancy has important long-term negative effects on the growth, development, behavior, and cognition of the infant, in addition to its fetal effects.

The most consistent predictors of fetal growth restriction are small maternal size, low maternal weight gain, history of previous low-birth-weight infant, and smoking (Kramer, 1987). It has long been hypothesized that reductions in birth weight associated with maternal smoking are in fact nutritionally mediated.

Early researchers suggested that much of the effect of maternal smoking during pregnancy was mediated through reduced maternal weight gain (e.g., Davies and Abernethy, 1976; Lancet, 1979; Rush, 1974, 1976). In particular, they attributed the comparatively lower gestational weight gain of smokers to lower caloric intake. Subsequent work showed that, among women at equivalent levels of smoking, growth restriction in the infants was inversely related to higher gestational weight gain and higher prepregnancy weight (Garn et al., 1979; Luke et al., 1981). Moreover, within maternal weight gain or prepregnancy weight categories, frequencies of LBW and absolute values of birth weight, length, and head circumference were related to the level of smoking (Meyer, 1978; Luke et al., 1981).

However, the apparent mediating effect of the interaction between smoking and nutrition was not observed in studies that reported smoking-related decreases in birth weights without differences in maternal weight gain (Abel, 1980). Naeye (1978, 1981a, b) reported that, at least among heavy smokers, maternal weight gains are independent of either fetal or placental weight. Similarly, Haworth and co-workers (1980) noted that infants of obese smokers still weigh significantly less than those of obese nonsmokers. In fact, some of the effects of smoking (e.g., increased placental size/placental ratios) are contrary to those described for moderate maternal malnutrition (Lechtig et al., 1975). Moreover, since the incidence of proportional rather than disproportional SGA increases with smoking, and since the effects involve lean body tissue rather than deposition of subcutaneous fat (D'Souza et al., 1981; Harrison et al., 1983), the hypothesis of a simple energy availability effect is probably partly inadequate.

Studies show that smokers, including pregnant women, do not generally eat less than nonsmokers or ex-smokers, even after controlling for socioeconomic status and height differences, and often eat more (Haste et al., 1990; McKenzie-Parnell et al., 1993; reviewed by Klesges et al., 1989; and Perkins, 1992). Thus, the lower weights and pregnancy weight gains of smokers are not necessarily due to appetite suppression or reduced intake of calories, and must therefore be explained by other mechanisms (IOM, 1990). One possibility is the chronic increase in metabolic rate observed in smokers (Perkins et al., 1989).

In general, smoking is associated with lower levels of vitamin E, vitamin C, beta-carotene, selenium, and B-complex vitamins (Preston, 1991). The concentration of vitamin C in amniotic fluid during the third trimester has been reported to be almost 10 times lower in smokers (0.33 mg/dl) versus 2.8 mg/dl in nonsmokers (Barrett et al., 1991). Both maternal serum and neonatal cord serum vitamin C, vitamin E, and beta-carotene levels are lower when the mother smokes, despite no differences in maternal intakes (Norkus et al., 1987)

Smoking has been reported to decrease production of breast milk in breastfeeding mothers (Hopkinson et al., 1992; IOM, 1991). The volume of breast milk was 20 percent less in breastfeeding mothers of postterm infants who smoked compared with breastfeeding mothers of postterm infants who did not smoke (Hopkinson et al., 1992). Furthermore, the volume of breast milk produced by breastfeeding mothers who smoked did not increase from 2 to 4 months postpartum.

Maternal Smoking as an Indicator of Health and Nutrition Benefit

If nutritional factors mediate the observed effects of maternal smoking during pregnancy on the growth and development of the fetus and infants, as has been hypothesized, the supplemental food and nutrition education provided by the WIC program could benefit pregnant women. The juices provided by the WIC food package may help maintain adequate levels of vitamin C.

Few studies in WIC populations have assessed whether WIC participation was beneficial in smokers versus nonsmokers, and results of several are equivocal (Rush et al., 1988b; Schramm, 1986; Stockbauer, 1987). However, the only randomized trial of the WIC program concluded that although there was not a significant difference in birth weight of infants born to all women studied, WIC participation was associated with a 176 g increase in birth weight of infants born to women who were heavy smokers (greater than 10 cigarettes per day), after adjusting for several covariates (Metcoff et al., 1985). A benefit of WIC participation for smokers (yes/no, as reported on birth certificates) was also reported by the observational 1988 New York State WIC program evaluation, but relationships varied according to type of financial coverage for delivery. Among women with private payment, WIC participation was associated with significantly reduced proportions of low birth weight and preterm deliveries for nonsmokers, but not smokers. However, WIC participation was associated with significant reductions in low birth weight and preterm delivery only among smokers in the "self-pay" group. Finally, WIC was significantly associated with better birth outcomes for both smokers and nonsmokers in the Medicaid group, and greater proportional decreases in low birth weight and preterm delivery were observed among the smokers (Bureau of Nutrition, 1990).

Many of the maternal food supplementation trials in populations where women rarely smoke but are at risk for other factors (e.g., poor nutritional status by anthropometric and biochemical criteria) have shown beneficial effects of supplementation on weight gains and birth weights (Adair and Pollitt 1985; Prentice 1991; Smith 1992). Since nutritional factors could be partially responsible for the low birth weight in the offspring of women who smoke, supplementary feeding of pregnant women who smoke may reduce their risk of delivering a low-birth-weight infant.

Several clinical trials of smoking cessation programs have reported some success in achieving smoking cessation (Ershoff et al., 1989; Mayer et al., 1990; Sexton, 1991). The 1990 Surgeon General's Report on Smoking and Health concluded that discontinuing smoking up to 30 weeks of gestation leads to increased birth weight compared to continuing to smoke (DHHS, 1990). The WIC program can help link participants with smoking cessation programs.

Use of Maternal Smoking as a Nutrition Risk Criterion in the WIC Program

According to 1992 state plans, 51 state WIC agencies include tobacco use as a nutrition risk criterion in the WIC for pregnant women (USDA, 1994). Cutoff values range from any tobacco use to smoking more than 20 cigarettes per day.

Recommendation for Maternal Smoking

Risks of *maternal smoking* to the health of mothers and their fetuses are well documented, and risks to breastfeeding infants have also been reported. Too few studies have been conducted to determine whether the WIC food package contributes to the amelioration of the toxic effects of cigarette smoking. However, consumption of nutritious foods is beneficial for other reasons, and the committee felt that both the education and referral components of the WIC program have the potential to benefit women who smoke during pregnancy and/or lactation. The committee strongly supports current public health policies recommending that women abstain from smoking during pregnancy. The lack of scientific evidence as to appropriate cutoff points relative to the potential for women who smoke during pregnancy or lactation from to benefit from the WIC program makes setting a cutoff point difficult. Therefore, as an interim approach, the committee recommends *maternal smoking* as a nutrition risk criterion for pregnant and lactating women in the state WIC program, with a cutoff of "any smoking." However, the committee recommends that this criterion be given lower priority, comparable to that of the predisposing risk category that is currently in use.[2]

The committee further recommends (1) that research be conducted to address the extent to which women who smoke benefit from the WIC program and the level of smoking that should be set as the cutoff point, if applicable, and (2) that USDA appoint an expert committee to provide guidance on cutoff points for cigarette smoking that will identify pregnant and lactating women who are most likely to benefit from the WIC program. Members of the expert committee should have expertise in maternal smoking and its assessment and treatment, public policy, nutrition, and epidemiology.

---

[2] Two committee members (Barbara Abrams and Barbara Devaney) preferred a recommendation of establishing higher cutoff points (such as > 10 cigarettes per day) and keeping the risk criterion at its current high priority level. This approach could more clearly delineate women whose smoking places them at higher risk of poor pregnancy and lactation outcomes and who would therefore be more likely to benefit from WIC program participation. However, if cigarette smoking at lower levels produces poor health outcomes, or if women underreport their smoking habit, using these higher cutoffs may exclude some women from the program who could benefit.

Alcohol and Illegal Drug Use

Prevalence of and Factors Associated with Alcohol Use

The 1988 National Maternal Infant Health Survey reported that 45 percent of women respondents consumed alcohol during the 3 months before they learned of their pregnancy. Nearly 21 percent reported consuming alcohol after learning that they were pregnant, 17 percent took three or fewer drinks per month during pregnancy, and 0.6 percent took six or more drinks per week during pregnancy (CDC, 1995a). Alcohol use was most prevalent among white, non-Hispanic women, followed by Hispanic and black women.

Alcohol Use as an Indicator of Nutrition and Health Risk

Infants are at risk from alcohol and illicit substances transmitted through the placenta and/or through breast milk. They are also at risk of nutritional deficits secondary to maternal nutrition deficits. Postnatally, the infant may also be at nutritional risk owing to the impaired ability of the mother to provide optimal care, including nutrition.

Alcohol is a rapidly absorbed drug that enters the fetal circulation and maternal milk. The safe amount of alcohol consumption during pregnancy is unknown. Pregnant women who consume greater than 6 fluid ounces of liquor daily (or the equivalent) have at least a 20 percent likelihood of delivering an infant with fetal alcohol syndrome (FAS) (Benson and Pernell, 1994). FAS is characterized by prenatal and postnatal growth restriction, distinct facial anomalies, and mental deficiency. Between 2 and 5 cases of FAS are estimated to occur per 1,000 live births (Bloss, 1994).

Adverse physical and neurobehavioral effects may also occur at lower levels of exposure to alcohol (Bloss, 1994). These effects range from spontaneous abortion to subtle behavioral effects in the offspring. Fetal growth restriction has been noted, although inconsistently, at levels of alcohol ingestion of 1 to 2 oz/day (Hanson et al., 1978; Little, 1977; Wright et al., 1983). Postnatal growth may be adversely affected in children who do not have full FAS.

Many animal studies have demonstrated a direct dose-response effect of alcohol on fetal growth and development (IOM, 1990), and malnutrition may be involved. Chronic alcoholics typically have an inadequate nutrient intake. In a prospective study of alcohol use during pregnancy, those with positive scores on the Michigan Alcoholic Screening Test had lower intakes of protein from meat and vegetable sources, dairy foods, cereal and breads, calcium, B vitamins, and vitamin D (Sokol et al., 1981). Heavy alcohol intake may interfere with nutrient absorption and lead to impaired nutrient metabolism by the liver. Specific deficiencies of zinc, vitamin A, folate, and thiamin may occur with chronic alcohol consumption, and one study suggests that maternal zinc deficiency may act as a co-teratogen with alcohol (Flynn et al., 1981).

During the breastfeeding period, excessive alcohol may be associated with failure to initiate the let-down reflex and with lethargy in the breastfed infant. Although a strong positive association has been reported between psychomotor development scores (Bayley Scales of Infant Development) and proxy measures of exposure to alcohol through breastfeeding (Little et al., 1989), the actual differences between exposure groups were minor. Maternal deficiencies (for example, of thiamin and folate) may be reflected in low intakes of these micronutrients by the breastfed infant.

Prevalence of and Factors Associated with Illegal Drug Use

A prospective study of consecutive prenatal patients from a poor inner-city population in 1989 reported that 18 percent had used cocaine during pregnancy (Zuckerman et al., 1989). Estimates of the prevalence of marijuana use during pregnancy have ranged from 10 to 27 percent in hospital-based studies (Hatch and Bracken, 1986; Linn et al., 1983; Zuckerman et al., 1989).

Illegal Drug Use as an Indicator of Nutrition and Health Risk

There is growing evidence that cocaine use during pregnancy is associated with both preterm delivery and fetal growth restriction as well as spontaneous abortion and abruptio placentae (IOM, 1990). Data on the influence of marijuana on pregnancy outcome in humans are limited and inconsistent. Adverse effects that have been reported include lower birth weight and body length; increased frequency of preterm delivery; higher rates of precipitate labor; increased risk of infant features compatible with FAS; and altered neural behavioral responses in neonates (IOM, 1990).

Head circumference and birth length are disproportionately decreased in infants when mothers use cocaine during their pregnancy (Zuckerman et al., 1989). Detection of cocaine in maternal urine is associated with decreased fetal fat, suggesting that cocaine may alter nutrient transfer to the fetus and fetal energy metabolism. High maternal serum values of cocaine, phencyclidine (PCP), and marijuana have been associated with decreased maternal serum levels of ferritin and folate. Cocaine is an appetite depressant and may reduce maternal intake of energy and nutrients. Marijuana may stimulate appetite, but there has been no consistent finding of increased maternal food intake during pregnancy. Detection of marijuana metabolites in maternal urine is associated with decreased fetal muscle mass, suggesting maternal-fetal hypoxia, which could be secondary to increased carboxyhemoglobinemia (IOM, 1990).

Among current users of alcohol or illicit substances, multiple substance use and smoking are common. It is quite likely, therefore, that the mother and infant can be at risk nutritionally from more than one drug substance.

Marijuana appears in the human milk as b-9-tetrahydrocannabinol, which is poorly absorbed but may cause lethargy and decreased feedings in the breastfed infant. Heroin and cocaine also appear in human milk and place the infant at considerable risk of toxicity.

Alcohol or Illegal Drug Use as Indicators of Nutrition and Health Benefit

If eaten, a balanced diet can help correct the nutrient shortfalls that are common among pregnant, lactating, or postpartum women who are abusing alcohol or illicit drugs. However, there is no convincing evidence that improved nutrition can counteract other adverse effects of alcohol or drugs.

The committee is unaware of studies on the effects of nutrition intervention in pregnant alcohol or cocaine users or in pregnant or postpartum substance users. In theory, linking substance users with medical care and social supports is a potentially beneficial intervention for the WIC program.

Use of Alcohol and Illegal Drug Use as Risk Indicators in the WIC Setting

History of alcohol or drug use through self-reports or written referrals are used to document these risks in the WIC setting. See Table 5-1 for state WIC agencies using these nutrition risk indicators. Cutoff points vary widely, from any use of alcohol or drug use through a history of drug use, to "addict" or "alcoholic."

Recommendations for Alcohol and Illegal Drug Use

Risks of *use of alcohol or illegal drugs*, or both, to the health of mothers and their fetuses are well documented, and risks to breastfeeding infants have also been reported. Too few studies have been conducted to determine whether the WIC food package contributes to the amelioration of the toxic effects of these substances. However, consumption of nutritious foods is beneficial for other reasons, and the committee felt that both the education and referral components of the WIC program have the potential to benefit women who use alcohol or illegal drugs during pregnancy and lactation. The committee strongly supports current public health policies recommending that women abstain from these substances during pregnancy. Setting a cutoff point is difficult because of the lack of scientific evidence relative to the potential for women who use alcohol or illegal drugs during pregnancy or lactation to benefit from the WIC program. Therefore, as an interim approach, the committee recommends *alcohol use* and *illegal drug use* as nutrition risk criteria for pregnant and lactating women in the state WIC program, with a cutoff of "any use." However, the committee recommends that these criteria be given lower priority, comparable to that of the predisposing risk category that is currently in use.[3]

The committee further recommends (1) that research be conducted to address the extent to which women who use alcohol or drugs benefit from the WIC program and the level of substance use that should be set as the cutoff point, if applicable, and (2) that USDA appoint an expert committee to provide guidance on cutoff points for alcohol and substance abuse that will identify pregnant and lactating women who are most likely to benefit from the WIC program. Members of the expert committee should have expertise in alcohol and substance abuse during pregnancy and lactation, assessment and treatment of alcohol and substance abuse, public policy, nutrition, and epidemiology.

Lead Poisoning

The persistence of lead in the environment is an ongoing public health problem. Major sources of lead exposure have included lead in gasoline, soldered cans, paint, and the soil. Within the past two decades, however, the amount of lead used in gasoline has decreased 99.8 percent, the amount in paint has been limited to less than 0.06 percent by weight, and lead-soldered food or beverage cans are no longer manufactured in the United States (Pirkle et al., 1994). The remaining sources of lead exposure are from residual deposits (in soil dust, old paint and plaster), occupational exposures, and lead-containing imported containers used for serving or storing food or beverages.

Lead poisoning (defined as a blood lead concentration of ≥ 10 µg/dl), although entirely preventable, is one of the worst environmental health threats to children in the United States (CDC, 1991; CEH-AAP, 1993). For women and children, pica can include the ingestion of lead-containing toxic substances (see also Chapter 6). Factors associated with lead poisoning include young age, male gender, low income, non-Hispanic black race/ethnicity, poor housing, homelessness, poor nutrition, limited child supervision, and family history of pica

---

[3] Three committee members (Barbara Abrams, Barbara Devaney, and Roy Pitkin) preferred a recommendation of establishing higher cutoff points for alcohol use and keeping the risk criteria for both drug and alcohol use at their current high priority level. The higher cutoff for alcohol use would more clearly delineate women whose level of alcohol use places them at higher risk of poor pregnancy and lactation outcomes and therefore would be more likely to benefit from WIC program participation. A higher cutoff could be based on a validated scale for assessing "problem drinking." For illegal drug use, they agree with the committee's cutoff of "any use."

(Pirkle et al., 1994; USDA, 1991b). Children's hand-to-mouth activities expose them to greater risk of lead poisoning.

Prevalence of and Factors Associated with Lead Poisoning

Data from phase one of NHANES III indicate substantial reductions in blood lead levels across all segments of the U.S. population between NHANES II and NHANES III (or, for Mexican Americans, between Hispanic HANES and NHANES III) (Pirkle et al., 1994). The percentage of all persons surveyed with blood lead concentrations greater than or equal to 10 µg/dl dropped from 77.8 to 4.3 percent. Among children 1 to 5 years of age, the prevalence of high blood lead concentrations dropped from 88.2 to 8.9 percent, among women from 66.7 to 1.8 percent, and among low-income (up to and 130 percent of the poverty level) individuals, from 78.6 to 8.8 percent. Data on the prevalence of lead poisoning among the WIC program population were not available to the committee.

Lead Poisoning as an Indicator of Nutrition and Health Risk

Lead ingested by pregnant women crosses the placenta and detrimentally affects the developing fetus. Mobilization of lead stored in bone occurs during lactation, but the kinetics of this lead release are not understood relative to the factors that might alter the rate or amount of transfer of lead from mother to nursing infant. In humans, umbilical cord blood lead concentration tends to equal to or be slightly lower than maternal blood lead concentrations (Goyer, 1990). During pregnancy, release of lead stores may increase the total dose presented to the fetus. One study found that lactating women over 30 years of age have higher levels of lead in their milk than younger women. Because bone serves as a reservoir for calcium during lactation, these higher lead levels may reflect the greater concentration of lead in mineralized tissue as a function of age (Silbergeld, 1990).

Lead increases blood pressure in adults (Harlan, 1988; Sharp et al., 1989). Analysis of data from NHANES II showed a significant linear association between blood lead concentrations and blood pressure. Additional analysis by Pirkle et al. (1985) showed that large initial increments in blood pressure occur at relatively low blood lead concentrations (range 7 to 34 µg/dl); this is followed by a leveling of blood pressure at higher blood lead concentrations.

Clinical investigations of the gastrointestinal absorption of lead among adults have produced inconsistent findings. Lead absorption has been estimated to be around 40 percent (Ziegler et al., 1978). Lead ingested during fasting is absorbed to a much greater extent than that ingested with food (Rabinowitz,

1980). The particular component of food intake that so dramatically reduces lead absorption largely remains to be identified. Inconsistencies in various lead absorption studies on adults were attributed to measurement techniques, timing and severity of deficiency, dietary factors, or related compensatory responses to the deficiencies. Deficiencies in such nutrients as iron, calcium, protein, and zinc increase the absorption of lead (Mahaffey, 1981, 1990; Needleman and Bellinger, 1991). In addition, studies have reported an inverse relationship between blood lead concentration and stature (Frisancho and Ryan, 1991; Schwartz et al., 1986).

The mechanism for the effects of lead on the central nervous system is unclear, but many studies have supported the fact that the mean intelligence quotients (IQ) achieved by children rise when elevated blood lead concentrations are reduced. The data do not, however, provide a threshold lead-IQ relationship. There is contradictory evidence whether blood lead concentrations of 10 to 25 µg/dl in infants or children are associated with decreased IQ scores or with deficits in particular cognitive processes (Davis and Svendsgaard, 1987; Mushak et al., 1989).

Long-term deficiency of iron in animals increases the absorption and biotoxicity of lead (CDC, 1991). Children who are iron deficient have significant delays in mental and motor development, but whether these developmental effects are additive or interactive with the effects from elevated blood lead concentrations needs to be determined (Wasserman et al., 1992). Severe lead poisoning in infants and children is associated with increased risk of coma, convulsions, and even death. Adverse effects of higher blood lead concentrations include damage to the central nervous system, kidneys, and hematopoietic system.

Lead Poisoning as an Indicator of Nutrition and Health Benefit

Adequate intake of calories, calcium, magnesium, iron, zinc, and various vitamins (e.g., thiamin, ascorbic acid, and vitamin E) is known to decrease the absorption of lead in adults and decrease children's susceptibility to the toxic effects of lead (Mahaffey, 1990). In conditions of lead exposure, however, nutrition factors will not prevent lead intoxication.

Mahaffey (1990) discussed the role of nutrition as an adjunct intervention in ameliorating the untoward health effects of lead and recommended that nutritional assessment and dietary intervention be a component of the strategy to minimize the neurobehavioral and cognitive impacts of chronic low-dose lead exposure. The primary benefits of participation in the WIC program for individuals with lead poisoning result from referrals to lead treatment programs and possibly supplemental food.

Use of Lead Poisoning as a Nutrition Risk Criterion in the WIC Setting

Health care providers report lead poisoning to WIC program staff. Table 5-1 lists numbers of state WIC agencies that use lead poisoning as a nutrition risk criterion in the WIC. Data on cutoff values used in the WIC program were not available to the committee.

Recommendation for Lead Poisoning

The risk of *lead poisoning* is well documented in women, infants, and children, and a practical clinical method for identifying this condition is available. There is empirical evidence and a theoretical basis that those with high lead concentrations can benefit from participation in the WIC program. Therefore, the committee recommends use of *lead poisoning* as a nutrition risk criterion for women, infants, and children in the WIC program, with the CDC cutoff value of ≥ 10 µg/dl.

SUMMARY

In general, most biochemical and medical risk criteria predict nutrition risk, with varying degrees of benefit. The most common concern of the committee was the lack of scientific justification for the generous cutoff points for biochemical and other medical risk criteria currently used by state WIC agencies. When evidence of risk and benefit was present, the committee found no reason that all states should not use scientifically justified nutrition risk criteria. Table 5-4 summarizes the committee's recommendations for biochemical and other medical risk indicators. In general, it should be assumed that any medical condition not mentioned in this chapter would be a suitable nutrition risk criterion if it causes ongoing impairment of self feeding, digestion, absorption, or utilization of nutrients.

Risk criteria for which there was risk and benefit only under specific conditions included *long-term drug-nutrient interactions*. The committee felt that this criterion is too vague to be useful in its current form and recommends that a listing of drugs for which there are clear drug-nutrient interactions or potential for misuse be developed. For *chronic and recurrent infections*, evidence of risk and benefit was available only for the chronic infections for which there were documented nutrition deficits, and the committee recommended that states should clearly define "chronic" or "recurrent" in determining cutoff points for these indicators. The committee recommends that the criterion *prematurity* be used only for infants and that the criterion *high parity* be discontinued.

REFERENCES

AAP-ACOG (American Association of Pediatrics, American College of Obstetrics and Gynecology). 1992. Guidelines for Perinatal Care, 3rd ed. Elk Grove, Ill.: AAP.

Abel, E.L. 1980. Smoking during pregnancy: A review of effects on growth and development of offsprings. Hum. Biol. 52:593–625.

Abrams, B., and V. Newman. 1991. Small-for-gestational-age birth: Maternal predictors and comparison with risk factors of spontaneous preterm delivery in the same cohort. Am. J. Obstet. Gynecol. 164:785–790.

Abrams, B., V. Newman, T. Key, and J. Parker. 1989. Maternal weight gain and preterm delivery. Obstet. Gynecol. 74:577–583.

Abrams, B., D. Duncan, and I. Hertz-Picciotto. 1993. A prospective study of dietary intake and acquired immune deficiency syndrome in HIV-Seropositive homosexual men. J. Acquired Immune Deficiency Syndromes 6:949–958.

ACOG (American College of Obstetrics and Gynecology). 1985. Standards for Obstetric-Gynecologic Services, 6th ed. Washington, D.C.: ACOG.

ACOG (American College of Obstetrics and Gynecology). 1989. Diagnosis and Management of Postterm Delivery. Technical Bulletin 130. Washington, D.C.: ACOG.

ACOG (American College of Obstetrics and Gynecology). 1995. Thyroid disease in pregnancy. ACOG Technical Bulletin 181. Washington, D.C.: ACOG.

Adair, L.S., and E. Pollitt. 1985. Outcome of maternal nutritional supplementation: A comprehensive review of the Bacon Chow study. Am. J. Clin. Nutr. 41:948–978.

Alexander, G.R., and C.C. Korenbrot. 1995. The role of prenatal care in preventing low birth weight. Future Child. 5(1):103–120.

American Cancer Society. 1995. Cancer Facts and Figures—1995. Atlanta: American Cancer Society.

American Diabetes Association. 1995. Medical Management of Pregnancy Complicated by Diabetes, 2nd ed. Alexandria, Va.: American Diabetes Association.

American Diabetes Association and American Dietetic Association. 1994. Nutrition recommendations and principles for people with diabetes mellitus. J. Am. Diet. Assoc. 94:504–506.

American Dietetic Association. 1994. Position of The American Dietetic Association and The Canadian Dietetic Association: Nutrition intervention in the care of persons with human immunodeficiency virus infection. J. Am. Diet. Assoc. 94:1042–1045.

Anderson, K.E., A.H. Conney, and A. Kappas. 1979. Nutrition and oxidative drug metabolism in man: Relative influence of dietary lipids, carbohydrate, and protein. Clin. Pharmacol. Ther. 26:493–501.

Backe, B. 1993. Maternal smoking and age. Effect on birth weight and risk for small-for-gestational age births. Acta Obstet. Gynecol. Scand. 72:172–176.

Balistreri, W.F. 1985. Neonatal cholestasis. J. Pediatr. 106:171–184.

Barness, L.A., ed. 1993. Pediatric Nutrition Handbook, 3rd ed. Elk Grove Village, Ill.: American Academy of Pediatrics, Committee on Nutrition.

Barrett, B.M., E. Gunter, and M. Wang. 1991. Ascorbic acid status in women who smoke during pregnancy. J. Amer. Diet. Assoc. 9:A–15.

Baum, M., L. Cassetti, P. Bonvehi, G. Shor-Posner, Y. Lu, and H. Sauberlich. 1994. Inadequate dietary intake and altered nutrition status in early HIV-1 infection. Nutrition 10:16–20.

Baxter, J., R.F. Hamman, T.K. Lopez, J.A. Marshall, S. Hoag, and C.J. Swenson. 1993. Excess incidence of known non-insulin-dependent diabetes mellitus (NIDDM) in Hispanics compared with non-Hispanic whites in the San Luis Valley, Colorado. Ethn. Dis. 3:11–21.

Beaulac-Baillargion, L., and C. Desrosiers. 1987. Caffeine-cigarette interaction on fetal growth. Am. J. Obstet. Gynecol. 157:1236–1240.

Behrman, R.E., ed. 1992. Nelson Textbook of Pediatrics, 14th ed. Philadelphia: W.B. Saunders.

Benson, R.C., and M.L. Pernell. 1994. Handbook of Obstetrics and Gynecology, 9th ed. New York: McGraw-Hill.

Beral, V. 1985. Long term effects of childbearing on health. J. Epid. Comm. Health 39:343–346.

Bergstein, J.M. 1992. Renal failure. Pp. 1352–1355 in Nelson Textbook of Pediatrics, 14th ed., R.E. Behrman and R.M. Kliegman, eds. Philadelphia: W.B. Saunders.

Berini, R.Y., and E. Kahn, eds. 1987. Clinical Genetics Handbook. Oradell, N.J.: Medical Economics Books.

Berkowitz, G.S. 1988. Smoking and pregnancy. Pp. 173–191 in Drug Use in Pregnancy, 2nd ed., J.R. Niebyl, ed. Philadelphia: Lea and Febiger.

Berkowitz, G.S., M.L. Skovron, R.H. Lapinski, and R.L. Berkowitz. 1990. Delayed childbearing and the outcome of pregnancy. N. Engl. J. Med. 322:659–664.

Bithoney, W.G., J. McJunkin, J. Michalek, J. Snyder, H. Egan, and D. Epstein. 1991. The effect of a multidisciplinary team approach on weight gain in nonorganic failure-to-thrive children. J. Dev. Behav. Pediatr. 12:254–258.

Bloss, G. 1994. The economic cost of FAS. Alcohol Health Res. World 18:53–54.

Bluestone, C.D., and R.J. Nozza. 1992. Inflammatory Diseases. Pp. 1608–1618 in Nelson Textbook of Pediatrics, 14th ed., R.E. Behrman and R.M. Kliegman, eds. Philadelphia: W.B. Saunders.

Bourgeois, F.J., and J. Duffer. 1990. Outpatient obstetric management of women with type I diabetes. Am. .J. Obstet. Gynecol. 163:1065–1072.

Bowers, E.J., R.F. Mayro, L.A. Whitaker, P.S. Pasquariello, D. LaRossa, and P. Randall. 1987. General body growth in children with clefts of the lip, palate, and craniofacial structure. Scand. J. Reconstr. Surg. Hand Surg. 21:7–14.

Boyle, J.T. 1995. Chronic Diarrhea. Chapter 287 in Nelson Textbook of Pediatrics, 15th ed., R.E. Behrman, R.M. Kliegman, and A. Arvin, eds. Philadelphia: W.B. Saunders.

Brody, D.J., and M.B. Bracken. 1987. Short interpregnancy interval: A risk factor for low birthweight. Am. J. of Perinatalogy 4:50–54.

Brooke, O.G., H.R. Anderson,. J.M. Bland, J.L. Peacock, and C.M. Stewart. 1989. Effects on birth weight of smoking, alcohol, caffeine, socioeconomic factors, and psychosocial stress. Br. Med. J. 298:795–801.

Brown, J.E., S.A. Kaye, and A.R. Folsom. 1992. Parity-related weight change in women. Int. J. Of Obesity 16:627–631.

Brunell, P.A. 1992. Hepatitis. Pp. 818–822 in Nelson Textbook of Pediatrics, 14th ed., R.E. Behrman and R.M. Kliegman, eds. Philadelphia: W.B. Saunders.

Buescher, P., L. Larson, M. Nelson, and A. Lenihan. 1993. Prenatal WIC participation can reduce low birth weight and newborn medical costs: A cost-benefit analysis of WIC participation in North Carolina. J. Am. Diet. Assoc. 93:163–166.

Bureau of Nutrition. 1990. The New York State WIC Evaluation: The association between prenatal WIC participation and birth outcomes. Albany: New York State Department of Health.

Burt, V.L., P. Whelton, E.J. Roccella, C. Brown, J.A. Cutler, M. Higgins, M.J. Horan, and D. Labarthe. 1995. Prevalence of hypertension in the U.S. adult population: Results from the Third National Health and Nutrition Examination Survey, 1988–1991. Hypertension 25:305–313.

Caan, B., D.M. Horgen, S. Margen, J.C. King, and N.P. Jewell. 1987. Benefits associated with WIC supplemental feeding during the interpregnancy interval. Am. J. Clin. Nutr. 45:29–41.

Casey, P.H., and W.C. Arnold. 1985. Compensatory growth in infants with severe failure to thrive. South Med. J. 78:1057–1060.

CDC (Centers for Disease Control and Prevention). 1989. CDC criteria for anemia in children and childbearing-aged women. Morbid. Mortal. Weekly Rep. 38:400–404.

CDC (Centers for Disease Control and Prevention). 1991. Preventing Lead Poisoning in Young Children: A Statement by the Centers for Disease Control. Atlanta: U.S. Department of Health and Human Services, Public Health Service.

CDC (Centers for Disease Control and Prevention). 1992. Recommendations for the use of folic acid to reduce the number of cases of spina bifida and other neural tube defects. Morbid. Mortal. Weekly Rep. 41(RR-14):1–7.

CDC (Centers for Disease Control and Prevention). 1994a. HIV/Aids Surveillance Report 5(4). Atlanta: U.S. Department of Health and Human Services.

CDC (Centers for Disease Control and Prevention). 1994b. HIV/AIDS Surveillance report 6(2). Atlanta: U.S. Department of Health and Human Services.

CDC (Centers for Disease Control and Prevention). 1995a. Sociodemographic and Behavioral Characteristics Associated with Alcohol Consumption During Pregnancy—United States, 1988. Morbid. Mortal. Weekly Rep. 44(13):261–264.

CDC (Centers for Disease Control and Prevention). 1995b. Update: AIDS among women—United States, 1994. Morbid. Mortal. Weekly Rep. 44:81–84.

CDC/NCHS (Centers for Disease Control and Prevention, National Center for Health Statistics). 1993. Advance report of final natality statistics, 1991. Monthly Vital Statistics Report 42(3S):1–48. Hyattsville, Md.: Public Health Service.

Cefalo, R.C., and M.K. Moos. 1988. Preconceptual Health Promotion: A Practical Guide. New York: Raven Press.

CEH-AAP (Committee on Environmental Health, American Academy of Pediatrics). 1993. Lead poisoning: From screening to primary prevention. Pediatrics 92:176–183.

Chachoua, A., R. Krigel, F. Lafleur, R. Ostreicher, M. Speer, L. Laubenstein, J. Wernz, P. Rubenstein, E. Zang, and A. Friedman-Kien. 1989. Prognostic factors and staging classifications of patients with epidemic Karposi's Sarcoma. J. Clin. Oncol. 7:774–780.

Cleland, J.C., and Z.A. Sathar. 1984. The effect of birth spacing on child mortality in Pakistan. Population Studies 38:401–418.

Cliver, S.P., R.L. Goldenberg, G.R. Cutter, H.J. Hoffman, R.L. Copper, S.J. Gotlieb, and R.O. Davis. 1992. The relationships among psychosocial profile, maternal size, and smoking in predicting fetal growth retardation. Obstet. Gynecol. 80:262–267.

Clugson, G.A., and B.S. Hetzel. 1994. Iodine. Pp. 252–263 in Modern Nutrition in Health and Disease, 8th ed., M.E. Shils, J.A. Olson, and M. Shike, eds. Philadelphia: Lea and Febiger.

COD-AAP (Committee on Drugs, American Academy of Pediatrics).1994. The transfer of drugs and other chemicals into human milk. Pediatrics 93:137–150.

COG-AAP (Committee on Genetics, American Academy of Pediatrics). 1991. Maternal phenylketonuria. Pediatrics 88:1284.

Cogswell, M.E., and R. Yip. 1995. The influence of fetal and maternal factors on the Distribution of Birthweight. Sem. Perinatology 19: 222–240.

Colditz, G.A., W.C. Willett, A. Rotnitzky, and J.E. Manson. 1995. Weight gain as a risk factor for clinical diabetes mellitus in women. Ann. Intern. Med. 122:481–486.

Cole, M.D., and K. Peevy. 1994. Hypoglycemia in normal neonates appropriate for gestational age. J. Perinatol. 14:118–120.

Coustan, D.R., M.W. Carpenter, P.S. O'Sullivan, and S.R. Carr. 1993. Gestational diabetes: Predictors of subsequent disordered glucose metabolism. Am J. Obstet. Gynecol. 168:1139–1145.

Coutsoudis, A., R.A. Bobat, H.M. Coovadia, L. Kuhn, W.Y. Tsai, and Z.A. Stein. 1995. The effects of vitamin A supplementation on the morbidity of children born to HIV-infected women. Am. J. Public Health 85:1076–1081.

Crofford, O.B. 1995. Diabetes control and complications. Annu. Rev. Med. 46:267–279.

Cunningham, F.G., P.C. MacDonald, K.J. Leveno, N.F. Gant, and L.C. Gilstrap, III. 1993. William's Obstetrics, 19th ed.. Norwalk, Conn.: Appleton and Lange.

Curry, M.A. 1990. Factors associated with inadequate prenatal care. J. Community. Health Nurs. 7:245–252.

Cystic Fibrosis Foundation. 1995. Cystic Fibrosis Foundation Patient Registry Annual Data Report, 1994. Bethesda, Md.: Cystic Fibrosis Foundation.

Davies, D.P., and M. Abernethy. 1976. Cigarette smoking in pregnancy: Associations with maternal weight gain and fetal growth. Lancet 1:385–387.

Davis, J.M., and D.J. Svendsgaard. 1987. Lead and child development. Nature 329:297–300.

Day, N., M. Cornelius, L. Goldschmidt, G. Richardson, N. Robles, and P. Taylor. 1992. The effects of prenatal tobacco and marijuana use on offspring growth from birth through 3 years of age. Neurotoxicol. Teratol. 14:407–414.

de Haas, J.H. 1975. Parental smoking. Its effects on fetus and child health. Eur. J. Obstet. Gynecol. Reprod. Biol. 5:283–296.

Devaney, B., L. Bilheimer, and J. Schore. 1990. The Savings in Medicaid Costs for Newborns and Their Mothers from Prenatal Participation in the WIC Program, vol. I. Office of Analysis and Evaluation, Food and Nutrition Service, U.S. Department of Agriculture. Washington, D.C.: U.S. Government Printing Office.

DHHS (U.S. Department of Health and Human Services). 1989. Reducing the Health Consequences of Smoking: 25 Years of Progress. A Report of the Surgeon General DHHS Publication No. (CDC) 89-8411. Washington D.C.: U.S. Government Printing Office.

DHHS (U.S. Department of Health and Human Services). 1990. 1990 Surgeon General's Report on Smoking and Health. Washington, D.C.: U.S. Government Printing Office.

DHHS (U.S. Department of Health and Human Services). 1994. Preventing Tobacco Use Among Young People. A Report of the Surgeon General. Washington, D.C.: U.S. Government Printing Office.

Diamond, A. 1995. The effect of a modest tyrosine deficiency on cognition: Children treated early and continuously for PKU. In A Healthy Body and a Health Mind? The Relationship Between Cognitive Function and Physical Illness. London: The Well Come Trust.

Drotar, D., and L. Sturm. 1992. Personality development, problem solving, and behavior problems among preschool children with early histories of nonorganic failure-to-thrive: A controlled study. J. Dev. Behav. Pediatr. 13:266–273.

D'Souza, S.W., P. Black, and B. Richards 1981. Smoking in pregnancy: Associations with skinfold thickness, maternal weight gain, and fetal size at birth. Br. Med. J. 282:1661–1663.

Edozien, J.C, B.R. Switzer, and R.B. Bryan. 1979. Medical evaluation of the Special Supplemental Food Program for Women, infants, and children. Am. J. Clin. Nutr. 32:677–692.

Eisen, G.M., and R.S. Sandler. 1994. Update on the epidemiology of IBD. Progress in Inflammatory Bowel Disease. Chrohn's and Colitis Foundation of America, Inc. 15:1–8.

Eisner, V., J.V. Brazie, M.W. Pratt et al. 1979. The risk of low birth weight. Am. J. Public Health 69:887–893.

Ekvall, S.W., ed. 1993. Pediatric Nutrition in Chronic Diseases and Developmental Disorders: Prevention, Assessment, and Treatment. New York: Oxford University Press.

Elwood, P.C., P.M. Sweetnam, O.P. Gray, D.P. Davies, and P.D. Wood. 1987. Growth of children from 0–5 years: With special reference to mother's smoking in pregnancy. Ann. Hum. Biol. 14:543–557.

English, P.B., and B. Eskenazi. 1992. Reinterpreting the effects of maternal smoking on infant birth weight and perinatal mortality: A multivariate approach to birth weight standardization. Int. J. Epidemiol. 21:1097–1105.

Epilepsy Foundation of America. 1993. Epilepsy Facts and Figures. Landover, Md.: Epilepsy Foundation of America.

Ershoff, D.H., P.D. Mullen, and V.P. Quinn. 1989. A randomized trial of a serialized self-help smoking cessation for pregnant women in an HMO. Am. J. Public Health 79:182–187.

Farahati, M., N. Bozorgi, and B. Luke. 1993. Influence of maternal age, birth-to-conception intervals and prior prenatal factors on perinatal outcomes. J. Reprod. Med. 38:751–756.

Ferris, A.M., and E.A. Reece. 1994. Nutrition consequences of chronic maternal conditions during pregnancy and lactation: Lupus and diabetes. Am. J. Clin. Nutr. 59(suppl.):465S–473S.

Ferris, A.M., C.K. Dalidowitz, C.M. Ingardia, E.A. Reece, F.D. Fumia, R.G. Jensen, and L.H. Allen. 1988. Lactation outcome in insulin-dependent diabetic women. J. Am. Diet. Assoc. 88:317–322.

Flynn, A., S.I. Miller, S.S. Martier, N.L. Golden, R.J. Sokol, and B.C. Del Villano. 1981. Zinc status of pregnant alcoholic women: A determinant of fetal outcome. Lancet 1:572–575.

Frank, D.A., and S.H. Zeisel. 1988. Failure to thrive. Pediatr. Clin. North Am. 35:1187–1206.

Fredricsson, B., and H. Gilljam. 1992. Smoking and reproduction: Short-and long-term effects and benefits of smoking cessation. Acta Obstet. Gynecol. Scand. 71:580–592.

Fretts, R.C., J. Schmittdiel, F.H. McLean, R.H. Usher, and M.B. Goldman. 1995. Increased maternal age and the risk of fetal death. New Engl. J. Med. 333:953–957.

Fried, P.A., and C.M. O'Connell. 1987. A comparison of the effects of prenatal exposure to tobacco, alcohol, cannabis and caffeine on birth size and subsequent growth. Neurotoxicol. Teratol. 9:79–85.

Frisancho, A.R., and A.S. Ryan. 1991. Decreased stature associated with moderate blood lead concentrations in Mexican-American children. Am. J. Clin. Nutr. 54:516–519.

GAO (U.S. General Accounting Office, Comptroller General of the United States). 1987. Prenatal Care: Medicaid Recipients and Uninsured Women Obtain Insufficient Care. A report to the Congress of the United States. HRD-87-137. Washington, D.C.: GAO.

Garn, S.M. 1985. Smoking and human biology. Hum. Biol. 57:505–523.

Garn, S.M. et al. 1979. Pregnant? No ifs, ands or butts. Res. Staff Phys. 25:152–162.

Gilstrap, L.C., and B.B. Little. 1992. Drugs and Pregnancy. New York: Elsevier.

Godsey, R.K., and R.B. Newman. 1991. Hyperemesis gravidarum: A comparison of single and multiple admissions. J. Reprod. Med. 36:287–290.

Goldstein, H. 1977. Smoking in pregnancy: Some notes on the statistical controversy. Bri. J. Prev. Soc. Med. 31:13–17.

Gonzalez, R. 1992. Urologic disorders in infants and children. Pp. 1359–1383 in Nelson Textbook of Pediatrics, 14th ed., R.E. Behrman and R.M. Kliegman, eds. Philadelphia: W.B. Saunders.

Gordon, A., and L. Nelson. 1995. Characteristics of WIC participants and nonparticipants: analysis of the national maternal health survey. Alexandria, Va.: U.S. Department of Agriculture, Food and Consumer Service, Office of Analysis and Evaluation.

Goyer, R.A. 1990. Transplacental transport of lead. Environ. Health Perspect. 89:101–105.

Hanson, J.W., A.P. Streissguth, and D.W. Smith. 1978. The effects of moderate alcohol consumption during pregnancy on fetal growth and morphogenesis. J. Pediatr. 92:457–460.

Harlan, W.R. 1988. The relationship of blood lead levels to blood pressure in the U.S. population. Environ. Health Perspect. 78:9–13.

Harrison, G.G. 1994. Editorial. Arch. Pediatr. Adolesc. Med. 148:1228–1229.

Harrison, G.G., R.S. Branson, and V.E. Vaucher. 1983. Association of maternal smoking with body composition of the newborn. Am. J. Clin. Nutr. 38:757–762.

Haste, F.M., O.G. Brooke, H.R. Anderson, J.M. Bland, A. Shaw, J. Griffin, and J.L. Peacock. 1990. Nutrient intakes during pregnancy: Observations on the influence of smoking and social class. Am. J. Clin. Nutr. 51:29–36.

Hatch, E.E., and M.B. Bracken. 1986. Effect of marijuana use in pregnancy on fetal growth. Am. J. Epidemiol. 124:986–993.
Haworth, J.C., J.J. Ellestad-Sayed, J. King, and L.A. Dilling. 1980. Relation of maternal cigarette smoking, obesity and energy consumption to infant size. Am. J. Obstet. Gynecol. 138:1185–1189.
Hebel, R.J., N.L. Fox, and M. Sexton. 1988. Dose-response of birth weight to various measures of maternal smoking during pregnancy. J. Clin. Epidemiol. 41:483–489.
Henderson, P., and G.A. Little. 1990. The detection and prevention of pregnancy-induced hypertension and preeclampsia. Pp. 479–500 in New Perspectives on Prenatal Care, I.R. Merkatz and J.E. Thompson, eds. New York: Elsevier.
Hobcraft, J.N., J.W. McDonald, and S.O. Rutstein. 1985. Demographic determinants of infant and child mortality. Population Studies 39:363.
Holmes, L.B. 1992. General clinical principles in genetic disorders. Pp. 274–276 in Nelson Textbook of Pediatrics, 14th ed., R.E. Behrman and R.M. Kliegman, eds. Philadelphia: W.B. Saunders.
Hopkinson, J.M., R.J. Schanler, J.K. Fraley, and C. Garza. 1992. Milk production by mothers of premature infants: Influence of cigarette smoking. Pediatrics 90:934–938.
Idjradinata, P., and E. Pollitt. 1993. Reversal of developmental delays in iron-deficient anaemic infants treated with iron. Lancet 341:1–4.
Infante-Rivard, C., and A. Fernandez. 1993. Otitis media in children: Frequency, risk factors, and research avenues. Epidemiologic Reviews 15:444–465.
IOM (Institute of Medicine). 1985. Preventing Low Birthweight. Report of the Committee to Study the Prevention of Low Birthweight, Division of Health Promotion and Disease Prevention. Washington, D.C.: National Academy Press.
IOM (Institute of Medicine). 1990. Nutrition During Pregnancy. Part I, Weight Gain; Part II, Nutrient Supplements. Report of the Subcommittee on Nutritional Status and Weight Gain During Pregnancy and Subcommittee on Dietary Intake and Nutrient Supplements During Pregnancy, Committee on Nutritional Status During Pregnancy and Lactation, Food and Nutrition Board. Washington, D.C.: National Academy Press.
IOM (Institute of Medicine). 1991. Nutrition During Lactation. Report of the Subcommittee on Nutrition During Lactation, Committee on Nutritional Status During Pregnancy and Lactation, Food and Nutrition Board. Washington, D.C.: National Academy Press.
IOM (Institute of Medicine). 1993. Iron Deficiency Anemia: Recommended Guidelines for the Prevention, Detection, and Management Among U.S. Children and Women of Childbearing Age. Report of the Committee on the Prevention, Detection, and Management of Iron Deficiency Anemia Among U.S. Children and Women of Childbearing Age, Food and Nutrition Board. Washington, D.C.: National Academy Press.
IOM (Institute of Medicine). 1995. The Best Intentions: Unintended Pregnancy and the Well-Being of Children and Families. Report of the Committee on Unintended Pregnancy, Division of Health Promotion and Disease Prevention. Washington, D.C.: National Academy Press.

Ito, M., H. Koyama, A. Ohshige, T. Maeda, T. Yoshimura, and H. Okamura. 1994. Prevention of preeclampsia with calcium supplementation and vitamin D_3 in an antenatal protocol. Int. J. Gyn. Obstet. 47:115–120.

Jacobson, J.L., S.W. Jacobson, and R.J. Sokol. 1994. Effects of prenatal exposure to alcohol, smoking, and illicit drugs on postpartum somatic growth. Alcohol Clin. Exp. Res. 18:317–323.

Jovanovic-Peterson, L., and C.M. Peterson. 1990. Dietary manipulation as a primary treatment for pregnancies complicated by diabetes. J. Am. Coll. Nutr. 9:320–325.

Kalmuss, D.S., and P.B. Namerow. 1994. Subsequent childbearing among teenage mothers: The determinants of a closely spaced second birth. Family Plann. Persp. 26:149–153, 159.

Kato, R., T. Oshima, and S. Tomizawa. 1968. Toxicity and metabolism of drugs in relation to dietary protein. Jpn. J. Pharmacol. 18:356–366.

Kennedy, E.T. 1986. A prenatal screening system for use in a community-based setting. J. Am. Diet. Assoc. 86:1372–1375.

Kennedy, E.T., and M. Kotelchuck. 1984. The effect of WIC supplemental feeding on birth weight: A case control analysis. Am. J. Clin. Nutr. 40:579–585.

Keusch, G.T. 1994. Nutrition and infection. Pp. 1241–1258 in Modern Nutrition in Health and Disease. 8th ed., M.E. Shils, J.A. Olson, and M. Shike, eds. Philadelphia: Lea and Febiger.

Kim, I., D.W. Hungerford, R. Yip, S.A. Kuester, C. Zyrkowski, and F.L. Trowbridge. 1992. Pregnancy Nutrition Surveillance System—United States, 1979–1990. CDC Surveillance Summaries. Morbid. Mortal. Weekly Rep. 41(no. SS-7):26–42.

Klebanoff, M.A., P.A. Koslowe, R. Kaslow, and G.G. Rhoads. 1985. Epidemiology of vomiting in early pregnancy. Obstet. Gynecol. 66:612.

Kleinman, J.C., M.B. Pierre, Jr., J.H. Madans, G.H. Land, and W.F. Sohramm. 1988. The effects of maternal smoking on fetal and infant mortality. Am. J. Epidemiol. 127:274–282.

Klesges, R.C., A.W. Meyers, L.M. Klesges, and M.E. La Vasque. 1989. Smoking, body weight, and their effects on smoking behavior: A comprehensive review of the literature. Psychol. Bull. 106:204–230.

Kline, J., Z.A. Stein, M. Susser, and D. Warburton 1977. Smoking: A risk factor for spontaneous abortion. N. Engl. J. Med. 297:793–796.

Kotchen, J.M., J. Holley, and T.A. Kotchen. 1989. Treatment of high blood pressure in the young. Semin. Nephrol. 9:296–303.

Kotchen, T.A., and J.M. Kotchen. 1994. Nutrition, diet, and hypertension. Pp. 1287–1297 in Modern Nutrition in Health and Disease. 8th ed., M.E. Shils, J.A. Olson, and M. Shike, eds. Philadelphia: Lea and Febiger.

Kotchen, T.A., J.M. Kotchen, and M.A. Boegehold. 1991. Nutrition and hypertension prevention. Hypertension 18:115–120.

Kramer, M.S. 1987. Determinants of low birth weight: Methodological assessment and meta-analysis. Bull. World Health Organ. 65:663–737.

Krebs, N.F., J.E. Westcott, N. Butler-Simon, and K.M. Hambidge. In press. Effects of a zinc supplement on growth of normal breast-fed infants. Experimental Biology.

Kritz-Silverstein, D., E. Barrett-Conner, and D.L. Wingard. 1989. The effect of parity on the later development of non-insulin-dependent diabetes mellitus or impaired glucose tolerance. N. Engl. J. Med. 321:1214–1219.

Krueger, L.E., R.W. Wood, P.H. Diehr, and C.L. Maxwell. 1990. Poverty and HIV seropositivity: The poor are more likely to be infected. AIDS 4:811–814.

Lancet. 1979. Smoking and intrauterine growth retardation. Lancet 1:536–537.

Lang, J.M., E. Lieberman, K.J. Ryan, and R.R. Monson. 1990. Interpregnancy interval and risk of preterm labor. Am. J. Epidemiol. 132:304–309.

Lechtig, A., C. Yarbrough, H. Delgado, R. Martorell, R.E. Klein, and M. Behar et al. 1975. Effect of moderate maternal malnutrition on the placenta. Am. J. Obstet. Gynecol. 123:191–201.

Lieberman, E., J.M. Lang, K.J. Ryan, R.R. Monson, and S.C. Schoenbaum. 1989. The association of inter-pregnancy interval with small for gestational age births. Obstet. Gynecol. 74:1–5.

Lifshitz, F., S. Friedman, M.M. Smith, C. Cervantes, B. Recker, and M. O'Connor. 1991. Nutritional dwarfing: A growth abnormality associated with reduced erythrocyte Na^+, $K^{(+)}$-ATPase activity. Am. J. Clin. Nutr. 54:997–1004.

Lincoln, R. 1986. Smoking and reproduction. Fam. Plann. Perspect. 18:79–84.

Linn, S., S.C. Schoenbaum, R.R. Monson, R. Rosner, P.C. Stubblefield, and K.J. Ryan. 1983. The association of marijuana use with outcome of pregnancy. Am. J. Public Health 73:1161–1164.

Little, R.E. 1977. Moderate alcohol use during pregnancy and decreased infant birth weight. Am. J. Public Health 67:1154–1156.

Little, R.E., K.W. Anderson, C.H. Ervin, R.B. Worthington, and S.K. Clarren. 1989. Maternal alcohol use during breast-feeding and infant mental and motor development at one year. N. Engl. J. Med. 321:425–430.

Lozoff, B., G.M. Brittenham, F.E. Viteri, A.W. Wolf, and J.J. Urrutia. 1982. The effects of short-term oral iron therapy on developmental deficits in iron-deficient anemia infants. J. Pediatr. 100:351–357.

Lozoff, B., E. Jimenez, and A.W. Wolf. 1991. Long-term developmental outcome of infants with iron deficiency. N. Engl. J. Med. 325:687–694.

LSRO (Life Sciences Research Office). 1991. Guidelines for the Assessment and Management of Iron Deficiency in Women of Childbearing Age, S.A. Anderson, ed. Bethesda, Md.: Federation of American Societies for Experimental Biology.

LSRO/FASEB (Life Sciences Research Office, Federation of American Societies for Experimental Biology). 1990. Nutrition and HIV Infection: A Review and Evaluation of the Extant Knowledge of the Relationship Between Nutrition and HIV Infection. Bethesda, Md.: LSRO/FASEB.

Luke, B., M.M. Hawkins, and R.H. Petrie. 1981. Influence of smoking, weight gain and pregravid weight-for-height on intrauterine growth. Am. J. Clin. Nutr. 34:1410–1417.

Luke B., T.R.B. Johnson, and R.H. Petrie. 1993. Clinical Maternal-Fetal Nutrition. New York: Little, Brown and Company.

Lutter, C.K., J-P. Habicht, J.A. Rivera, and R. Martorell. 1992. The relationship between energy intake and diarrhoeal disease in their effects on child growth: Biological model, evidence, and implications for public health policy. Food Nutr. Bull. 14(1):36–42.

MacArthur, C., and E.G. Knox. 1988. Smoking in pregnancy: Effects of stopping at different stages. Br. J. Obstet. Gynaecol. 95:551–555.

MacLeod, S., and J.L. Kiely. 1988. The effects of maternal age and parity on birthweight: A population-based study in New York City. Int. J. Gynecol. Obstet. 26:11–19.

Mahaffey, K.R. 1981. Nutritional factors in lead poisoning. Nutr. Rev. 39:353–362.

Mahaffey, K.R. 1990. Environmental lead toxicity: Nutrition as a component of intervention. Environmental Health Perspectives 89:75–78.

Malloy, M.H., J.C. Kleinman, J.M. Bakewell, W.F. Schramm, and G.H. Land. 1989. Maternal smoking during pregnancy: No association with congenital malformations in Missouri 1980–1983. Am. J. Public Health 79:1243–1246.

Mayer, J.P., B. Hawkins, and R. Todd. 1990. A randomized evaluation of smoking cessation interventions for pregnant women at a WIC clinic. Am. J. Public Health 80:76–78.

McCormick, M.C. 1985. The contribution of low birth weight to infant mortality and childhood morbidity. N. Engl. J. Med. 312:82–90.

McKenzie-Parnell, J.M., P.D. Wilson, W.R. Parnell, G.F. Spears, and M.F. Robinson. 1993. Nutrient intake of Dunedin women during pregnancy. New Zealand Med. Journal 106:273–276.

McKinney, R.E., Jr., and J.W. Robertson. 1993. Effects of human immunodeficiency virus infection on the growth of young children. Duke Pediatric AIDS Clinical Trials Unit. J. Pediatr. 123:579–582.

Merchant, K., and R. Martorell. 1988. Frequent reproductive cycling: does it lead to nutritional depletion of mothers? Prog. Food Nutr. Sci. 12:339–369.

Merchant, K., R. Martorell, and J. Haas. 1990. Maternal and fetal responses to the stresses of lactation concurrent with pregnancy and of short recuperative intervals. Am. J. Clin. Nutr. 52:280–288.

Metcoff, J., P. Costiloe, W.M. Crosby, S. Dutta, H.H. Sandstead, D. Milne, C.E. Bodwell, and S.H. Majors. 1985. Effect of food supplementation (WIC) during pregnancy on birth weight. Am. J. Clin. Nutr. 41:933–947.

Meyer, M.B. 1978. How does maternal smoking affect birth weight and maternal weight gain? Evidence from the Ontario Perinatal Mortality Study. Am. J. Obstet. Gynecol. 131:888–893.

Miller, J.E. 1989. Determinants of intrauterine growth retardation: Evidence against maternal depletion. J. Biosoc. Sci. 21: 235–243.

MMWR (Morbidity and Mortality Weekly Report). 1992. Recommendations for the use of folic acid to reduce the number of cases of spina bifida and other neural tube defects. Morbid. Mortal. Weekly Rep. 41:1–7.

Moffatt, M.E.K., S. Longstaffe, J. Besant, and C. Dureski. 1994. Prevention of iron deficiency and psychomotor decline in high-risk infants through use of iron-fortified infant formula: A randomized clinical trial. J. Pediatr. 125:527–534.

MRC Vitamin Study Research Group. 1991. Prevention of neural tube defects: Results of the Medical Research Council Vitamin Study. Lancet 338:131–137.

Mushak, P., J.M. Davis, A.F. Crocetti, and L.D. Grant. 1989. Prenatal and postnatal effects of low-level lead exposure: Integrated summary of a report to the U.S. Congress on childhood lead poisoning. Environ. Res. 50:11–36.

Naeye, R.L. 1978. Effects of maternal cigarette smoking on the fetus and placenta. Br. J. Obstet. Gynaecol. 85:732–737.

Naeye, R.L. 1981a. Nutritional/nonnutritional interactions that affect the outcome of pregnancy. Am. J. Clin. Nutr. 34:727–731.

Naeye, R.L. 1981b. Influence of maternal cigarette smoking during pregnancy on fetal and childhood growth. Obstet. Gynecol. 57:18–21.

Naeye, R.L. 1992. Effects of maternal cigarette smoking on the fetus and neonate. Pp. 77–91 in Disorders of the Placenta, Fetus, and Neonate: Diagnosis and Clinical Significance. St. Louis, Mo.: Mosby Year Book.

National Commission on AIDS. 1992. The Challenge of HIV/AIDS in Communities of Color. Washington, D.C.: National Commission on AIDS.

NCHS (National Center for Health Statistics) and S.J. Ventura. 1989. Trends and variations in first births to older women, 1970–1986. Vital and Health Statistics. Series 21. No. 47. DHHS publication no. (PHS) 89–1925. Washington, D.C.: U.S. Government Printing Office.

Needleman, H.L., and D. Bellinger. 1991. The health effects of low level exposure to lead. Annu. Rev. Public Health 12:111–140.

Neubauer, S.H., A.M. Ferris, C.G. Chase, J. Fanelli, C.A. Thompson, C.J. Lammi-Keefe, R.M. Clark, R.G. Jensen, R.B. Bendel, and K.W. Green. 1993. Delayed lactogenesis in women with insulin-dependent diabetes mellitus. Am. J. Clin. Nutr. 58:54–60.

Newell, M.L., and C. Peckham. 1994. Vertical transmission of HIV infection. Acta. Pediatr. Suppl. 400:43–45.

Norkus, E.P., H. Hsu, and M.R. Cehelsky. 1987. Effect of cigarette smoking on the vitamin-C status of pregnant women and their offspring. Ann. N.Y. Acad. Sci. 498:500–501.

NRC (National Research Council). 1982. Diet, Nutrition, and Cancer. Report of the Committee on Diet, Nutrition and Cancer, Food and Nutrition Board, Commission on Life Sciences. Washington, D.C.: National Academy Press.

NRC (National Research Council). 1989. Diet and Health: Implications for Reducing Chronic Disease Risk. Report of the Committee on Diet and Health, Food and Nutrition Board, Commission on Life Sciences, Institute of Medicine. Washington, D.C.: National Academy Press.

Olsen, J., A. da C. Pereira, and S.F. Olsen. 1991. Does maternal tobacco smoking modify the effect of alcohol on fetal growth? Am. J. Public Health 81:69–73.

Paneth, N.S. 1995. The problem of low birth weight. Future Child. 5(1):19–34.

Parker, J., and B. Abrams. 1993. Differences in postpartum weight retention between black and white mothers. Obstet. Gynecol. 81:768–91.

Peacock, J.L., J.M. Bland, and H.R. Anderson. 1991. Effects on birth weight of alcohol and caffeine consumption in smoking women. J. Epidemiol. Community Health 45:159–163.

Perkins, K.A., L.H. Epstein, B.L. Marks, R.L. Stiller, and R.G. Jacob. 1989. The effect of nicotine on energy expenditure during light physical activity. New Engl. J. Med. 320:898–903.

Perkins, K.A. 1992. Effects of tobacco smoking on caloric intake. Br. J. Addict. 87:193–205.

Phelps, L. 1991. Nonorganic failure to thrive: Origins and psychoeducational implications. School Psychol. Rev. 20:417–427.

Pirkle, J.L., J. Schwartz, J.R. Landis, and W.R. Harlan. 1985. The relationship between blood lead levels and blood pressure and its cardiovascular risk implications. Am. J. Epidemiol. 121:246–258.

Pirkle, J.L., D.J. Brody, E.W. Gunter, R.A. Kramer, D.C. Paschal, K.M. Flegal, and T.D. Matte. 1994. The decline in blood lead levels in the United States: The National Health and Nutrition Examination Surveys. J. Am. Med. Assoc. 272:284–291.

Platt, L.D., R. Koch, C. Azen, W.B. Hanley, H.L. Levy, R. Matalon, B. Rouse, E. de la Cruz, and C.A. Walla. 1992. Maternal phenylketonuria collaborative study, obstetric aspects and outcome: The first 6 years. Am. J. Obstet. Gynecol. 166:1150–1162.

Pollitt, E. 1993. Iron deficiency and cognitive function. Ann. Rev. Nutr. 13:521–537.

Pollitt, E. 1994. Poverty and child development: Relevance of research in developing countries to the United States. Child Dev. 65:283–295.

Pollitt, E., P. Hathirat, N.J. Kotchabhakdi, L. Missell, and A. Valyasevi. 1989. Iron deficiency and educational achievement in Thailand. Am. J. Clin. Nutr. 50:687–697.

Powell, G.F. 1988. Nonorganic failure to thrive in infancy: An update on nutrition, behavior, and growth. J. Am. Coll. Nutr. 7:345–353.

Prentice, A.M. 1991. Can maternal dietary supplements help in preventing infant malnutrition? Acta Paediatr. Scand. Suppl. 374:67–77.

Preston, A.M. 1991. Cigarette smoking and nutritional implications. Prog. Food Nutr. Sci. 15:183–217.

Pruitt, A.B. 1992. Systemic Hypertension. Pp. 1222–1227 in Nelson Textbook of Pediatrics, 14th ed., R.E. Behrman and R.M. Kliegman, eds. Philadelphia: W.B. Saunders.

Rabinowitz, M.B., J.D. Kopple, and G.W. Wetherill. 1980. Effect of food intake and fasting on gastrointestinal lead absorption in humans. Am. J. Clin. Nutr. 33:1784–1788.

Rawlings, J.S., V.B. Rawlings, and J.A. Read. 1995. Prevalence of low birth weight and preterm delivery in relation to the interval between pregnancies among white and black women. N. Engl. J. Med. 332: 69–74.

Repke, J.T. 1994. Calcium and vitamin D. Clin. Obstet. Gynecol. 37:550–557.

Roe, D.A. 1994. Diet, nutrition, and drug reactions. Pp. 1399–1416 in Modern Nutrition in Health and Disease, 8th ed., M.E. Shils, J.A. Olson, and M. Shike, eds. Philadelphia: Lea and Febiger.

Rohr, F.J., H.L. Levy, and V.E. Shih. 1985. Inborn errors of metabolism. In Nutrition in Pediatrics, W.A. Walker and J.B. Watkins, eds. New York: Little, Brown, and Company.

Rosenberg, I.H., and J.B Mason. 1994. Inflammatory bowel disease. Pp. 1043–1049 in Modern Nutrition in Health and Disease, 8th ed., M.E. Shils, J.A. Olson, and M. Shike, eds. Philadelphia: Lea and Febiger.

Rothman, K.J., L.L. Moore, M.R. Singer, U.S.D.T. Nguyen, S. Mannino, and A. Milunsky. 1995. Teratogenicity of high vitamin A intake. New Engl. J. Med. 333:1369–1373.

Ruff, A.J. 1994. Breastmilk, breastfeeding, and transmission of viruses to the neonate. Semin. Perinatol. 18:510–516.

Rush, D. 1974. Examination of the relationship between birth weight, cigarette smoking during pregnancy and maternal weight gain. J. Obstet. Gynaecol. Br. Commonw. 81:746–752.

Rush, D. 1976. Cigarette smoking during pregnancy: The relationship with depressed weight gain and birth weight. An updated report. Pp. 161–172 in Birth Defects: Risks and Consequences, S. Kelly, E.B. Hook, D.T. Janerich, and I.H. Porter, eds. New York: Academic Press.

Rush, D., and K.R. Callaghan. 1989. Exposure to passive cigarette smoking and child development: A critical review. Ann. N.Y. Acad. Sci. 562:74–100.

Rush, D., J. Leighton, N.L. Sloan, J.M. Alvir, D.G. Horvitz, W.B. Seaver, G.C. Garbowski, S.S. Johnson, R.A. Kulka, J.W. Devore, M. Holt, J.T. Lynch, T.G. Virag, M.B. Woodside, and D.S. Shanklin. 1988a. The National WIC Evaluation: Evaluation of the Special Supplemental Food Program for Women, Infants, and Children. VI. Study of infants and children. Am. J. Clin. Nutr. 48:484–511.

Rush, D., N.L. Sloan, J. Leighton, J.M. Alvir, D.G. Horvitz, W.B. Seaver, G.C. Garbowski, S.S. Johnson, R.A. Kulka, M. Holt, J.W. Devore, J.T. Lynch, M.B. Woodside, and D.S. Shanklin. 1988b. The National WIC Evaluation: Evaluation of the Special Supplemental Food Program for Women, Infants, and Children. V. Longitudinal study of pregnant women. Am. J. Clin. Nutr. 48:439–483.

Saavedra, J.M., R.A. Henderson, J.A. Perman, N. Hutton, R.A. Livingston, and R.H. Yolken. 1995. Longitudinal assessment of growth in children born to mothers with human immunodeficiency virus infection. Arch. Pediatr. Adolesc. Med. 149:497–502.

Samet, J.M., E.M. Lewit, and K.E. Warner. 1994. Involuntary smoking and children's health. Future Child. 4(3):94–114.

Sampson, H.A. 1994. Food allergy. Pp. 1391–1398 in Modern Nutrition in Health and Disease, 8th ed., M.E. Shils, J.A. Olson, and M. Shike, eds. Philadelphia: Lea and Febiger.

Schaller, J.G. 1992. Nonrheumatic conditions mimicking rheumatic diseases of childhood. Pp. 637–640 in Nelson Textbook of Pediatrics, 14th ed., R.E. Behrman and R.M. Kliegman, eds. Philadelphia: W.B. Saunders.

Scholl, T.O., M.L. Hediger, R.L. Fischer, and J.W. Shearer. 1992. Anemia vs. iron deficiency: Increased risk of preterm delivery in a prospective study. Am. J. Clin. Nutr. 55:985–988.

Schramm, W.F. 1986. Prenatal participation in WIC related to Medicaid costs for Missouri newborns: 1982 update. Public Health Rep. 101:607–615.

Schwartz, J., C. Angle, and H. Pitcher. 1986. Relationship between childhood blood lead levels and stature. Pediatrics. 77:281–8.

Seidman, D.S., P. Ever-Hadani, and R. Gale. 1990. Effect of maternal smoking and age on congenital anomalies. Obstet. Gynecol. 76:1046–1050.

Semba, R.D., W.T. Caiaffa, N.M. Graham, S. Cohn, and D. Vlahov. 1995. Vitamin A deficiency and wasting as predictors of mortality in human immunodeficiency virus-infected injection drug users. J. Infectious Dis. 171:1196–1202.

Semba, R.D., P.G. Miotti, J.D. Chiphangwi, A.J. Saah, J.K. Canner, G.A. Dallabetta, and D.R. Hoover. 1994. Maternal vitamin A deficiency and mother-to-child transmission of HIV-1. Lancet 343:1593–1597.

Seshadri, S., and T. Gopaldas. 1989. Impact of iron supplementation on cognitive functions in preschool and school-aged children: The Indian experience. Am. J. Clin. Nutr. 50(suppl.):675–686.

Sexton, J.F. 1991. Smoking interventions during pregnancy. Pp. 153–165 in Advances in the Prevention of Low Birth weight: An International Symposium, H. Berendes, S. Kessel, and S. Yaffe, eds. Washington, D.C.: National Center for Education in Maternal and Child Health.

Shandling, B. 1992. Congenital and perinatal anomalies of the gastrointestinal tract and intestinal obstruction. Pp. 948–964 in Nelson Textbook of Pediatrics, 14th ed., R.E. Behrman and R.M. Kliegman, eds. Philadelphia: W.B. Saunders.

Sharp, D.S., J. Osterloh, C.E. Becker, B. Bernard, A.H. Smith, J.M. Fisher, S.L. Syme, B.L. Holman, and T. Johnston. 1989. Blood pressure and blood lead concentrations in bus drivers. Environ. Health Perspect. 78:131–137.

Shaughnessy, A.F., and Slawson, D.C. 1994. Complications of IDDM. J. Fam. Pract. 38:632–633.

Shaw, G.M., E.J. Lammer, C.R. Wasserman, C.D. O'Malley, and M.M. Tolarova.1995. Risks of orofacial clefts in children born to women using multvitamins containing folic acid periconceptionally. Lancet 346:393–396.

Shils, M.E., J.A. Olson, and M. Shike, eds. 1994. Modern Nutrition in Health and Disease, 8th ed. Philadelphia: Lea and Febiger.

Shiono, P.H., M.A. Klebanoff, and G.G. Rhoads. 1986a. Smoking and drinking during pregnancy: Their effects on preterm birth. J. Am. Med. Assoc. 255:82–84.

Shiono, P.H., M.A. Klebanoff, and H.W. Berendes. 1986b. Congenital malformations and maternal smoking during pregnancy. Teratology 34:65–71.

Shiono, P.H., and R.E. Behrman. 1995. Low birth weight: Analysis and recommendations. Future Child. 5(1):4–18.

Silbergeld, E.K. 1990. Implications of new data on lead toxicity for managing and preventing exposure. Environ. Health Perspect. 89:49–54.

Singhal, P.K., M. Singh, V.K. Paul, A.K. Deorari, M.G. Ghorpade, and A. Malhotra. 1992. Neonatal hypoglycemia: Clinical profile and glucose requirements. Indian Pediatr. 29:167–171.

Sloan, A.E., and M.E. Powers. 1986. A perspective on popular perceptions of adverse reactions to foods. J. Allergy Clin. Immunol. 78:127–133.

Smith, N.C. 1992. Detection of the fetus at risk. Eur. J. Clin. Nutr. 46:S1–S5.

Soewondo, S., M. Husaini, and E. Pollitt. 1989. Effects of iron deficiency on attention and learning processes in preschool children: Bandung, Indonesia. Am. J. Clin. Nutr. 50(suppl.):667–674.

Sokol, R.J., S.I. Miller, S. Debanne, N. Golden, G. Collins, J. Kaplan, and S. Martier. 1981. The Cleveland NIAAA prospective alcohol-in-pregnancy study: The first year. Neurobehav. Toxicol. Teratol. 3:203–209.

Souba, W.W., and D.W. Wilmore. 1994. Diet and nutrition in the care of the patient with surgery, trauma, and sepsis. Pp. 1207–1240 in Modern Nutrition in Health and Disease, 8th ed., M.E. Shils, J.A. Olson, and M. Shike, eds. Philadelphia: Lea and Febiger.

Sperling, M.A. 1992. Hypoglycemia. Pp. 409–419 in Nelson Textbook of Pediatrics, 14th ed., R.E. Behrman and R.M. Kliegman, eds. Philadelphia: W.B. Saunders.

Spiers, P.S., and L. Wang. 1976. Short pregnancy interval, low birthweight, and the sudden infant death syndrome. Am. J. Epidemiol. 104:15–21.
Springer, N.S., K. Bischoping, C.M. Sampselle, F.L. Mayes, and B.A. Petersen. 1992. Using early weight gain and other nutrition-related risk factors to predict pregnancy outcomes. J. Am. Diet Assoc. 92:217–219.
Stockbauer, J.W. 1987. WIC prenatal participation and its relation to pregnancy outcomes in Missouri: A second look. Am. J. Public Health 77:813–818.
Taffel, S.M. 1989. Trends in low birth weight: United States, 1975–1985. Centers for Disease Control, National Center for Health Statistics. Vital and Health Statistics. Series 21. No. 48. Washington, D.C.: U.S. Government Printing Office.
Tang, A.M., N.M.H. Graham, A.J. Kirby, L.D. McCall, W.C. Willet, and A.J. Saah. 1993. Dietary micronutrient intake and risk of progression to acquired immunodeficiency syndrome (AIDS) in human immunodeficiency virus type 1 (HIV-1)-infected homosexual men. Am. J. Epidemiol. 138:937–951.
Tinker, L.F. 1994. Diabetes mellitus: A priority health care issue for women. J. Am. Diet. Assoc. 94:976–985.
Torun, B., and F. Chew. 1994. Protein-energy malnutrition. Pp. 950–976 in Modern Nutrition in Health and Disease, 8th ed., M.E. Shils, J.A. Olson, and M. Shike, eds. Philadelphia: Lea and Febiger.
Ulmer, H.U., and E. Goepel. 1988. Anemia, ferritin and preterm labor. J. Perinat. Med. 16:459–465.
USDA (U.S. Department of Agriculture). 1987. Estimation of Eligibility for the WIC Program: Report of the WIC Eligibility Study. Summary of Data, Methods, and Findings. Office of Analysis and Evaluation, Food and Nutrition Service. Contract No. 53-3198-3-138. Washington, D.C.: USDA.
USDA (U.S. Department of Agriculture). 1991a. Evidence for Effects of Timing of Prenatal Care and Nutritional Supplementation on Pregnancy Outcome. Report no. 7 in Technical Papers: Review of WIC Nutrition Risk Criteria. Prepared for the Food and Nutrition Service by the Department of Family and Community Medicine, College of Medicine, University of Arizona, Tucson. Washington, D.C.: USDA.
USDA (U.S. Department of Agriculture). 1991b. Pica and Lead Exposure in Infants and Children: Health and Nutritional Risk Implications. Report no. 14 in Technical Papers: Review of WIC Nutritional Risk Criteria. Prepared for the Food and Nutrition Service by the Department of Family and Community Medicine, College of Medicine, University of Arizona, Tucson. Washington, D.C.: USDA.
USDA (U.S. Department of Agriculture). 1994. Study of WIC Participant and Program Characteristics, 1992. Background Data. Office of Analysis and Evaluation, Food and Nutrition Service. Washington, D.C.: USDA.
U.S. Department of Commerce. 1993. Statistical Abstract of the United States, 1993. Lanham, Md.: Bernan Press.
Valway, S., W. Freeman, S. Kaufman, T. Welty, S.D. Helgerson, and D. Gohdes. 1993. Prevalence of diagnosed diabetes among American Indians and Alaskan Natives, 1987. Estimates from a national outpatient data base. Diabetes Care 16:271–276.
Van den Eeden, S.K., M.R. Karagas, J.R. Daling, and T.L. Vaughan. 1990. A case-control study of maternal smoking and congenital malformations. Paediatr. Perinat. Epidemiol. 4:147–155.

Van den Elzen, H.J., J.W. Wladimiroff, T.E. Overbeek, C.D. Morris, and D.E. Grobbee. 1995. Calcium metabolism, calcium supplementation and hypertensive disorders of pregnancy. Eur. J. Obstet. Reprod. Biol. 59:5–16.

Ventura, S.J., J.A. Martin, S.M. Taffel, T.J. Mathews, and S.C. Clarke. 1995. Advance report of final natality statistics, 1993. Monthly vital statistics report, vol. 44, no. 3 supplement. Hyattsville, Md.: Centers for Disease Control and Prevention, National Center for Health Statistics.

Walter, T., I. De Andraca, P. Chadud, and C.G. Perales. 1989. Iron deficiency anemia: Adverse effects on infant psychomotor development. Pediatrics. 84:7–17.

Walravens, P.A., A. Chakar, R. Mokni, J. Denise, and D. Lemonnier. 1992. Zinc supplements in breastfed infants. Lancet 340:683–685.

Wasserman, G., J.H. Graziano, P. Factor-Litvak, D. Popovac, N. Morina, A. Musabegovic, N. Vrenezi, S. Capuni-Paracka, V. Lekic, E. Preteni-Redjepi et al. 1992. Independent effects of lead exposure and iron deficiency anemia on developmental outcome at age 2 years. J. Pediatr. 121:695–703.

Watkins, W., and E. Pollitt. In press. Iron deficiency and cognition among school age children. Proceedings of the 1995 PAHO meeting, Kingston, Jamaica.

Welling, P.G. 1977. Influence of food and diet on gastrointestinal drug absorption: A review. J. Pharmacokinet. Biopharm. 5:291–334.

Wen, S.W., R.L. Goldenberg, G.R. Cutter, H.J. Hoffman, S.P. Cliver, R.O. Davis, and M.B. DuBard. 1990. Smoking, maternal age, fetal growth, and gestational age at delivery. Am. J. Obstet. Gynecol. 162:53–58.

WHO (World Health Organization). 1978. Arterial Hypertension: Report of a WHO Expert Committee. Technical Rep. Ser. 628. Geneva: WHO.

Williamson, D.F., J. Madans, E. Pamuk, K.M. Flegal, J.S. Kendrick, and M.K. Serdula. 1994. A prospective study of childbearing and 10-year weight gain in U.S. white women 25 to 45 years of age. Int. J. Obes. 18:561–569.

Wilmore, D.W. 1977. The Metabolic Management of the Critically Ill. New York: Plenum Medical Book Company.

Winkvist, A., K.M. Rasmussen, and J-P. Habicht. 1992. A new definition of maternal depletion syndrome. Am. J. Public Health 82:691–694.

Witwer, M.B. 1990. Prenatal care in the United States: Reports call for improvements in quality and accessibility. Fam. Plann. Perspect. 22:31–35.

Wolke, D., D. Skuse, and B. Mathisen. 1990. Behavioral style in failure-to-thrive infants: A preliminary communication. J. Pediatr. Psychol. 15:237–254.

Wright, J.T., E.J. Waterson, I.G. Barrison, P.J. Toplis, I.G. Lewis, M.G. Gordon, K.D. MacRae, N.F. Morris, and I.M. Murray-Lyon. 1983. Alcohol consumption, pregnancy, and low birth weight. Lancet 1:663–665.

Yerushalmy, J. 1971. The relationship of parents' cigarette smoking to outcome of pregnancy—implications as to the problem of inferring causation from observed associations. Am. J. Epidemiol. 93:443–456.

Yip, R., I. Parvanta, K. Scanlon, E.W. Borland, C.M. Russell, and F.L. Trowbridge. 1992. Pediatric nutrition surveillance system—United States, 1980–1991. Morbid. Mortal. Weekly Rep. 41(SS-7):1–24.

Zeiger, R.S., and S. Heller. 1995. The development and prediction of atopy in high-risk children: Follow-up at age seven years in a prospective randomized study of combined maternal and infant food allergen avoidance. J. Allergy Clin. Immunol. 95:1179–1190.

Ziegler, E.E., B.B. Edwards, R.L. Jensen, K.R. Mahaffey, and S.J. Fomon. 1978. Absorption and retention of lead by infants. Pediatr. Res. 12:29–34.

Zlatnik, F.J., and L.F. Burmeister. 1977. Low "gynecologic age": An obstetric risk factor. Am. J. Obstet. Gynecol. 128:183–186.

Zuckerman, B., D.A. Frank, R. Hingson, H. Amaro, S.M. Levenson, H. Kayne, S. Parker, R. Vinci, K. Aboagye, L.E. Fried, H. Cabral, R. Timperi, and H. Bauchner. 1989. Effects of maternal marijuana and cocaine use on fetal growth. N. Engl. J. Med. 320:762–768.

6

Dietary Risk Criteria

The third category of nutrition risk criteria used in the WIC program (the Special Supplemental Nutrition Program for Women, Infants, and Children) is *dietary deficiencies that impair or endanger health, such as inadequate dietary patterns assessed by a 24-hour dietary recall, dietary history, or food frequency checklist* (7 CFR Subpart C, Section 246.7(e)(2)(iii)). In general, dietary risk criteria are used to certify pregnant and breastfeeding women and infants at nutrition risk as demonstrated by inadequate dietary pattern under priority IV, children under priority V, and nonbreastfeeding postpartum women under priority VI. For the WIC program to work most effectively to *prevent* the occurrence of overt problems of dietary origin, methods are needed to identify behaviors or conditions related to diet that can lead to overt nutrition problems. Dietary risk criteria are intended to do this.

This chapter addresses the evidence that dietary risk criteria are valid indicators of nutrition and health risk and of an individual's potential to benefit from participation in the WIC program. In addition, the chapter addresses methods by which dietary risk is assessed in the WIC program setting and the validity of those assessments. Chapters 4 and 5 cover many of the adverse effects of dietary inadequacy.

Dietary assessments are routinely carried out by all WIC programs as a basis for nutrition education—whether or not the assessments are used to certify an individual. These assessments provide a tool for individualizing nutrition education (and sometimes the food package itself and health care referrals). Thus, dietary assessment is an important part of the benefit package of the WIC program. The multiple roles of dietary assessment need to be considered because time and resources are expended in a dietary assessment. If its only role were in determining program eligibility, yield of benefit would be central. However, the dietary assessment has extra value since it forms an essential part of the intervention package.

State and local WIC programs use a variety of criteria for dietary risk in the certification of participants. Most agencies report assessing dietary quality for women using categories of moderately inadequate, severely inadequate, deficient, or excessive for energy intake, nutrient intake, or food group consumption. Recently, some states have proposed the use of hunger or food insecurity as a dietary risk criterion.

This chapter places dietary risks into three categories: (1) inappropriate dietary patterns, (2) inadequate diet, and (3) food insecurity. The first two categories are consistent with nutrition risk criteria specified by the WIC program. Food insecurity is a proposed new category. A list of the risk criteria used by state WIC agencies appears in Table 6-1. A summary of broad cate

TABLE 6-1 Summary of Broad Dietary Risk Criteria in the WIC Program and Use by States

Risk Criterion	States Using[a] Pregnant Women	Infants	Children
Inappropriate dietary patterns	—	44	48
Excessive consumption of sugar, fat, or sodium	11	—	—
Insufficient or excessive calories	14	—	—
Inappropriate use of nursing bottle	—	27	28
Inappropriate introduction to solids/foods	—	23	9
Excessive/insufficient vitamins/minerals	11	13	11
Excessive caffeine intake	—	—	—
Pica	33	20	22
Inadequate diet	—	44	48
Moderately inadequate	42	—	—
Seriously inadequate	40	—	—
Food insecurity	1	1	1

NOTE: Dashes indicate that the criterion was not reported for that population.

[a] Data for postpartum women were not readily available.

SOURCE: Adapted from USDA (1994).

gories of risk criteria as predictive of risk or benefit appears in Table 6-2. The names of some of the risk criteria used by this committee differ from some of those reported by state WIC agencies to increase specificity.

INAPPROPRIATE DIETARY PATTERNS

As used by WIC state agencies, the term *inappropriate dietary pattern* encompasses many dietary risk criteria (see Table 6-1). These include overall descriptors of dietary patterns, developmentally or age-inappropriate patterns of feeding, and identification of the ingestion of specific inappropriate substances. This section addresses the major nutrition risk criteria for an inappropriate dietary pattern.

Dietary Patterns That Fail to Meet Dietary Guidelines for Americans

Dietary Guidelines for Americans (USDA/DHSS, 1995) is designed to help Americans over 2 years of age to consume diets that will meet nutrient requirements, promote health, support active lives, and reduce chronic disease risks. These guidelines suggest the following goals for daily fat intake: no more than 30 percent of total calories from fat, less than 10 percent of calories from saturated fat, less than 300 mg of cholesterol, and less fat from animal sources. The guidelines recommend using sugar in moderation and choosing a diet moderate in salt and sodium. The Food Guide Pyramid, which is incorporated in

TABLE 6-2 Summary of Broad Dietary Risk Criteria as Predictive of Risk or Benefit Among Women, Infants, and Children

Risk Criterion[a]	Women Risk	Women Benefit	Infants Risk	Infants Benefit	Children Risk	Children Benefit
Inappropriate diet	✓	✓			✓	✓
Inappropriate infant feeding[a]			✓	✓		
Caffeine intake	0	?			?	?
Pica	✓	?			✓	✓
Inadequate diet	✓[b]	✓[b]	✓	✓	✓[b]	✓[b]
Food insecurity	✓	✓	✓	✓	✓	✓

NOTE: ✓ = predictive of risk or benefit; ? = no evidence; 0 = evidence, but no effect; blank = not applicable to that group.

[a] Guidelines also apply to children 1 to 2 years of age.
[b] Current assessment methods are inadequate for targeting.

the *Dietary Guidelines,* recommends numbers of servings from each of five food groups. These recommendations include eating 6 to 11 servings of grain products; 3 to 5 servings of vegetables; 2 to 4 servings of fruits; 2 to 3 servings of meat, fish, poultry, or legumes; and 2 to 3 servings of milk products daily (USDA, 1995).

Prevalence of Dietary Patterns That Fail to Meet Dietary Guidelines for Americans

Information about dietary patterns of low-income women and children has been obtained using data from the second National Health and Nutrition Examination Survey (NHANES II), a nationally representative sample of individuals surveyed from 1976 to 1980 (USDA, 1987). In that study, a "food group deficiency" for the individual was defined as an average daily intake (in number of servings per day) of any one of the food groups that fell below the following cutoffs:

Food Group	Children	Pregnant Women
Bread and Cereals	less than 4	less than 3
Fruits and Vegetables	less than 4	less than 3
Milk and Dairy	less than 3	less than 2
Meat and Protein	less than 2	less than 1

By applying these cutoffs to data from a 24-hour recall and a weekly-food-frequency recall, almost 60 percent of low-income women ages 12 to 49 years and 43 percent of children ages 12 months to 5 years were identified as having a dietary risk (called an inappropriate dietary pattern). No strong age relationships were found, but women younger than 18 years had a slightly lower dietary risk than older women (56 versus 60 percent). In children, the prevalence of inappropriate dietary patterns increased steadily with age, from 40 percent of those ages 1 to 2 years to 46 percent of those ages 4 to 5 years.

Using data from the 1989–1991 Continuing Surveys of Food Intakes by Individuals, Krebs-Smith and co-workers (1995) report a mean daily fruit and vegetable intake of 3.6 servings daily for individuals from households earning less than $10,000 per year, and increasing mean fruit and vegetable intake with increased household income. Over a 3-day period, 63 percent of individuals from households earning less than $10,000 per year consumed less than one serving of fruit per day, and 14 percent consumed less than one serving of vegetables per day.

Other studies have focused on the degree to which individuals of all income levels follow the Dietary Guidelines for fat and cholesterol intake. For children, identification of fat and cholesterol intakes exceeding the Dietary Guidelines is relevant only for those ages 2 years and older (USDA, 1995). Data from Phase I of the third National Health and Nutrition Examination Survey (NHANES III) (McDowell et al., 1994; CDC, 1994) and from the 1987–1988 National Food Consumption Survey (Johnson et al., 1994) indicate that the mean fat intake (expressed as a percentage of total dietary energy intake) remains above the recommended 30 percent for women ages 12 to 49 years and for children ages 3 to 5 (approximately 34 and 33 percent, respectively) (Johnson et al., 1994; Kennedy and Goldberg, 1995), regardless of income. The data show slightly higher fat intakes (average 36 percent of energy) by non-Hispanic black women.

Mean dietary cholesterol intakes for women and children were below the recommended daily consumption of 300 mg/day (McDowell et al., 1994); only 13 percent of children under 5 years had 3-day cholesterol intakes exceeding 300 mg.

About one-quarter of children had daily sodium intakes in excess of the recommended 2,400 mg.

Dietary Patterns That Fail to Meet Dietary Guidelines for Americans as an Indicator of Nutrition and Health Risk

Women. Dietary patterns that fail to meet Dietary Guidelines may provide lower than recommended amounts of essential nutrients. The fewer the number of servings from a food group, the greater the chance that nutrient intake will not cover nutrient needs. Such dietary patterns are associated with long-term risk of chronic diseases that are ordinarily diagnosed in middle age. These risks, however, are real and profound (Pennington, 1991). Cardiovascular disease, primarily atherosclerotic heart disease, is the most prevalent cause of death among postmenopausal women. Hypertension, a clear risk factor for both heart disease and stroke, is aggravated by high sodium intakes in sodium-sensitive individuals. A large body of literature supports the conclusions that chronically high intakes of total fat, saturated fat, and cholesterol contribute to risk of cardiovascular disease, heart attack, and premature mortality and that the relatively lower risk of cardiovascular disease enjoyed by women compared to men essentially disappears after menopause. High fat intake may also increase risk of certain kinds of cancer, such as breast cancer and colon cancer (Clifford and Kramer, 1993). Low intake of fruits and vegetables is associated with increased risk of many types of cancer (Graham et al., 1991; Landa et al., 1994; Shibata et al., 1992; Steinmetz et al., 1994; Tavani and LaVecchia, 1995). Low intake of milk products may contribute to later risk of osteoporosis (NIH, 1994). These are active research areas.

Children. As for women, dietary patterns that are low in basic food groups may provide lower than recommended nutrient intakes. Considerable controversy exists over the relevance to children of guidelines to reduce fat, saturated fat, and cholesterol consumption (Olson, 1995). Early concerns focused on case reports of the ill effects of overzealous restriction of dietary fat in children's diets by some health-conscious parents (Lifschitz and Moses, 1989; Pugliese et al., 1983). In those studies, the adverse effects on growth and nutrition status were likely due to failure to meet energy needs. Two recent studies addressed the adequacy of diets with fat intakes at a level of 30 percent of total calories for young children. One obtained multiple days of dietary data from 215 3- to 4-year-olds (Shea et al., 1993), and one studied 106 4-year-old Canadian children (Gibson et al., 1993). Both indicate that adequate energy intake, nutrient intake, and growth are quite possible with fat intakes at or slightly below 30 percent of total calories provided that low-fat dairy products are included in the diet.

Children with high serum cholesterol concentrations tend to continue to have high concentrations as adults (Lauer and Clarke, 1990). Data from two studies (Newman et al., 1991; PDAY Research Group, 1990) indicate that the earliest development of atherosclerotic lesions of the aorta in children appears to be related to concentrations of low-density lipoprotein and very-low-density lipoprotein cholesterol. Data from the Bogalusa Heart Study indicate that children with higher serum cholesterol concentrations have significantly higher fat intakes than children with lower serum cholesterol concentrations (Nicklas et al., 1989). The American Heart Association, the National Cholesterol Education Program, and the American Academy of Pediatrics all agree that dietary fat intake for children over the age of 2 years should average 30 percent of total calories and should be coupled with adequate dietary energy for growth and activity (CN-AAP, 1992b; DHHS, 1991).

Failure to Meet the Dietary Guidelines for Americans as an Indicator of Nutrition and Health Benefit

Increasing intake of fruits (including juices) and vegetables is associated with increased intake of vitamins A, C, and folate as well as many other micronutrients important to growth, reproduction, and health. The standard WIC package provides the equivalent of about one serving of vitamin C-rich fruit juice daily. High intake of calcium-rich milk products may reduce risk of developing preeclampsia (Repke, 1994). Milk products make a major contribution to supplying the calcium and other nutrients needed for growth, pregnancy, and breastfeeding. The standard WIC package provides the equivalent of three or more servings of milk daily.

Pregnancy and the early postpartum period may represent periods in women's lives when they are especially receptive to education and when they may be motivated to improve their own health and that of their families. However, the committee is aware of no studies that have addressed the effects of dietary change during pregnancy and the postpartum period on long-term dietary patterns in adult women. The opportunity to reach women with effective nutrition education can be used to provide and reinforce messages about the potential long-term health benefits of following the Dietary Guidelines and using the Food Pyramid (USDA, 1992).

The benefits from assessment and education to improve the composition of the diet to more closely approximate the Dietary Guidelines (USDA, 1995) for children older than 2 years of age are less clear, but following the guidelines clearly promotes a healthful diet, and the WIC food package can help achieve that goal.

Failure to Meet Dietary Guidelines for Americans as a Risk Indicator in the WIC Setting

Table 6-1 lists some parts of *Dietary Guidelines for Americans* (e.g., excessive consumption of sugar, fat, or sodium) that are used as nutrition risk criteria by WIC state agencies. Many states use a food group approach and categorize shortfalls in food group intake as dietary inadequacies rather than as inappropriate diet.

Tools and Cutoff Points to Assess Dietary Patterns That Fail to Meet the Dietary Guidelines for Americans

In the WIC program, data on dietary patterns are usually derived from brief 24-hour recalls or questions about the frequency of intake of food groups (Gardner et al., 1991). It is relatively easy to hand-tally numbers of servings from food groups, to compare the results with the recommended number of servings, and to use the results in nutrition education tailored to WIC program participants. Results from two food group scoring methods suggest that screening diets for food group consumption provides meaningful information about their quality (Guthrie and Scheer, 1981; Kant et al., 1991; Krebs-Smith and Clark, 1989), but the committee could find no evidence on which to single out the most effective method of comparing intake with the Dietary Guidelines. The North Dakota WIC program adopted, as its standard dietary assessment method, a computerized food frequency questionnaire that provides information about food group consumption and an index of nutritional quality (J. R. Rice, North Dakota Department of Health, personal communication, 1995).

Some evidence indicates that it is possible to identify dietary patterns with relatively high fat content through short assessment questionnaires. A number of investigators have developed and conducted validity studies on brief assessment instruments to identify individuals with high fat intakes (e.g., Ammerman et al., 1991; Block et al., 1989; Coates et al., 1995; Heller et al., 1981; Hopkins et al., 1989; Kinlay et al., 1991; Knapp et al., 1988; Kristal et al., 1989, 1990; Van Assema et al., 1992). Some of these are simplified, targeted food frequency-type instruments. Others focus on behaviors associated with fat intake. Scores obtained using these short questionnaires have compared favorably with estimates from multiple food records or more extensive questionnaires.

The committee is not aware of similar short instruments for identifying high sodium intakes. However, a brief screen for fruit, vegetable, and fiber intake is available (Serdula et al., 1993).

Cholesterol intake can be assessed with questions regarding the usual number of servings of the few concentrated sources of these compounds.

In general, brief dietary assessment instruments offer significant time and cost advantages relative to traditional nutrient-based dietary approaches. Carefully designed instruments have often been shown to be as good as more complex methods in ranking individuals and identifying high or low levels of intake of a limited number of food groups or nutrients. They are, however, likely to be quite population specific, especially those that rely on eating and food preparation behaviors to identify extremes of intake (Thompson and Byers, 1994). Moreover, such instruments may have limited usefulness as nutrition education tools.

Recommendations for Dietary Patterns That Fail to Meet Dietary Guidelines for Americans

The risk of *dietary patterns that fail to meet Dietary Guidelines* is well documented for adults. The potential for benefit from participation in the WIC program is good on theoretical grounds. Therefore, the committee recommends use of *failure to meet Dietary Guidelines* as a nutrition risk criterion. The committee believes that any cutoff points would be arbitrary. The more generous the cutoff points, the higher the false positive rate and the lower the yield of benefit.

In addition, the committee recommends research to develop practical dietary assessment instruments to identify those who fail to meet Dietary Guidelines and to test their validity in WIC program subgroups.

Vegetarian Diets

Vegetarian diets usually include at least a few kinds of foods of animal origin, most commonly eggs and dairy products. Vegan diets are complete vegetarian diets. That is, they exclude the use of animal foods of any type.

Prevalence of Vegetarian Diets

Liberal vegetarian diets are becoming much more common, with one survey finding 13.5 percent of U.S. households claiming at least one vegetarian member. This represents an eight-fold increase in vegetarianism between 1979 and 1992 (Johnston, 1994). The prevalence of vegans in the United States has been estimated from less than 1 percent (Vegetarian Resource Group, 1994) to as much as 5 to 6 percent (Johnston, 1994) of the population. The prevalence of adherence to various kinds of vegetarian diets among families with young children is not known. When the definition is restricted vegan diets, the prevalence is probably quite low.

Vegetarian Diets as an Indicator of Nutrition and Health Risk

Liberal vegetarian diets that include dairy products and eggs are generally high in essential nutrients and unlikely to pose health risks. In fact, vegetarian eating practices have been associated with good health (USDA, 1995). However, there is clear evidence that strict adherence to vegan diets places women and their infants at nutrition and health risk. Unless specially fortified foods are consumed, the diet lacks vitamins B_{12} and D, as reviewed in *Nutrition During Lactation* (IOM, 1991). Vitamin B_{12} deficiency has been found in breastfed infants of vegan mothers, and infants may develop clinical signs of deficiency before their mothers do. The more limited the diet, the greater the risk of serious nutrient deficiencies (Haddad, 1994). Inadequate energy intake may also occur if the diet is very high in bulk and low in fat.

Children reared in strict vegan families that permit no animal products at all are at risk of poor growth and, in northern parts of the United States, where insufficient exposure to sunlight may occur, vitamin D-deficiency rickets (Dwyer, 1991). Other nutrient deficiencies include vitamin B_{12} and sometimes calcium.

Vegetarian Diets as an Indicator of Nutrition and Health Benefit

Education is the principal intervention for most women and children at risk because of a vegan eating pattern. The eggs, milk, and cheese in the food package would not be consumed.

Tools and Cutoff Points to Assess Vegetarian Diets

Vegetarian and/or vegan diets in women and children can be assessed by asking a few well-targeted questions.

Recommendation for Vegetarian Diets

The risk from unfortified *vegan diets* is well documented. The potential to benefit from participation in the WIC program is expected to be good on theoretical grounds. Therefore, the committee recommends use of vegan dietary practices as a nutrition risk criterion for women, infants, and children.

Highly Restrictive Diets

Highly restrictive diets are diets that are very low in calories, that severely limit intake of important food sources of nutrients (e.g., fruit and nut diets), or otherwise involve high-risk eating patterns. A vegan diet is a type of restrictive diet that is covered in the previous section.

Prevalence of Highly Restrictive Diets

The prevalence of highly restrictive diets was unavailable to the committee but is believed to be quite low.

Highly Restrictive Diets as an Indicator of Nutrition and Health Risk

Highly restrictive diets severely limit nutrient intake, may interfere with growth if taken regularly, and, if very low in calories, may lead to a number of adverse physiological effects. Highly restrictive diets pose particular risks during pregnancy and lactation (IOM, 1990, 1991). For example, regular intake of fewer than 1,500 kcal may impair the milk production of lactating women (Strode et al., 1986).

Highly Restrictive Diets as an Indicator of Nutrition and Health Benefit

Given the clear health and nutrition risks associated with highly restrictive diets and the motivation of most women to optimize their own and their infant's health during the critical periods targeted by the WIC program, one might predict a good potential for benefit from WIC program participation. Essentially no evidence in the published literature supports this conclusion, however, perhaps because the prevalence of the patterns mentioned is low enough to make systematic study difficult.

Tools and Cutoff Points to Assess Highly Restrictive Diets

Several conditions indicating highly restrictive diets in women are assessed by asking a few well-targeted questions (e.g., see IOM, 1992). Dieting is so prevalent among U.S. women that it likely requires some specific probing to identify high-risk behaviors such as prolonged fasting, purging, or very low calorie diets.

Recommendation for Highly Restrictive Diets

There is theoretical evidence that *highly restrictive diets* pose health and nutrition risks. Potential for benefit from participation in the WIC program is expected to be good on theoretical grounds. Therefore, the committee recommends use of *highly restrictive diets* as a risk criterion in the WIC program.

Inappropriate Infant Feeding

Infant feeding practices include breastfeeding habits, the type of formula or milk fed, and the timing and contents of the supplemental foods and fluids introduced. The Committee on Nutrition of the American Academy of Pediatrics (CN-AAP) has set forth recommendations for feeding healthy infants (CN-AAP, 1980, 1992a, 1993), which are summarized briefly below.

During infancy, breast milk or an appropriate formula is the major source of nutrients. Breastfeeding is the preferred method of feeding infants (CN-AAP, 1993; IOM, 1991). Pediatricians and family physicians generally recommend the use of iron-fortified formulas if infants are fed formula (Fomon, 1993). American Academy of Pediatrics guidelines help breastfeeding mothers know that they are providing sufficient milk for their baby's health and growth (CN-AAP, 1993).

Infants should not be fed whole cow milk, skim milk, 1 or 2 percent fat milk, or evaporated milk formulas during the first 12 months of life (CN-AAP, 1992a, 1993). Solid foods should be introduced when an infant is able to sit with support and the infant has good control of the head and neck, usually at 4 to 6 months of age (CN-AAP, 1993). Solid foods of appropriate consistency should be started one at a time at weekly intervals to identify any food intolerance. Infants need dependable sources of iron after 4 to 6 months of age.

Prevalence of Inappropriate Infant Feeding

Over time, infant feeding practices have gradually become more consistent with the recommendations and guidelines of CN-AAP. Breastfeeding of newborns was twice as common in 1990 as it was in 1970 (CN-AAP, 1993), the feeding of cow milk to infants under 4 months of age is much less common (Fomon, 1987), and the feeding of solid foods to infants under 2 months of age is infrequent today (CN-AAP, 1993).

Nevertheless, data from national population-based surveys show that there is room for improvement of infant feeding practices. Data from the 1988 National Maternal and Infant Health Survey (NMIHS) show that only 24 percent of low-income infants and 32 percent of higher-income infants had feeding practices consistent with CN-AAP guidelines throughout their first 6 months. These percentages are so low largely because cow milk and solid foods are introduced before the age of 4 months. However, in the first month of life, guidelines were met by 85 percent of low-income infants participating in the WIC program, 89 percent of low-income infants not participating in WIC program, and 94 percent of higher-income infants (Gordon and Nelson, 1995).

Despite strong recommendations for breastfeeding by CN-AAP, infant formula tends to be the milk source chosen for most U.S. infants over much of their first year. In 1990, approximately half of all infants started breastfeeding while they were in the hospital (CN-AAP, 1993). However, the percentage of breastfeeding infants declined to 18 percent at age 6 months and to 6 percent by age 12 months.

Despite strong recommendations to the contrary, cow milk is fed to many infants, especially in the second 6 months of life. The percentage of infants fed either whole cow milk or evaporated milk formulas rose: from 5 percent at 6 months to 79 percent at 12 months of age (CN-AAP, 1993). The use of reduced-fat cow milk is also common. Market research data collected by Ross Laboratories during the early 1980s showed that of the infants ages 8 to 13 months consuming cow milk, 42 percent were fed reduced-fat milk (Fomon, 1987). Data were not available on the prevalence of other inappropriate infant feeding practices.

Inappropriate Infant Feeding as an Indicator of Nutrition and Health Risk

Most empirical evidence on the effects of inappropriate infant feeding focuses on the use of cow milk and shows that its use during the first 12 months is associated with at least two adverse outcomes. First, infants fed cow milk have poorer iron status, a higher prevalence of iron deficiency anemia, lower plasma iron concentrations, lower transferrin saturation concentrations, and lower plasma ferritin concentrations than those fed infant formula (Penrod et al., 1990). In part, this may be due to increased intestinal blood loss compared with infants fed formula (Wilson, 1984; Woodruff, 1983; Ziegler et al., 1990). Evidence also suggests that cow milk inhibits the availability of iron from such other dietary sources as infant cereals, most likely because of the high concentrations of calcium and phosphorus and the low concentration of ascorbic acid in cow milk (CN-AAP, 1993).

Second, infants fed cow milk have higher than recommended intakes of sodium, potassium, chloride, and protein and lower than recommended intakes of linoleic acid and vitamin E (CN-AAP, 1993; Martinez et al., 1985). The median potential renal solute load of diets of infants fed cow milk is substantially higher than that of diets of infants fed formula (Ernst et al., 1990; Martinez et al., 1985). In early infancy, diets high in potential renal solute load lead to dehydration more rapidly during episodes of fever and diarrhea.

The use of reduced-fat cow milk exacerbates the risks associated with cow milk, primarily because larger volumes are necessary to meet the energy needs of infants. Infants fed low-fat or skim milk tend to have inadequate food energy and linoleic acid intakes and very high protein intakes and potential renal solute loads (Ernst et al., 1990; Fomon, 1993).

Breastfed infants and infants who are fed formula that is not fortified with iron are subject to iron deficiency if they do not obtain adequate iron from solid foods or supplemental iron.

There are no known nutritional advantages to introducing solid foods before 4 to 6 months of age (CN-AAP, 1958, 1993). Although little evidence exists to document poor outcomes resulting from the early introduction of solid foods into infant diets, studies in developing countries clearly document the risk in environments in which sanitation is poor. The recommendation to delay the introduction of solid foods to U.S. infants generally reflects knowledge of the development of gastrointestinal function and nutrition needs (Weaver and Lucas, 1991). Adding such foods as infant cereals to bottles rather than spoon feeding is not recommended as this deprives children of the opportunity to learn to feed themselves (CN-AAP, 1993). This also increases risks from poor sanitation in young infants.

Other examples of inappropriate infant feeding practices include improper dilution of formula, feeding of sugar-based beverages (e.g., fruit flavored drinks) or other foods low in nutrient density in place of formula, and lack of sanitation in the preparation of nursing bottles. Such practices can lead to severely impaired growth, dehydration (from concentrated formula), and/or gastrointestinal infections. Infrequent breastfeeding as the sole source of nutrients can lead to serious undernutrition and dehydration.

Inappropriate Infant Feeding as an Indicator of Nutrition and Health Benefit

Although the evidence is indirect, by and large it suggests that educational efforts and food supplementation can improve infant feeding practices. Probably the strongest evidence comes from reviewing the trends in infant feeding discussed above, which show increased breastfeeding, decreased feeding of cow milk, and later introduction of solid foods for all U.S. infants (Fomon, 1993). In addition, data from the Pediatric Nutrition Surveillance System indicate that the prevalence of anemia among white low-income infants has decreased significantly over time, a finding largely attributed to improvements in status resulting from infants' participation in public health programs, especially the WIC program (Yip et al., 1992). Other studies also found that infant participation in the WIC program was associated with increased serum iron content and a lower incidence of iron deficiency anemia (Edozien et al., 1979; Miller et al., 1985).

Limited information is available on the effects of the WIC program and other nutrition education programs on the diets of low-income infants. A study among Hmong women at several WIC sites showed that a short-term nutrition education intervention increased the number of women who initiated breastfeeding and the duration of their breastfeeding (Tuttle and Dewey, 1995).

An early study (Edozien et al., 1979), subsequently corroborated by the National WIC Evaluation (Rush, 1988), found that WIC program participation was associated with higher iron and vitamin C intakes—nutrients supplied by the iron-fortified cereal and formula and the vitamin C-rich juices in the infant food package. Gordon and Nelson (1995) found that mothers of infant WIC participants and of income-eligible nonparticipants followed the CN-AAP guidelines to a similar extent during the first 4 months of feeding. Mothers of WIC infants were significantly more likely than mothers of income-eligible nonparticipants, however, to follow the CN-AAP guidelines in the fifth and sixth months, primarily because they were less likely to feed their infants cow milk in these months.

Tools and Cutoff Points to Assess Inappropriate Infant Feeding in the WIC Setting

Almost all states use inappropriate infant feeding as a nutrition risk criterion for infants. In general, inappropriate intake is assessed by either a 24-hour recall or specially targeted questions about infant feeding practices. In a field test of the impact of the WIC program on the growth and development of children, Puma and colleagues (1991) documented the inadequacies of using 24-hour recalls for assessing the dietary intakes of infants. These investigators examined infant feeding by asking a set of questions on breastfeeding, the type of milk or formula being used, the type of solid foods being consumed, and when these foods were introduced into infant diets. Similarly, the 1988 NMIHS included a series of questions on infant feeding practices that could be used in the WIC program setting to assess infant feeding practices (Gordon and Nelson, 1995).

Recommendation for Inappropriate Infant Feeding

Risks from most *inappropriate infant feeding practices* described above are well documented. Acceptable methods are available for identifying these practices. The potential for benefit from participation in the WIC program is expected to be good based on theoretical and indirect empirical evidence. Therefore, the committee recommends use of selected *inappropriate infant feeding practices* as risk criteria for use by all states, as listed in Table 6-3.

Inappropriate Use of Nursing Bottle

Rampant dental caries affecting the primary teeth of infants and young children can result from the practice of allowing the child to fall asleep with a bottle filled with a fermentable liquid (fruit juice, milk, or other beverage with added sugar). This form of caries is known by several names, including nursing bottle caries, baby bottle tooth decay, and nursing bottle syndrome.

Prevalence of Inappropriate Use of Nursing Bottle

Data on the prevalence of baby bottle tooth decay are inadequate because young children do not usually receive routine dental care or examinations. Reports have indicated that 2.5 to 14 percent of U.S. preschool age children show evidence of extensive tooth decay (Derkson and Ponti, 1982; Johnsen,

TABLE 6-3 Summary of Broad Dietary Risk Criteria and Committee Recommendations for the Specific WIC Population

Risk Criterion	Committee Recommendation	Pregnant Women	Postpartum Women Lactating	Postpartum Women Nonlactating	Infants	Children
Failure to meet Dietary Guidelines	Use; develop valid assessment tools	✓	✓	✓		✓
Vegan diets	Use	✓	✓	✓		✓
Other vegetarian diets	Do not use					
Highly restrictive diets	Use	✓	✓	✓		✓
Inappropriate infant feeding	Use				✓	
Early introduction of solid foods	Use				✓	
Feeding cow milk during 1st 12 months	Use				✓	
No dependable source of iron after 4–6 months	Use				✓	
Improper dilution of formula	Use				✓	
Feeding other foods low in essential nutrients	Use				✓	
Lack of sanitation in preparation of nursing bottles	Use				✓	
Infrequent breastfeeding as sole source of nutrients	Use				✓	
Inappropriate use of nursing bottle	Use				✓	

Excessive caffeine intake	Do not use			✓
Pica	Use	✓		
Inadequate diet	Do not use; use diet recall or FFQ to tailor nutrition education; develop valid assessment tools		✓	✓
Food insecurity	Use; develop valid assessment tools	✓	✓	

NOTE: ✓ = subgroup for which the recommendation applies; FFQ = food frequency questionnaire.

1984; Johnsen et al., 1984). Some subgroups are at higher risk, including low-income children and American-Indian children (Broderick et al., 1989; Nowjack and Gift, 1990).

Inappropriate Use of Nursing Bottle as an Indicator of Nutrition and Health Risk

The maxillary anterior teeth are affected first and most severely because of their prolonged and repeated exposure (Dilley et al., 1980; Fass, 1962; Fomon, 1993; Johnsen, 1984; Johnsen et al., 1984; Marks, 1951; Ripa, 1978). The fermentation of carbohydrates on the surface of the tooth produces organic acids that demineralize and destroy enamel, with subsequent tooth decay. Generally, many teeth are involved, the decay develops rapidly, and the decay occurs on surfaces normally thought to be at low risk for decay (Ripa, 1988).

If inappropriate use of the nursing bottle persists, the child is at substantial risk of painful toothaches, costly dental treatment, loss of primary teeth, and, sometimes, developmental lags in eating and chewing ability. Moreover, if the child continues to be bottle-fed well beyond the usual weaning period, there is a risk of decay of permanent teeth.

Inappropriate Use of Nursing Bottle as an Indicator of Nutrition and Health Benefit

Inappropriate use of nursing bottles is relatively easily identified in the WIC program setting and is most appropriately corrected with educational intervention. The potential for health, nutrition, and economic benefits from effective intervention is substantial.

Recommendation for Inappropriate Use of Nursing Bottle

The risk from *inappropriate use of nursing bottles* is well documented. The potential to benefit from participation in the WIC program is expected to be high based on theoretical evidence. Therefore, the committee recommends use of the nutrition risk criterion *inappropriate use of nursing bottle* by state WIC programs.

Inappropriate Diets in Children

Some state WIC programs use additional criteria for inappropriate diets for children including high intake of sugar or of high-calorie, low-nutrient snacks, use of skim or low-fat milk before age 2 years, and self-feeding difficulties. These are not discussed further since they are covered in other sections of the report. See the section "Dietary Patterns that Fail to Meet Dietary Guidelines for Americans" in this chapter and "Central Nervous System Disorders" in Chapter 5.

Excessive Caffeine Intake

Caffeine is a plant alkaloid found in coffee, tea, cocoa, cola beverages and some other soft drinks, chocolate, and over-the-counter medications including cold tablets, allergy and analgesic preparations, appetite suppressants, and stimulants (Dalvi, 1986; Watkinson and Fried, 1985). Chocolate and other confectioneries contain only minor amounts of caffeine.

Prevalence of Excessive Caffeine Intake

Women. Estimated average caffeine intakes during pregnancy for U.S. and Canadian women range from 99 to 270 mg/day (Beaulac-Baillargeon and Desrosiers, 1986; Graham, 1978; Srisuphan and Bracken, 1986; Tebbutt et al., 1984), and the prevalence of caffeine use during pregnancy has been estimated to range from 69 to 79 percent (Graham, 1978; Srisuphan and Bracken, 1986) to 90 to 98 percent (Beaulac-Baillargeon and Desrosiers, 1986; Hill, 1973; Watkinson and Fried, 1985). Heavier caffeine consumption among pregnant women has been found to be related to less formal education, older maternal age, greater gravity and parity, alcohol use, and cigarette smoking (Beaulac-Baillargeon and Desrosiers, 1986; Istvan and Martarazzo, 1984; Linn et al., 1982; Srisuphan and Bracken, 1986; Watkinson and Fried, 1985).

Children. The prevalence of high caffeine intakes in children served by the WIC program is unknown, but it is clear from the available data (Ellison et al., 1995) that almost all school age children consume some caffeine-containing beverages (e.g., soft drinks, iced tea, cocoa) and foods.

Excessive Caffeine as an Indicator of Nutrition and Health Risk

Women. Although substantial evidence indicates that caffeine in large doses is teratogenic in animals, there is no convincing evidence that it is associated with birth defects in humans (IOM, 1990). The available evidence is equivocal about whether consuming relatively large amounts of either caffeine or coffee reduces birth weight, increases the risk of spontaneous abortion (IOM,

1990; Armstrong et al., 1992; McDonald et al., 1992a, b), contributes to nutrient inadequacy (Morck et al., 1983; Pecoud et al., 1975; Watkinson and Fried, 1985), or has other adverse effects (Massey and Hollingbery, 1988a, b; Munoz et al., 1988). Caffeine consumed by lactating women passes into their milk. If the dose is sufficiently high, it may cause irritability in the infant (IOM, 1990).

Although the preponderance of current evidence is that women who ingest caffeine during pregnancy or lactation do not put their fetuses or infants at serious risk, there are recommendations to moderate such intake during these periods (FDA, 1980; IOM, 1990, 1991).

Children. Health or nutrition risks resulting from high levels of caffeine consumption by children are not clear. A variety of behavioral and metabolic abnormalities have been attributed to caffeine intake, but the results of the few studies are inconsistent (Ellison et al., 1995).

Excessive Caffeine Intake as an Indicator of Nutrition and Health Benefit

Without evidence of risk, there can be no evidence of benefit related to high caffeine consumption by women or children.

Tools and Cutoff Points to Assess Caffeine Intake

Caffeine intake can be assessed with questions regarding the usual number of servings of the few concentrated sources of these compounds.

Recommendation for Excessive Caffeine

Because of lack of evidence of nutrition risk, the committee recommends discontinuation of use of *excessive caffeine intake* as nutrition risk criterion by state WIC agencies.

Pica

Pica is a perceived craving for and ingestion of nonfood items, including, but not limited to, clay, starch (laundry and cornstarch), ice or freezer frost, dirt, and paint chips. Although pica is a long-standing dietary practice, little research on pica has been conducted over the last decade (Edwards et al., 1994; Horner, et al., 1991; Lacey, 1990). Reid (1992) identified pica as a culturally prescribed behavior in some groups.

Prevalence of Pica

Women. In the United States, pica has been observed primarily among low-income southern black pregnant women (Horner, et al., 1991). The true prevalence is unknown. In a cohort of 553 pregnant women in an urban environment, Edwards and colleagues (1994) found that 3 percent self-reported that they ate freezer frost, about 4 percent said that they ate ice, and over 1 percent reported that they ate starch. In this same group of women, 28 percent stated that they had seen others in their social network (mothers, other relatives, and pregnant women) eat nonfood items. Older studies reported higher prevalences (approximately 30 percent) of pica among pregnant women (Keith et al., 1968). A link between hunger and pica has been discussed because starch, in particular, offers a source of bulk and calories (Edwards et al., 1994).

Children. Since ingestion of lead-contaminated paint is the most common form of pica among young children, the prevalence of pica among young children can be indirectly inferred from the prevalence of elevated concentrations of lead in blood. See the section "Lead Poisoning" in Chapter 5.

Pica as an Indicator of Nutrition and Health Risk

Geophagy (eating clay or dirt) during pregnancy and as a traditional practice in the United States, South America, and Africa has been interpreted as offering beneficial anti-diarrheal properties or protection to prevent gastric distress (Vermeer, 1979, 1985) through the chemical binding properties of the clay matrix. The potential chelating action of the clay particles also is thought to bind minerals and hence to be a contributing cause of nutrient deficiencies (Arcasoy et al., 1978).

Many of the data on the health risks of pica are quite old, and the quality of the data is variable. The ingestion of significant amounts of clay or starch has been associated with a variety of poor pregnancy outcomes, including toxemia (Edwards et al., 1964; O'Rourke et al., 1967), maternal death (Key et al., 1981), prematurity (Sage, 1962), and low birth weight and poor functional status of infants (Edwards et al., 1964). Cases of toxemia, hypertension, and intestinal obstruction have been reported for women practicing pica during pregnancy (NRC, 1983).

The strongest and most persistent association of nutrition risk with pica is anemia in women. There has been a long debate over the direction of the association: whether anemia predisposes a woman to pica (Crosby, 1982; Keith et al., 1968, 1970), or whether anemia is the consequence of pica (Reid, 1992). The ingestion of large amounts of laundry starch or clay may not by itself inhibit the absorption of iron, but it may displace foods that contain iron (NRC,

1983; Talkington et al., 1969). Low intake of iron, folate, pyridoxine, magnesium, and zinc has been reported for women who were actively practicing pica (Edwards et al., 1994).

Pica as an Indicator of Nutrition and Health Benefit

Two studies report that craving for nonfood substances could be reduced or corrected with iron therapy (Lanzkowsky, 1959; Reynolds et al., 1977). Once pica is identified, the WIC program's food package, nutrition education, and referral for health care all offer the potential for nutrition and health benefit. The supplemental foods provided through the WIC program supply critical nutrients, but they cannot be expected to prevent adverse effects of the ingestion of lead or clay.

Tools and Cutoff Points to Assess Pica

Pica can be identified through specific questioning about consumption of specific nonfood substances. However, since the practice is widely known to be viewed negatively by health professionals, it may be underreported. For children, questions should be directed toward hand-to-mouth activity and environmental lead exposure.

Recommendation for Pica

The risk of *pica* is very high in children because of its link with lead poisoning (see Chapter 5). The potential for benefit from nutrition education and referral for children is expected to be good on theoretical grounds. The risk of *pica* for women is less well documented. The committee recommends use of *pica* as a nutrition risk criterion for children by all state WIC programs and for pregnant women in areas where the prevalence is high enough to justify it.

INADEQUATE DIET

Dietary inadequacy can be defined as food or nutrient intake insufficient to meet a specified percentage of Recommended Dietary Allowances (RDAs)—the nutrient intake recommendations of the Food and Nutrition Board, National Academy of Sciences (NRC, 1989).

Prevalence of Inadequate Diets

Existing data do not permit definitive statements about the prevalence of inadequate dietary intake among low-income women, infants, or children. Limitations arise from inconsistent definitions for an inadequate diet, unknown variations in the degree of undersampling of the poorest households, and more serious methodologic issues stemming from the inherent limitations of practical survey methods for measuring usual dietary intakes (Willett, 1990). There is indisputable evidence that the prevalence of diets that are low in nutrients when compared with the RDAs is very high among the population of women and children eligible for the WIC program. However, there is no other evidence of widespread nutrient deficiencies. Moreover, having a mean nutrient intake below the RDAs does not necessarily indicate the presence or likelihood of nutrition and health problems. When survey data are examined to estimate the prevalence of individual diets that fall below a specified percent of the RDA, the estimates of true low intake are known to be inflated (NRC, 1986). However, a higher prevalence of low nutrient intake for low-income groups than for higher-income groups is cause for concern, especially if there is other evidence of nutrient deficiencies among the low-income groups.

Cook and Martin (1995), using 1986 data from the Continuing Survey of Food Intake by Individuals (CSFII), examined the prevalence of nutrient intake below 70 percent of the RDA (averaged over 4 days of data collected over a 1-year period) for children ages 1 to 5 years defined as poor (household income < 130 percent of federal poverty guidelines) and nonpoor (household income ≥ 130 percent of federal poverty guidelines). Prevalence of low intakes ranged from 1.5-fold to several-fold higher for poor than for nonpoor children. Prevalence estimates exceeded 15 percent for low intakes of energy, vitamin C, and vitamin B_6 by poor children and 30 percent for vitamin E, iron, and zinc. However, data on weight-for-height of young children suggest that an energy deficit is an uncommon problem (see Chapter 4).

Similarly, among 3- to 5-year-old children in NHANES II, there were significant differences between poor and nonpoor children in the estimated prevalences of very low intakes (< 50 percent of the RDA) for vitamins A and C, calcium, and food energy. The relative risk of low intake among poor children ranged from approximately 1.3 to almost twice that among nonpoor children (Cook and Martin, 1995).

Inadequate Diet as an Indicator of Nutrition or Health Risk

There is no doubt that substantial nutrition and health risks result from diets that are truly inadequate in nutrients among pregnant and lactating women, infants, and young children. The adverse health consequences of specific nutrient deficiencies in pregnant and lactating women and in infants and young children are well documented (CN-AAP, 1993; IOM, 1990, 1991; NRC, 1989). Iron deficiency, the most common micronutrient deficiency among U.S. women and children, may increase the risk of low birth weight and pregnancy complications in pregnant women (IOM, 1990), result in reduced cognitive and intellectual functioning and development in infants and young children, and impair general well-being, work performance, and physical activity at all ages (Pollitt, 1994, 1995). Inadequate intake of folate around the time of conception has now been convincingly shown to increase the risk of neural tube defects (NTD), one of the most common congenital abnormalities—especially in women with a previously affected pregnancy (CDC, 1991; MRC Vitamin Study Research Group, 1991).

If intake of one or more vitamins or minerals is chronically very low, serious overt deficiency diseases can develop (e.g., rickets resulting from vitamin D deficiency). Suboptimal nutrient intakes may increase long-term impacts on morbidity and on risks of heart disease and cancer (Block, 1991; Knekt et al., 1991; Olson, 1993; Steinberg et al., 1992).

Among lactating women, low maternal intakes may have relatively little effect on the concentrations of iron, copper, zinc, calcium, and folate in breast milk but may lead to depleted maternal stores of these nutrients (IOM, 1991). Such depletion of stores compromises the mother's nutritional status, the health of subsequent infants, or both. Long-term deficiency of vitamin B_{12} intake by a lactating woman can lead to vitamin B_{12} deficiency in the infant (see the section "Vegetarian Diets").

Inadequate Diet as an Indicator of Nutrition and Health Benefit

A major goal of the WIC program is to improve the quality and sufficiency of diets consumed by low-income pregnant, postpartum, and breastfeeding women, infants, and children who are at nutrition risk. The nutritious foods provided by the WIC program can help correct subclinical deficiency states and replenish stores of many nutrients. The supplemental food package provided through the WIC program consists of foods chosen because they are concentrated sources of a number of nutrients believed to be in short supply in the diets of low-income women and children.

Evaluations of the WIC program indicate that the program has had positive and measurable effects in reducing the prevalence of iron deficiency anemia (Yip et al., 1987, 1992) and the incidence of low and very low birth weight (Devaney et al., 1992; Edozien et al., 1979; Kennedy et al., 1982; Metcoff et al., 1985). These reductions are likely mediated wholly or in part through dietary improvement. In addition, the program has been shown to be effective in improving dietary quality among children (Rush, 1988). Nutrition assessment and education in the program focus on diet in the prevention or amelioration of nutrition problems. Several studies of WIC program participants and other groups have shown nutrition education to be effective in changing both knowledge and attitudes about nutrition (Johnson and Johnson, 1985; Navaie et al., 1994), and such nutrition-related behaviors as meal planning, shopping, and food preparation (Koblinsky et al., 1992).

Use of Inadequate Diet as a Risk Indicator in the WIC Setting

Table 6-1 provides information about the use of inadequate diets as a nutrition risk criterion by WIC state agencies. The most often cited risk criteria are deficiencies in vitamins A, C, and D; iron; protein; and/or calcium (not shown). Many WIC programs report using "inadequate or excessive calorie intake" as a risk criterion. The RDA cutoff points reported to be used by WIC agencies in 1992 ranged from 66 to 100 percent of the RDA.

Tools and Cutoff Points to Assess Inadequate Diets

Dietary assessment is used to obtain presumptive evidence of dietary deficiencies or excesses in individuals. Self-report of recent or usual intake is the only practical approach in the WIC program setting. For women and children, the most commonly used instrument for assessment of dietary inadequacy in the WIC program is some type of food frequency questionnaire (FFQ), a 24-hour recall of food intake, or both.

The actual instruments used vary widely (Gardner et al., 1991), as do the guidelines for interpretation of the information obtained, including definitions of inadequacy. Twenty-four-hour recall data on food intake are generally interpreted either in terms of food groups (see previous section "Inappropriate Dietary Patterns") or in terms of the Recommended Dietary Allowances (RDA) (NRC, 1989).

Most FFQs used by the WIC program examine patterns of food intake and do not produce estimates of nutrient intake. Recently, FFQs have been developed that can provide computer-generated estimates of nutrient intakes and then compare them to the RDAs (Jacobson et al., 1990; USDA, 1994). Either a 24-hour recall of food intake or a food frequency questionnaire (FFQ) may be useful for nutrition education purposes, but each has different limitations when used as the basis for estimating adequacy of nutrient intake. Since 24-hour recalls or FFQs are methods currently in use in WIC programs, the performance of these measures in identifying inadequate diets among individuals is briefly reviewed.

Twenty-four-hour recalls. The major factor constraining the ability to infer usual intake from a recall of recent food intake (last 24 hours or the previous day's intake) is within-person variation in food intake over time, including day-to-day variation and periodic variation (e.g., day-of-the-week effects, effects related to the timing of household income, and seasonal effects) (Beaton et al., 1979; LSRO/FASEB, 1986; NRC, 1986). The ratio of within-person to between-person variance in nutrient intake from food intake data collected by a 24-hour recall is large enough that a single 24-hour period cannot be used with any reliability to assess the usual intakes of individuals. Single 24-hour recall data can be used to describe the mean intakes of populations or groups of people if the sample is large enough; the limitation is in the extrapolation of the data to the probability of the risk of deficiency or excess for an individual. For most nutrients, within-person variation can be reduced if the individual's mean of many days is used, but the number of days is so large as to be impractical in the WIC setting.

Food frequency assessments. Food frequency questionnaires or interviews theoretically provide relatively stable estimates of usual intakes because they cover an extended period: in the WIC program this is typically the previous week or month. With a food frequency instrument, a prespecified list of foods is used and the respondent is asked to estimate the frequency of consumption of each item. Compared with diet recalls, FFQs are less subject to omissions because of incomplete recall. Some FFQs ask the respondent to estimate usual portion sizes.

Most of the methodologic development and validation of food frequency instruments has been within the context of chronic disease epidemiology, rather than with attention to considerations of targeting. The Block FFQ (Block et al., 1986) was developed on the basis of 24-hour dietary recall collected from adults in NHANES II, including the major food sources of energy and 17 nutrients and incorporating the usual portion sizes of those foods. Validation studies of the original (100-item) version of the Block FFQ have been reported for a variety of adult groups (Block et al., 1990, 1992; Coates et al., 1991; Mares-Perlman et al., 1993; Sobell et al., 1989). Two new versions, one for children and one for women, have been developed and tested for use in WIC (USDA, 1994).

A second widely used food frequency questionnaire, available in several versions, was developed at Harvard University by Willett and others (Willett, 1990) and has been modified for several specific populations. The food lists were drawn from food records collected from participants in several different pilot studies. Validation studies have been reported for female nurses (Salvini et al., 1989; Willett et al., 1985, 1987), male health professionals (Feskanich et al., 1993; Rimm et al., 1992), low-income pregnant women (Suitor et al., 1989), and children (Stein et al., 1992). The Harvard FFQ has been adapted for use in the WIC program and tested for practicality in Massachusetts (M. Rodan, Georgetown University, personal communication, 1995). It provides an index of nutritional quality and information about food patterns, but it was intentionally designed not to automatically generate estimates of absolute nutrient intakes. (These estimates can be accessed for data analysis, however.)

Recently, Block and colleagues (USDA, 1994) completed a systematic validation study of both the Harvard and the Block FFQs with more than 600 individuals (pregnant, breastfeeding, and postpartum nonbreastfeeding women and children ages 1 to 5 years) within the WIC program setting. The sample included approximately equal numbers of black, Hispanic, and white subjects. These subjects were recruited from sites in four geographic areas of the country (Northeast, Pacific, South, and Midwest). Study participants completed either the Harvard FFQ or the Block FFQ, three nonconsecutive 24-hour dietary recalls (by telephone), and a second food frequency questionnaire. The multiple 24-hour dietary recall data were used as the standard of comparison for the nutrients targeted by the WIC program: protein, vitamin A, vitamin C, iron, and calcium. In addition, total energy intake was estimated.

The Block FFQ performed better than the Harvard FFQ for black and white women. For the Block FFQ, correlations with nutrient estimates from the three diet recalls were equal to or greater than 0.4, and the Block FFQ also showed more statistically significant ranking agreements by quartile than did the Harvard FFQ (six versus two). Neither FFQ performed well for Hispanic women or for children of any ethnic background. On the basis of that work, the authors recommended further research to develop appropriate food frequency questionnaires or methods of administration for Hispanic women. For children, they recommended further development and validation of a brief set of questions for assessing appropriate dietary intakes (USDA, 1994).

For black and white women, the Block FFQ performed as well as validated FFQs that are widely used in epidemiologic studies. Correlations of approximately 0.6, while considered acceptable for epidemiologic studies, result in much misclassification (and thus low yield of risk). Moreover, a substantial fraction (up to 15 to 20 percent) of WIC participants appear to have difficulty completing FFQs appropriately, with gross overestimation of intake the most common problem (P. Pehrsson, Nutrient Data Laboratory, USDA Agricultural Research Service, personal communication, 1995; Suitor et al., 1989; USDA, 1994).

Interpretation of Nutrient Intake Data

When data from a 24-hour recall or a quantitative food frequency assessment are to be converted to estimates of nutrient intakes, they must be processed through a computerized program that matches data on foods and serving sizes to data on the nutrient composition of food items. Increasingly, nutrient analysis software is becoming available in clinic-adapted forms. However, to date, only the North Dakota WIC program has computerized its system for collecting dietary data. Thus, comparison of calculated nutrient intake values with a standard such as the RDAs is impractical as an eligibility criterion in most settings.

Block's recent study, which analyzed data from multiple nonconsecutive days of intake recall, indicates that if intake of a single nutrient below 100 percent of the RDA were used as a cutoff point, essentially all of the women eligible for WIC program participation on the basis of income would be considered at risk (USDA, 1994). However, except for energy, RDAs are set high enough to provide for adequate estimated intakes for essentially all of the healthy population; thus, the majority of the population will have adequate intakes at levels below the RDAs.

The use of self-reported food intake, whether by 24-hour recalls or food frequency methods, is not a valid method of estimating calorie intake. Whether the dietary information is obtained by 24-hour recalls or FFQs, heavy adults and adolescents fairly consistently underreport their total energy intakes, and mothers may overreport the energy intakes of their young children. More appropriate ways to identify inadequate energy intake are assessment of weight-for-height and change in weight, and asking questions designed to elicit information about access to food.

Recommendations for Inadequate Diet

There is no doubt that if true inadequate nutrient intake could be identified with sensitivity and specificity, *inadequate diet* would constitute a high priority nutrition risk criterion. If the usual intake of any of the nutrients targeted by the WIC program is truly low, there is also no doubt that the WIC program's food package and nutrition education would result in a nutrition and health benefit. However, the assessment tools currently in use for identifying usual nutrient intakes have very low yield. That is, of the individuals identified to have a nutrition risk, a high proportion may not actually be at risk for inadequate diet. Moreover, a high proportion of false negatives is also likely.

Therefore, the committee recommends discontinuation of use of *inadequate diet* as a nutrition risk criterion. For similar reasons, the committee recommends discontinuation of *excessive caloric intake* as a nutrition risk criterion. Nonetheless, the value of collecting information about food intake as a basis for well-targeted nutrition education in the WIC program provides strong support for continued use of diet assessment. Research is urgently needed to develop practical and valid assessment tools for the identification of inadequate diets.

FOOD INSECURITY

Definition of Food Insecurity

The term *food security* was first used in the international development literature in the 1960s. By the mid-1980s, national and regional definitions reflected concern about the food security of households, recognizing that limited access to food supplies at the level of the household (consumption unit) is a primary determinant of malnutrition (Maxwell and Frankenberger, 1992; Bickel et al., 1995). Attention was directed to the generally understood but ill-defined concept of "hunger," and the multiple social and health effects of poverty (Mayer, 1990). During the 1980s, several groups conducted substantial theoretical and empirical work from which to develop measurement tools for hunger and risk of hunger (Campbell, 1991; FCS, 1994; Margen and Neuhauser, 1987; Mayer, 1990, and accompanying papers; Radimer et al., 1990, 1992; Wehler et al., 1992). The important theoretical contribution of these efforts was the concept and empirical demonstration of hunger as an active "managed process" of adaptation and coping (Radimer et al., 1990, 1992). This concept was congruent with the work in international contexts that described a sequence of progressively less reversible management decisions by which households cope with food scarcity and shortage (Maxwell and Frankenberger, 1992).

The incorporation of the concern with household-level "hunger" into the notion of household-level food insecurity in the United States was articulated clearly for the first time by a Life Sciences Research Organization expert panel in 1990. This panel clearly defined food security, food insecurity, and hunger in the U.S. context, as follows (LSRO/FASEB, 1990):

Food Security is access ... at all times to enough food for an active, healthy life and includes at a minimum: a) the ready availability of nutritionally adequate and safe foods, and b) the assured ability to acquire acceptable foods in socially acceptable ways.

Food Insecurity exists whenever the availability of nutritionally adequate and safe foods or the ability to acquire acceptable foods in socially acceptable ways is limited or uncertain.

Hunger, in its meaning of the uneasy or painful sensation caused by a lack of food, is in this definition a potential, although not necessary, consequence of food insecurity. Malnutrition is also a potential, although not necessary, consequence of food insecurity.

Since the federal definition of poverty is based on the ability to purchase the USDA Thrifty Food Plan with no more than one-third of the household's income, households with incomes below the poverty level might be considered by definition to be suffering from food insecurity. In some areas, high relative costs of such other necessities as housing and utilities place individuals at risk of food insecurity even if their incomes are considerably above the official poverty level. In a recent analysis of the 1986 CSFII, Cook and Martin (1995) demonstrated a higher prevalence of low energy intakes (< 50 percent of the RDA) among children ages 3 to 5 years in households with incomes less than 130 percent of the federal poverty level versus those in households with incomes higher than that cutoff.

Prevalence of Food Insecurity

The prevalence of food insecurity is assumed to be high based on the income eligibility criteria for WIC participation. The concept of food insecurity as a measurable and scalable continuum rather than as a dichotomous variable underlies current efforts to develop adequate tools to measure prevalence. A basic question on food security was included in the 1977–1978 NFCS, when for the first time respondents were asked to describe the food eaten in their household as "enough and the kind we wanted to eat"; "enough, but not always the kind we wanted to eat"; "sometimes not enough to eat"; and "often not enough to eat." This question has also been incorporated in the CSFII surveys. NHANES III incorporated a modification of the question plus some indicators adapted from the work by Wehler and colleagues (Briefel and Woteki, 1992).

In 1992, the National Nutrition Monitoring and Related Research Program recommended that the USDA and the National Center for Health Statistics develop a standardized mechanism, instrument, and associated methodologies for defining and obtaining data on the prevalence of "food insecurity" or "food insufficiency" in the United States (*Federal Register* 58(32):752–806). In response to this and earlier mandates, an instrument was developed that includes a series of questions designed to measure food shopping behavior (all households). For those households with income and expenditure patterns that indicate risk of food insecurity, the instrument includes sections on food sufficiency, coping mechanisms and food scarcity, and concern about food sufficiency. The aim was to develop a scaled, ordinal measure of the degree of household food insecurity that would lead to empirically based categories of (1) food secure households; (2) mild (Level 1) food insecurity; (3) more serious (Level 2) food insecurity; and, (4) severe (Level 3) food insecurity. The data for validation of this tool were collected as part of the supplement to the Current Population Survey by the Bureau of the Census in April 1995. Analyses of those data are not available at this writing but should provide a basis for prevalence estimates in the population and in various subgroups. No data on the proportion of WIC program participants who meet any particular criterion for food insecurity, beyond the income levels that certify them for participation in the program, were available to the committee.

Food Insecurity as a Predictor of Nutrition and Health Risk

Few published data directly link measures of household food insecurity to dietary quality or indices of malnutrition. However, food insecurity is a logical mediating variable between poverty and poor dietary quality and indices of malnutrition (particularly iron deficiency) that are strongly related to poverty. Available data indicate that homeless individuals, among whom food insecurity is almost certain, have diets low in dairy products, fruits and vegetables, and whole grains (Cohen et al., 1992). The 1989–1991 CSFII showed somewhat lower total energy intakes and a higher proportion of dietary energy from fat in children from less food-secure households (Kennedy and Goldberg, 1995).

Aside from the direct linkages of food insecurity with poor diet and poor nutrition status, food insecurity likely leads to preventable non-nutrition-related health risks. When income is sufficiently low that food cannot be reliably purchased in sufficient quantities, other unessential expenditures are bound to be curtailed by households. Thus, needed medical care, especially for preventive services for women and children may not be sought even if there is no direct charge, because of transportation costs, lost wages, or other factors.

Food insecurity itself may be regarded as a poor nutrition outcome, apart from the dietary, nutrition, and health risks that it may create (Campbell, 1991). The right to access to adequate food, particularly for children, has been codified in numerous international documents and declarations (Eide et al., 1992; Kent, 1993), including the United Nations Children's Fund's "Declaration on the Rights of the Child," to which the United States became a signatory in early 1995.

Food Insecurity as a Predictor of Nutrition and Health Benefit

The WIC program is designed specifically to provide enhanced nutrition and health care during vulnerable periods of growth and development. It is logical to assume that the benefit from food, nutrition education, and referrals will be greatest for individuals residing in households where the food supply is least assured and least adequate.

Limited data from the United States and other countries indicate that infants and young children tend to be relatively protected by families during periods when food is in short supply because adults and older children in the household tend to make food available by decreasing their food intakes (Harrison and Muramoto, 1994; Neumann et al., 1989; Radimer et al., 1992). The provision of adequate and nutritious food to infants through the WIC program, and the provision of food supplements for their mothers and young siblings, spares the household's resources and thus may benefit all household members, even those who do not partake directly of the WIC program's food package.

Assessing Food Insecurity in the WIC Setting

In 1992, only one state WIC agency (Montana) reported using hunger or food insecurity as a criterion for WIC program eligibility (Montana WIC Program Policy Statement, 1992).

Tools and Cutoff Points to Assess Food Insecurity

In the WIC setting, the focus should be on identification of individuals truly experiencing hunger or at risk for hunger through intermittent or continuing household food insecurity of a moderate or severe degree. Available brief assessment tools and the rapidly evolving work on measurement tools related to food insecurity provide resources for the WIC program to consider when developing such tools for the WIC population. Development and validation of appropriate assessment tools for the WIC setting should have high priority.

Recommendations for Food Insecurity

Food insecurity presents risks of malnutrition and unhealthful dietary patterns in both the present and the future. Furthermore, food insecurity can be considered a concern in its own right. Because of the fundamental relationship of food availability to nutrition and health, the committee assumes that identification of true food insufficiency in the WIC program setting would ordinarily result in certification for eligibility of those who are at nutrition and health risk. The potential to benefit from WIC participation is expected to be high on theoretical grounds. Therefore, the committee recommends use of *food insecurity* as a risk criterion and further research to specify better the overall yield of benefit and the components of that yield.

SUMMARY

Assessment of dietary intake and eating practices is integral to the WIC program. Such assessment focuses attention on food and diet as central to health, provides a basis to tailor the educational and referral components of WIC program interventions, and may be used as a basis for determining program eligibility. See Table 6-3 above for the committee's recommendations for dietary risk criteria.

Review of data on use of the food frequency questionnaire or 24-hour recall of food intake to identify nutrient inadequacy indicates the yields of these techniques are likely to be quite low. Thus, the committee recommends that they not be used for this purpose in the WIC program, but modifications of these tools may be useful for identifying inappropriate diet. Since the whole-diet approach to assessment focuses attention on diet in relation to health and provides a basis for nutrition education, use of diet recalls or food frequency questionnaires is recommended for this purpose.

Given the limitations of the methods used for the assessment of dietary risks, research efforts should be undertaken to develop, refine, and validate practical assessment tools that can be used to detect *inappropriate diet, inadequate diet,* and *food insecurity* in the context of the WIC program.

REFERENCES

Ammerman, A.S., P.S. Haines, P.F. DeVellis, D.S. Strogatz, T.C. Keyserling, R.J. Simpson, Jr., and D.S. Siscovik. 1991. A brief dietary assessment to guide cholesterol reduction in low-income individuals: Design and validation. J. Am. Diet. Assoc. 91:1385–1390.

Arcasoy, A., A.O. Cavdar, and E. Babacan. 1978. Decreased iron and zinc absorption in Turkish children with iron deficiency and geophagia. Acta Haemat. 60:76–84.

Armstrong, B.G., A.D. McDonald, and M. Sloan. 1992. Cigarette, alcohol, and coffee consumption and spontaneous abortion. Am. J. Public Health 82:85–87.

Beaton, G.H., J. Milner, P. Corey, V. McGuire, M. Cousins, B. Stewart, M. de Ramos, D. Hewitt, B. Grambasch, N. Kassim, and J.A. Little. 1979. Sources of variance in 24-hour dietary recall data: Implications for nutrition study design and interpretation. Am. J. Clin. Nutr. 32:2546–2559.

Beaulac-Baillargeon, L., and C. Desrosiers. 1986. Profile of the consumption of caffeine, cigarettes and alcohol by women in Quebec during pregnancy. Union Med. Can. 115:813–817, 821.

Bickel, G., M. Andrews, and B. Klein. 1995. Measuring the food security of the American people: The Food Security Supplement to the Current Population Survey. Forthcoming, Food and Consumer Services, U.S. Department of Agriculture.

Block, G. 1991. Vitamin C and cancer prevention: The epidemiologic evidence. Am. J. Clin. Nutr. 53:270S–282S.

Block, G., A.M. Hartman, C.M. Dresser, M.D. Carroll, J. Gannon, and L. Gardner. 1986. A data-based approach to diet questionnaire design and testing. Am. J. Epidemiol. 124:453–469.

Block, G., C. Clifford, M.D. Naughton, M. Henderson, and M. McAdams. 1989. A brief dietary screen for high fat intake. J. Nutr. Educ. 21:199–207.

Block, G., M. Woods, A. Potosky, and C. Clifford. 1990. Validation of a self-administered diet history questionnaire using multiple diet records. J. Clin. Epidemiol. 43:1327–1335.

Block, G., F.E. Thompson, A.M. Hartman, F.A. Larkin, and K.E. Guire. 1992. Comparison of two dietary questionnaires validated against multiple dietary records collected during a 1-year period. J. Am. Diet. Assoc. 92:686–693.

Briefel, R.R., and C.E. Woteki. 1992. Development of food sufficiency questions for the Third National Health and Nutrition Examination Survey. J. Nutr. Educ. 24:24S–28S.

Broderick, E., J. Maby, D. Robertson, and J. Thompson. 1989. Baby bottle tooth decay in Native American Children in Head Start centers. Public Health Rep. 104:50–54.

Campbell, C.C. 1991. Food insecurity: A nutritional outcome or a predictor variable? J. Nutr. 121:408–415.

CDC (Centers for Disease Control). 1991. Use of folic acid for prevention of spina bifida and other neural tube defects—1983–1991. Morbid. Mortal. Weekly Rep. 40:513–516.

CDC (Centers for Disease Control). 1994. Daily dietary fat and total food-energy intakes—NHANES III, Phase 1, 1988–1991. J. Am. Med. Assoc. 271:1309.

Clifford, C., and B. Kramer. 1993. Diet as risk and therapy for cancer. Med. Clin. N. Am. 77:725–744.

CN-AAP (Committee on Nutrition, American Academy of Pediatrics). 1958. On the feeding of solid foods to infants. Pediatrics 21:685–692.

CN-AAP (Committee on Nutrition, American Academy of Pediatrics). 1980. On the feeding of supplemental foods to infants. Pediatrics 65:1178–1181.

CN-AAP (Committee on Nutrition, American Academy of Pediatrics). 1992a. The use of whole cow's milk in infancy. Pediatrics 89:1105–1109.

CN-AAP (Committee on Nutrition, American Academy of Pediatrics). 1992b. Statement on cholesterol. Pediatrics 90:469–472.

CN-AAP (Committee on Nutrition, American Academy of Pediatrics). 1993. Pediatric Nutrition Handbook, 3rd ed., L.A. Barness, ed. Elk Grove Village, Ill.: American Academy of Pediatrics.

Coates, R.J., J.W. Eley, G. Block, E.W. Gunter, A.L. Sowell, C. Grossman, and R.S. Greenberg. 1991. An evaluation of a food frequency questionnaire for assessing dietary intake of specific carotenoids and vitamin E among low-income black women. Am. J. Epidemiol. 134:658–671.

Coates, R.J. M.K. Serdula, T. Byers, A. Mokdad, S. Jewell, S.B. Leonard, C. Ritenbaugh, P. Newcomb, J. Mares-Perlman, N. Chavez et al. 1995. A brief, telephone-administered food frequency questionnaire can be useful for surveillance of dietary fat intakes. J. Nutr. 125:1473–1483.

Cohen, B.E., N. Chapman, and M.R. Burt. 1992. Food sources and intake of homeless persons. J. Nutr. Educ. 24:45S–51S.

Cook, J.T., and K.S. Martin. 1995. Differences in Nutrient Adequacy Among Poor and Non-Poor Children. Boston: Center on Hunger, Poverty and Nutrition Policy, Tufts University School of Nutrition.

Crosby, W.H. 1982. Clay ingestion and iron deficiency anemia. Ann. Intern. Med. 97:465.

Dalvi, R.R. 1986. Acute and chronic toxicity of caffeine: A review. Vet. Hum. Toxicol. 28:144–150.

Derkson, G.D., and P. Ponti. 1982. Nursing bottle syndrome, prevalence and etiology in a non-fluoridated city. J. Can. Dent. Assoc. 48:389–393.

Devaney, B., L. Bilheimer, and J. Schore. 1992. Medicaid costs and birth outcomes: The effects of prenatal WIC participation and the use of prenatal care. J. Policy Anal. Manage. 11:573–592.

DHHS (U.S. Department of Health and Human Services). 1991. Report of the Expert Panel on Blood Cholesterol Levels in Children and Adolescents. DHHS publication No. 91-2732. September. Washington, D.C.: USDHHS.

Dietz, W.H., Jr., and J.T. Dwyer. 1983. Nutritional implications of vegetarianism for children. Pp. 179–188 in Textbook of Pediatric Nutrition, R.M. Suskind, ed. New York: Raven Press.

Dilley, G.J., D.H. Dilley, and J.B. Machen. 1980. Prolonged nursing habits: A profile of patients and their families. J. Dent. Child. 47:102–108.

Edozien, J.C., B.R. Switzer, and R.B. Bryan. 1979. Medical evaluation of the Special Supplemental Food Program for Women, Infants and Children. Am. J. Clin. Nutr. 32:677–692.

Edwards, C.H., A.A. Johnson, E.M. Knight, U.J. Oyemade, O.J. Cole, O.E. Westney, S. Jones, H. Laryea, and L.S. Westney. 1994. Pica in an urban environment. J. Nutr. 954S–962S.

Edwards, E.H., S. McDonald, J.R. Mitchell, L. Jones, L. Mason, and L. Trigg. 1964. Effect of clay and cornstarch on women and their infants. Am. Diet. Assoc. 44:109–115.

Eide, A., A. Oshaug, and W.B. Eide. 1992. Food security and the right to food in international law and development. Transnational Law and Contemporary Problems 1:415–467.

Ellison, C., M.R. Singer, L.L. Moore, U.D.T. Nguyen, E.J. Garrahie, and J.K. Marmor. 1995. Current caffeine intake of young children: Amount and sources. J. Am. Diet. Assoc. 95:802–804.

Ernst, J.A., M.S. Brady, and K.A. Rickard. 1990. Food and nutrient intake of 6- to 12- month old infants fed formula or cow milk: A summary of four national surveys. J. Pediatr. 117:S86–S100.

Fass, E.N. 1962. Is bottle feeding of milk a factor in dental caries? J. Dent. Child. 29:245–251.

FCS (Food and Consumer Service, U.S. Department of Agriculture). 1994. Conference on Food Security Measurement and Research: Papers and Proceedings. Washington D.C.

FDA (U.S. Food and Drug Administration). 1980. Caffeine and pregnancy. FDA Drug Bull. 10:19–20.

Feskanich, D., E.B. Rimm, E.L. Giovannucci, G.A. Colditz, M.J. Stampfer, L.B. Litin, and W.C. Willett. 1993. Reproducibility and validity of food intake measurements from a semiquantitative food frequency questionnaire. J. Am. Diet. Assoc. 93:790–796.

Fomon, S.J. 1987. Reflections on infant feeding in the 1970s and 1980s. Am. J. Clin. Nutr. 46:171–182.

Fomon, S.J. 1993. Nutrition of Normal Infants. St. Louis, Mo.: Mosby-Year Book, Inc.

Gardner, J.P., C.J. Suitor, J. Witschi, and Q. Wang. 1991. Dietary Assessment Methodology for Use in the Special Supplemental Food Program for Women, Infants and Children (WIC). Report to the U.S. Department of Agriculture. Boston: Harvard School of Public Health, July 1991.

Gibson, R., C. MacDonald, R.D. Smit-Vanderkoov, C.E. McLennan, and N. Mercer. 1993. Dietary fat patterns of some Canadian preschool children in relation to indices of growth, iron, zinc and dietary status. J. Can. Diet. Assoc. 54:33–37.

Gordon, A., and L. Nelson. 1995. Characteristics and Outcomes of WIC Participants and Nonparticipants: Analysis of the 1988 National Maternal and Infant Health Survey. Alexandria, Va.: Mathematica Policy Research, Inc., January 1995.

Graham, D.M. 1978. Caffeine: Its identity, dietary sources, intake and biological effects. Nutr. Rev. 36:97–102.

Graham, S., R. Hellmann, J. Marshall, J. Freudenheim, J. Vena, M. Swanson, M. Zielezny, T. Nemoto, N. Stubbe, and T. Raimondo. 1991. Nutritional epidemiology of postmenopausal breast cancer in western New York. Am. J. Epidemiol. 134:552–566.

Guthrie, H.A., and J.C. Scheer. 1981. Validity of a dietary score for assessing nutrient adequacy. J. Am. Diet. Assoc. 78:240–245.

Haddad, E.H. 1994. Development of a vegetarian food guide. Am. J. Clin. Nutr. 59:1248S–1254S.

Harrison, G.G., and M. L. Muramoto. 1994. Relationship of food security to dietary quality and nutritional status in highland Lesotho. Abstracts of the American Public Health Association, Washington D.C.

Heller, R.F., H.D. Pedoe, and G. Rose. 1981. A simple method of assessing the effect of dietary advice to reduce plasma cholesterol. Prev. Med. 10:364–370.

Hill, R.M. 1973. Drugs ingested by pregnant women. Clin. Pharmacol. Ther. 14:654–659.

Hopkins, P.N., R.R. Williams, H. Kuida, B.M. Stults, S.C. Hunt, G.K. Barlow, and K.O. Ash. 1989. Predictive value of a short dietary questionnaire for changes in serum lipids in high-risk Utah families. Am. J. Clin. Nutr. 50:292–300.

Horner, R.D., C.J. Lackey, and K. Warren. 1991. Pica practices of pregnant women. J. Amer. Diet. Assoc. 91:34–38.

IOM (Institute of Medicine). 1990. Nutrition During Pregnancy. Part I, Weight Gain; Part II, Nutrient Supplements. Report of the Subcommittee on Nutritional Status and Weight Gain During Pregnancy and Subcommittee on Dietary Intake and Nutrient Supplements During Pregnancy, Committee on Nutritional Status During Pregnancy and Lactation, Food and Nutrition Board. Washington, D.C.: National Academy Press.

IOM (Institute of Medicine). 1991. Nutrition During Lactation. Report of the Subcommittee on Nutrition During Lactation, Committee on Nutritional Status During Pregnancy and Lactation, Food and Nutrition Board. Washington, D.C.: National Academy Press.

IOM (Institute of Medicine). 1992a. Nutrition During Pregnancy and Lactation: An Implementation Guide. Report of the Subcommittee for a Clinical Application Guide, Committee on Nutritional Status during Pregnancy and Lactation, Food and Nutrition Board. Washington, D.C.: National Academy Press.

Istvan, J., and J.D. Matarazzo. 1984. Tobacco, alcohol and caffeine use: A review of their interrelationships. Psychol. Bull. 95:301–326.

Jacobson, H.N., D.L. Taren, and V.L. Innis. 1990. The Development, Testing, and Evaluating of a Computer-Assisted Food Intake Assessment for the Florida WIC Program. Final Report. Tampa, Fla.: Department of Community and Family Health, College of Public Health, University of Florida.

Johnsen, D.C. 1984. Dental caries patterns in preschool children. Dent. Clin. North Amer. 28:3–20.

Johnsen, D.C., D.W. Schultz, D.B. Schubot, and M.V.V. Easley. 1984. Caries patterns in Head Start children in a fluoridated community. J. Publ. Health Dent. 44:61–66.

Johnson, R.K., H. Guthrie, H. Smiciklas-Wright, and M.Q. Wang. 1994. Characterizing nutrient intakes of children by sociodemographic factors. Public Health Rep. 109:414–420.

Johnson, D.W., and R.T. Johnson, eds. 1985. Nutrition Education: A Model for Effectiveness, a Synthesis of Research. J. Nutr. Educ. 17(suppl. 2)

Johnston, P.K. 1994. Preface to Proceedings of Second International Congress on Vegetarian Nutrition. Am. J. Clin. Nutr. 59:Svii.

Kant, A.K., A. Schatzkin, G. Block, R.G. Ziegler, and M. Nestle. 1991. Food group intake patterns and associated nutrient profiles of the U.S. population. J. Am. Diet. Assoc. 91:1532–1537.

Kennedy, E.T., and J. Goldberg. 1995. What are American Children Eating? Implications for Public Policy. Nutr. Rev. 53:111–126.

Kennedy, E.T., S. Gershoff, R. Reed, and J. Austin. 1982. Evaluation of the effect of WIC supplemental feeding on birthweight. J. Am. Diet. Assoc. 80:220–227.

Kent, G. 1993. Children's right to adequate nutrition. Int. J. Child. Rights 1:133–154.

Keith, L., E.R. Brown, and G. Rosenberg. 1970. Pica: The unfinished story. Background: Correlation with anemia and pregnancy. Perspect. Biol. Med. 626–632.

Keith, R.H., H. Evenhouse, and A. Webster. 1968. Amylophagia during pregnancy. Obstet. and Gynecol. 32:415–418.

Key, T.C., E.O. Harger, and J.M. Miller. 1981. Geophagia as cause of maternal death. Obstet. Gynecol. 60:525–526.

Kinlay, S., R.F. Heller, and J.A. Halliday. 1991. A simple score and questionnaire to measure group changes in dietary fat intake. Prev. Med. 20:378–388.

Knapp, J.A., H.P. Hazuda, S.M. Haffner, E.A. Young, and M.P. Stern. 1988. A saturated fat/cholesterol avoidance scale: Sex and ethnic differences in a biethnic population. J. Am. Diet. Assoc. 88:172–177.

Knekt, P., A. Aromaa, J. Maatela, R.K. Aaran, T. Nikkari, M. Hakama, T. Hakulinen, R. Peto, and L. Teppo. 1991. Vitamin E and cancer prevention. Am. J. Clin. Nutr. 53:283S–286S.

Koblinsky, S.A., J.F. Gutherie, and L. Lynch. 1992. Evaluation of a nutrition education program for Head Start parents. J. Nutr. Educ. 24:4–13.

Krebs-Smith, S.M., D.A. Cook, A.F. Subar, L. Cleveland, and J. Friday. 1995. U.S. adults' fruit and vegetable intakes, 1989 to 1991: A revised baseline for the Healthy People 2000 Objective. Am. J. Public Health 85:1623–1629.

Kristal, A.R., A.L. Shattuck, H.J. Henry, and A.S. Fowler. 1989. Rapid assessment of dietary intake of fat, fiber and saturated fat: Validity of an instrument suitable for community intervention research and nutritional surveillance. Am. J. Health Prom. 4:288–295.

Kristal, A.R., A. Shattuck, and H.J. Henry. 1990. Patterns of dietary behavior associated with selecting diets low in fat: Reliability and validity of a behavioral approach to dietary assessment. J. Am. Diet. Assoc. 90:214–220.

Lacey, E.P. 1990. Broadening the perspective of pica: Literature review. Public Health Rep. 105:29–35.

Landa, M.C., N. Frago, and A. Tres. 1994. Diet and the risk of breast cancer in Spain. Eur. J. Cancer Prev. 3:313–320.

Lanzkowsky, P. 1959. Investigation into the aetiology and treatment of pica. Arch. Dis. Child. 34:140–148.

Lauer, R.M., and W.R. Clarke. 1990. Use of cholesterol measurements in childhood for the prediction of adult hypercholesterolemia. The Muscatine Study. J. Am. Med. Assoc. 264:3034–3038.

Lifshitz, F., and N. Moses. 1989. Growth failure: A complication of dietary treatment of hypercholesterolemia. Am. J. Dis. Child. 143:527–542.

Linn, S., S.C. Schoenbaum, R.R. Monson et al. 1982. No association between coffee consumption and adverse outcomes of pregnancy. New Engl. J. Med. 306: 141–145.

LSRO/FASEB (Life Sciences Research Office, Federation of American Societies for Experimental Biology). 1986. Guidelines for Use of Dietary Intake Data, S.A. Anderson, ed. Bethesda, Md.: LSRO/FASEB.

LSRO/FASEB (Life Sciences Research Office, Federation of American Societies for Experimental Biology). 1990. Core indicators of nutritional state for difficult to sample populations, S.A. Anderson, ed. J. Nutr. 120(11S):1559–1600.

Mares-Perlman, J.A., B.E. Klein, R. Klein, L.L. Ritter, M.R. Fisher, and J.L. Freudenheim. 1993. A diet history questionnaire ranks nutrient intakes in middle-aged and older men and women similarly to multiple food records. J. Nutr. 123:489–501.

Margen, S., and L. Neuhauser. 1987. Hunger Surveys in the United States: Report of a Workshop. Berkeley, Calif.: University of California.

Marks, E.F. 1951. Infant feeding relative to the incident of dental caries. Am. J. Dent. 55:129–131.

Martinez, G.A., A.S. Ryan, and D.J. Malec. 1985. Nutrient intakes of American infants and children fed cow's milk or infant formula. Am. J. Dis. Child. 139:1010–1018.

Massey, L.K., and P.W. Hollingbery. 1988a. Acute effects of dietary caffeine and aspirin on urinary mineral excretion in pre- and postmenopausal women. Nutr. Res. 8:848–851.

Massey, L.K., and P.W. Hollingbery. 1988b. Acute effects of dietary caffeine and sucrose on urinary mineral excretion of healthy adolescents. Nutr. Res. 8:1005–1912.

Maxwell, S., and T Frankenberger. 1992. Household Food Security: Concepts, Indicators, Measurements. A Technical Review. New York and Rome: UNICEF and IFAD.

Mayer, J. 1990. Hunger and undernutrition in the United States. J. Nutr. 120:919–923.

McDonald, A.D., B.G. Armstrong, and M. Sloan. 1992a. Cigarette, alcohol, and coffee consumption and congenital defects. Am J Public Health 82:91–93.

McDonald, A.D., B.G. Armstrong, and M. Sloan. 1992b. Cigarette, alcohol, and coffee consumption and prematurity. Am J Public Health 82:87–90.

McDowell, M.A., R.R. Briefel, K. Alaimo, A.M. Bischof, C.R. Caughman, M.D. Carroll, C.M. Loria, and C.L. Johnson. 1994. Energy and Macronutrient Intakes of Persons Ages 2 Months and Over in the United States: Third National Health and Nutrition Examination Survey, Phase 1, 1988–1991. Advance Data, No. 255. Hyattsville, Md.: National Center for Health Statistics.

Metcoff, J., P. Costiloe, W.M. Crosby, S. Dutta, H.H. Sandstead, D. Milne, C.E. Bodwell, and S.H. Majors. 1985. Effect of food supplementation (WIC) during pregnancy on birth weight. Am. J. Clin. Nutr. 41:933–947.

Miller, V., S. Swaney, and A. Deinard. 1985. Impact of the WIC program on the iron status of infants. Pediatrics 74:100–105.

Montana WIC Program. 1992. Policy Statement. Policy No. C-1. Effective date July 1, 1992. Health Services Division, Montana Department of Health and Environmental Sciences.

Morck, T.A., S.R. Lynch, and J.D. Cook. 1983. Inhibition of food iron absorption by coffee. Am. J. Clin. Nutr. 37:416–420.

MRC Vitamin Study Research Group. 1991. Prevention of neural tube defects: Results of Medical Research Council Vitamin Study. Lancet 338:131–137.

Munoz, L.M., B. Lonnerdal, C.L. Keen, and K.G. Dewey. 1988. Coffee consumption as a factor in iron deficiency anemia among pregnant women and their infants in Costa Rica. Am. J. Clin. Nutr. 48:645–651.

Navaie, M., D. Glik, and K. Saluja. 1994. Communication effectiveness of postnatal nutrition education in a WIC program. J. Nutr. Educ. 26:211–217.

Neumann, C., R. Trostle, M. Baksh, D. Ngare, and N. Bwibo. 1989. Household response to the impact of drought in Kenya. Food and Nutrition Bulletin 11:21–33.

Newman, W.P., III, W. Wattigney, and G.S. Berenson. 1991. Autopsy studies in US children and adolescents: Relationship of risk factors to atherosclerotic lesions. Ann. N.Y. Acad. Sci. 623:16–25.

Nicklas, T.A., R.P. Rarris, S.R. Srinivasan, L. S. Webber, and G.S. Berenson. 1989. Nutritional studies in children and implications for change: The Bogalusa Heart Study. J. Adv. Med. 2:451–474.

NIH (National Institutes of Health). Optimal Calcium Intake. NIH Consensus Statement. 1994. National Institutes of Health 12:1–31.

Nowjack-Raymer, R., and H.C. Gift. 1990. Contributing factors to maternal and child oral health. J. Public Health Dent. 50:370–378.

NRC (National Research Council). 1983. Alternative Dietary Practices Nutritional and Abuse. Report of the Committee on Nutrition of the Mother and Preschool Child, Food and Nutrition Board, Commission on Life Sciences. Washington, D.C.: National Academy Press.

NRC (National Research Council). 1986. Nutrient Adequacy: Assessment Using Food Consumption Surveys. Report of the Subcommittee on Criteria for Dietary Evaluation, Coordinating Committee on Evaluation of Food Consumption Surveys, Food and Nutrition Board, Commission on Life Sciences. Washington, D.C.: National Academy Press.

NRC (National Research Council). 1989. Recommended Dietary Allowances, 10th ed. Report of the Subcommittee on the Tenth Edition of the RDAs, Food and Nutrition Board, Commission of Life Sciences. Washington, D.C.: National Academy Press.

Olson, J.A. 1993. Vitamin A and carotenoids as antioxidants in a physiological context. J. Nutr. Sci. Vitaminol-Tokyo. 39:S57–S65.

Olson, R.E. 1995. The dietary recommendations of the American Academy of Pediatrics. Am. J. Clin. Nutr. 61:271–273.

O'Rourke, D.E., J.G. Quinn, J.O. Nicholson, and H.H. Gibson. 1967. Geophagia during pregnancy. Obstet. Gynecol. 29:581–584.

PDAY Research Group. 1990. Relationship of atherosclerosis in young men to serum lipoprotein cholesterol concentrations and smoking. A preliminary report from the Pathobiological Determinants of Atherosclerosis in Youth (PDAY) Research Group. J. Am. Med. Assoc. 264:3018–3024.

Pecoud, A., P. Donzel, and J.L. Schelling. 1975. Effect of foodstuffs on the absorption of zinc sulfate. Clin. Pharmacol. Ther. 17:469–474.

Pennington, J.A.T. 1991. Macronutrient intake in relation to nutritional standards. Pp. 139–158 in Monitoring Dietary Intakes, I. Macdonald, ed. New York: Springer-Verlag.

Penrod, J.C., K. Anderson, and P.B. Acosta. 1990. Impact on iron status of introducing cow's milk in the second six months of life. J. Pediatr. Gastroenterol. Nutr. 10:462–467.

Pollitt, E. 1994. Poverty and child development: Relevance of research in developing countries to the United States. Child Dev. 65:283–295.

Pollitt, E. 1995. Functional significance of the covariance between protein energy malnutrition and iron deficiency anemia. J Nutr. 125:2272S–2277S.

Pugliese, M.T., F. Lifshitz, G. Grad, P. Fort, and M. Marks-Katz. 1983. Fear of obesity: A cause of short stature and delayed puberty. N. Engl. J. Med. 309:513–518.

Puma, M., J. DiPietro, J. Rosenthal, D. Connell, D. Judkins, and M.K. Fox. 1991. Study of the Impact of WIC on the Growth and Development of Children: Field Test. Vol. I: Feasibility Assessment. Cambridge, Mass.: Abt Associates.

Radimer, K.L., C. M. Olson, and C.C. Campbell. 1990. Development of indicators to assess hunger. J Nutr. 120:1544–1548.

Radimer, K.L., C.M. Olson, J.C. Greene, C.C. Campbell, and J-P. Habicht. 1992. Understanding hunger and developing indicators to assess it in women and children. J. Nutr. Edu. 24:36S–44S

Reid, R.M. 1992. Cultural and medical perspective on geophagia. Med. Anthro. 13:337–351.

Repke, J.T. 1994. Calcium and vitamin D. Clin. Obstet. Gynecol. 37:550–557.

Reynolds, R.D., H.J. Binder, M.B. Miller, W.Y. Chang, and S. Horan. 1977. Pagophagia and iron deficiency anemia. Ann. Intern. Med. 69:435–440.

Rimm, E.B., E.L. Giovannucci, M.J. Stampfer, G.A. Colditz, L.B. Litin, and W.C. Willett. 1992. Reproducibility and validity of an expanded self-administered semiquantitative food frequency questionnaire among male health professionals. Am. J. Epidemiol. 135:1114–1126.

Ripa, L.W. 1978. Nursing habits and dental decay in infants: "Nursing bottle caries." J. Dent. Child. 45:274–275.

Ripa, L.W. 1988. Nursing caries: A comprehensive review. Pediatr. Dent. 10:268–282.

Rush, D. 1988. The National WIC Evaluation: An Evaluation of the Special Supplemental Food Program for Women, Infants, and Children. Research Triangle Park, N.C.: Research Triangle Institute.

Sage, J.D. 1962. The practice, incidence and effect of starch eating on Negro women at Temple University Medical Center. Master's Thesis. Temple University, Philadelphia, Pa.

Salvini, S., D.J. Hunter, L. Sampson, M. J. Stampfer, G.A. Colditz, B. Rosner, and W.C. Willett. 1989. Food-based validation of a dietary questionnaire: The effects of week-to-week variation in food consumption. Int. J. Epidemol. 18:858–867.

Serdula, M., R. Coates, T. Byers, A. Mokdad, S. Jewell, N. Chavez, J. Mares-Perlman, P. Newcomb, C. Ritenbaugh, F. Treiber, and G. Block. 1993. Evaluation of a brief telephone questionnaire to estimate fruit and vegetable consumption in diverse study populations. Epidemiology 4:455–463.

Shea, S., C.E. Basch, A.D. Stein, I.R. Contento, M. Irigoyen, and P. Zybert. 1993. Is there a relationship between dietary fat and stature or growth in children three to five years of age? Pediatrics 92:579–586.

Shibata, A., A. Paganini-Hill, R.K. Ross, and B.E. Henderson. 1992. Intake of vegetables, fruits, beta-carotene, vitamin C and vitamin supplements and cancer incidence among the elderly: A prospective study. Br. J. Cancer 66:673–679.

Sobell, J., G. Block, P. Koslowe, J. Tobin, and R. Andres. 1989. Validation of a retrospective questionnaire assessing diet 10–15 years ago. Am. J. Epidemiol. 130:173–187.

Srisuphan, W., and M.B. Bracken. 1986. Caffeine consumption during pregnancy and association with late spontaneous abortion. Am. J. Obstet. Gynecol. 154:14–20.

Stein, A.D., S. Shea, C.E. Basch, I.R. Contento, and P. Zybert. 1992. Consistency of the Willett semiquantitative food frequency questionnaire and 24-hour dietary recalls in estimating nutrient intakes of preschool children. Am. J. Epidemiol. 135:667–677.

Steinberg, D. and Workshop Participants. 1992. Antioxidants in the prevention of human atherosclerosis. Summary of the proceedings of a National Heart, Lung, and Blood Institute Workshop. Circulation 85:123–129.

Steinmetz, K.A., L.H. Kushi, R.M. Bostick, A.R. Folsom, and J.D. Potter. 1994. Vegetables, fruit, and colon cancer in the Iowa Women's Health Study. Am. J. Epidemiol. 139:1–15.

Strode, M.A., K.G. Dewey, and B. Lönnerdal. 1986. Effects of short-term caloric restriction on lactational performance of well-nourished women. Acta Paediatr. Scand. 75:222–229.

Suitor, C.J., J. Gardner, and W.C. Willett. 1989. A comparison of food frequency and diet recall methods in studies of nutrient intake of low-income pregnant women. J. Am. Diet. Assoc. 89:1786–1794.

Talkington, K.M., N.E. Gant, D.E. Scott, and J.A. Pritchard. 1969. Effect of ingestion of starch and some clays on iron absorption. Am. J. Obstet. Gynecol. 108:262–267.

Tavani, A., and C. La-Vecchia. 1995. Fruit and vegetable consumption and cancer risk in a Mediterranean population. Am J Clin Nutr. 61:1374S–1377S.

Tebbutt, I.H., A.J. Teare, J.H. Meek, K.A. Mallett, and D.F. Hawkins. 1984. Caffeine, theophylline and theobromine in pregnancy. Biol. Res. Pregnancy Perinatol. 5:174–176.

Thompson, F.E., and T. Byers. 1994. Dietary Assessment Resource Manual. J. Nutr. 124:2245S–2317S.

Tuttle, C.R., and K.G. Dewey. 1995. Impact of breastfeeding promotion program for Hmong women at selected WIC sites in Northern California. J. Nutr. Educ. 27:69–74.

USDA (U.S. Department of Agriculture). 1987. Estimation of Eligibility for the WIC Program: Report of the WIC Eligibility Study. Summary of Data, Methods, and Findings. Office of Analysis and Evaluation, Food and Nutrition Service. Contract No. 53-3198-3-138. Washington, D.C.: USDA.

USDA (U.S. Department of Agriculture). 1992. The Food Guide Pyramid. U.S. Department of Agriculture Home and Garden Bulletin No. 252. Washington, D.C.: USDA.

USDA (U.S. Department of Agriculture). 1994. WIC Dietary Assessment Validation Study. Final Report. Contract No. 53-3198-2-032. September. Washington, D.C.: USDA.

USDA(U.S. Department of Agriculture) Human Nutrition Information Service. Dietary Guidelines Advisory Committee. 1995. Report of the Dietary Guidelines Advisory Committee on the dietary guidelines for Americans, 1995, to the Secretary of Health and Human Services and the Secretary of Agriculture, prepared for the Committee by the Agricultural Research Service. Washington, D.C.: Dietary Guidelines Advisory Committee, USDA.

Van Assema, P., J. Brug, G. Kok, and H. Brants. 1992. The reliability and validity of a Dutch questionnaire on fat consumption as a means to rank subjects according to individual fat intake. Eur. J. Cancer Prev. 1:375–380.

Vermeer, D.E., and D.A. Frate. 1979. Geophagia in rural Mississippi: Environmental and cultural contexts and nutritional implications. Am. J. Clin. Nutr. 32:2129–2135.

Vermeer, D.E., and R.E. Ferrell. 1985. Nigerian geophagical clay: A traditional antidiarrheal pharmaceutical. Science 227:634–636.

Vegetarian Resource Group. 1994. How Many Vegetarians are There? Press Release June 24, 1994.

Watkinson, B. and P.A. Fried. 1985. Maternal caffeine use before, during and after pregnancy and effects upon offspring. Neurobehav. Toxicol. Teratol. 7:9–17.

Weaver, L.T., and A. Lucas. 1991. Development of Gastrointestinal Structure and Function. In Neonatal Nutrition and Metabolism, W.W. Hay, ed. St. Louis, Mo.: Mosby Year Book.

Wehler, C., R. Scot, and J. Anderson. 1992. The Community Childhood Hunger Identification Project: A model of domestic hunger–demonstration project in Seattle, Washington. J. Nutr. Educ. 24:29S–35S.

Willett, W. 1990. Nutritional Epidemiology. New York: Oxford University Press.

Willett, W.C., L. Sampson, M.J. Stampfer, B. Rosner, C. Bain, J. Witschi, C.H. Hennekens, and F.E. Speizer. 1985. Reproducibility and validity of a semiquantitative food frequency questionnaire. Am. J. Epidemiol. 122:51–65.

Willett, W.C., R.D. Reynolds, S. Cottrell-Hoehner, L. Sampson, and M.L. Browne. 1987. Validation of a semi-quantitative food frequency questionnaire: Comparison with a 1-year diet record. J. Am. Diet. Assoc. 87:43–47.

Wilson, J.F. 1984. Whole cow's milk, age, and gastrointestinal bleeding. Pediatrics 73:879–880.

Woodruff, C. 1983. Breast-feeding or infant formula should be continued for 12 months. Pediatrics 71:984–985.

Yip, R., N.J. Binkin, L. Fleshood, and F.L. Trowbridge. 1987. Declining Prevalence of Anemia Among Low-Income Children in the United States. J. Am. Med. Assoc., 258:1619–1623.

Yip, R., I. Parvanta, K. Scanlon, E.W. Borland, C.M. Russell, and F.L. Trowbridge. 1992. Pediatric Nutrition Surveillance System—United States, 1980–1991. Morbid. Mortal. Weekly Rep. 41(SS-7):1–24.

Ziegler, E.E., S.J. Fomon, S.E. Nelson, C.J. Rebouche, B.B. Edwards, R.R. Rogers, and L.J. Lehman. 1990. Cow milk feeding in infancy: Further observations on blood loss from the gastrointestinal tract. J. Pediatrics 116:11–18.

7

Predisposing Nutrition Risk Criteria

A final category of nutrition risk criteria used in the WIC program (Special Supplemental Nutrition Program for Women, Infants, and Children) is *conditions that predispose persons to inadequate nutrition patterns or nutritionally related medical conditions* (7 CFR Subpart 2, Section (d)(2)(iv)). In general, predisposing risk criteria are used to certify women, infants, and children for participation in the WIC program under Priority VII. In the face of funding constraints, however, individuals eligible for participation in the WIC program under Priority VII often are not served by the program. Yet, of all of the nutrition risk criteria discussed in this report, predisposing nutrition risk criteria may support most clearly the preventive nature of the WIC program.

Legislatively, the use of predisposing risk criteria has an interesting history. The Child Nutrition Amendments in 1978 (Public Law 95-627) expanded the definition of nutrition risk to *include predisposing conditions including, but not limited to, alcoholism and drug addiction....* Subsequent changes in regulations added homelessness and migrancy as specific predisposing nutrition risk criteria. Since health professionals have recently come to consider alcoholism and drug addiction as medical risks, these criteria too are now generally used as medical risk criteria to place individuals in one of the top three priorities. The Food and Consumer Service (FCS, administrative home to the WIC program at the U.S. Department of Agriculture [USDA]) has not considered homelessness, migrancy, or most other predisposing nutrition risk criteria as conditions that warrant placement of individuals in one of the top three priorities without a documented nutrition or medical risk (*Federal Register*, 59(66): 16, 146–16, 149).

The category of *predisposing conditions* poses a challenge to the committee's analysis of the scientific basis of the nutrition risk criteria. A large number of behavioral, cultural, nutrition, and medical conditions can place individuals at risk of poor nutrition status, and states have used considerable latitude in defining predisposing nutrition risk criteria. In addition to *homelessness* and *migrancy*, other predisposing risks used to certify the eligibility of individuals for participation in the WIC program include *passive smoking, low maternal education, young caregiver, battering, child of a mentally retarded parent*, and *child abuse and neglect*. This chapter summarizes the scientific evidence for these predisposing nutrition risk criteria. Table 7-1 presents the number of states using each of these predisposing risk criteria for women, infants, and children. Table 7-2 provides a summary of these criteria as predictors of nutrition risk and of benefit from WIC program participation.

This chapter does not cover *caretaker physically disabled* or *inadequate facilities for food preparation or storage*. Physical disability is a broad term covering widely varying conditions, most of which are compatible with appropriate child care. Apart from homelessness, the committee did not find a scientific basis on which to review the relationship between food preparation facilities and nutrition risk or benefit.

TABLE 7-1 Summary of Predisposing Risk Criteria in the WIC Program and Use by States

Risk Criterion	States Using Pregnant Women[a]	Infants	Children
Homelessness	1	—	—
Migrancy	—	21	20
Passive smoking	3	—	—
Low level of maternal education and illiteracy	2	—	—
Young caregiver	—	6	0
Maternal depression	—	—	—
Battering	7	—	—
Child abuse or neglect	—	9	7
Child of a mentally retarded parent	—	35	26

NOTE: Dashes denote that the criterion was not reported for that population.

[a] Data for postpartum women were not readily available.

SOURCE: Adapted from USDA (1992).

TABLE 7-2 Summary of Predisposing Risk Criteria as Predictive of Risk or Benefit Among Women, Infants, and Children

Risk Criterion	Women Risk	Women Benefit	Infants Risk	Infants Benefit	Children Risk	Children Benefit
Homelessness	✓	?	✓	?	✓	?
Migrancy	✓	?	✓	?	✓	?
Passive smoking	✓[a]	?	✓[a]	0	✓[a]	?
Low level of maternal education and illiteracy	✓	?	✓	?	✓	?
Maternal depression	✓	?	✓	?	✓	?
Battering	✓	?				
Child abuse or neglect			✓	?	✓	?
Child of a young caregiver			✓	?	✓	?
Child of a mentally retarded parent			✓	✓	✓	✓

NOTE: ✓ = predictive of risk or benefit; ? = no evidence; 0 = evidence, but no effect; blank = not applicable to the group.

[a] Health risk only, no evidence of nutrition risk.

The committee's recommendations for predisposing nutrition risk criteria are summarized in Table 7-3.

HOMELESSNESS

Until recently, *homelessness* by itself was not accepted as a valid nutrition risk criterion for eligibility for participation in the WIC program. Homeless women, infants, and children were eligible for the WIC program only if they had some other documented nutrition risk. However, based on the recommendations of the National Advisory Council on Maternal, Infant, and Fetal Nutrition (USDA, 1992), recent final regulations for participation in the WIC program (*Federal Register*, April 19, 1995) added homelessness and migrancy to the predisposing nutrition risk criteria for the WIC program. The regulations place individuals who are eligible solely on the basis of homelessness or migrancy under Priority VII. However, state WIC agencies, at their discretion, may place these individuals in priority groups as follows: pregnant or breastfeeding women and infants in Priority IV; children in Priority V; and postpartum women in Priority VI.

TABLE 7-3 Summary of Dietary Risk Criteria and Committee Recommendations for the Specific WIC Population

Risk Criterion	Committee Recommendation	Pregnant Women	Postpartum Women Lactating	Postpartum Women Nonlactating	Infants	Children
Homelessness	Use	✓	✓	✓	✓	✓
Migrancy	Use	✓	✓	✓	✓	✓
Passive smoking	Do not use					
Low level of maternal education or illiteracy	Use	✓	✓	✓	✓	✓
Maternal depression	Add	✓	✓	✓	✓	✓
Battering	Use	✓	✓	✓		
Child abuse or neglect	Use				✓	✓
Child of a young caregiver	Use				✓	✓
Child of a mentally retarded parent	Use				✓	✓

NOTE: ✓ = subgroup to which the recommendation applies.

Prevalence of and Factors Associated with Homelessness

The definition of a homeless individual used by the WIC program is broad:

a woman, infant or child who lacks a fixed and regular nighttime residence; or whose nighttime residence is: a supervised publicly or privately operated shelter (including a welfare hotel, a congregate shelter, or a shelter for victims of domestic violence) designated to provide temporary living accommodation; an institution that provides a temporary residence for individuals intended to be institutionalized; a temporary accommodation in the residence of another individual; or a public or private place not designed for, or ordinarily used as, a regular sleeping accommodation for human beings (*Federal Register*, 59(66):16,146–16,149).

Estimates of the number of homeless people vary widely because of ambiguities in the definition of homelessness and lack of a reliable counting method. During the 1980s, point-prevalence estimates of homelessness in the United States ranged from 350,000 to more than 3 million (USDA, 1991). Owing to inevitable design problems, surveys that actually try to count the number of homeless individuals generally provide smaller estimates than do other methods of estimating prevalence (Link et al., 1994). This recent study reports lifetime (any time) and 5-year prevalence estimates of homelessness that are significantly higher than previous point-prevalence estimates: (1) a lifetime combined prevalence of all types of homelessness of 14.0 percent (26 million individuals); (2) a 5-year (1985 to 1990) prevalence of all types of homelessness of 4.6 percent (8.5 million individuals); and (3) a lifetime prevalence of *literal homelessness* (sleeping in shelters, abandoned buildings, bus and train stations, etc.) of 7.4 percent (13.5 million individuals). Comparison of these 5-year and lifetime prevalence estimates with the earlier point-prevalence estimates of homelessness suggests a fluid process with people flowing in and out of homelessness.

Despite controversy over the absolute numbers, there is consensus that the number of homeless individuals increased steadily during the 1980s (Rossi et al., 1987). During this period several surveys of local areas found that between 30 and 50 percent of the homeless were families with children, usually headed by single women with at least one child under 18 years (Bassuk et al., 1986; Miller and Lin, 1988; New York Coalition for the Homeless, 1986; U.S. Conference of Mayors, 1984, 1986, 1987).

A variety of risk factors are associated with homelessness. Weitzman (1989) suggests that pregnancy and recent birth are precipitating factors for homelessness. Homeless women, especially homeless pregnant women, are more likely than housed low-income women to have alcohol problems, to use drugs, and to smoke (Becker et al., 1992; Fischer, 1991; Jaffee et al., 1992). Homeless women are also likely to be victims of domestic violence; 33 to 89 percent of all homeless women are estimated to have experienced abuse at some point during their life (Bassuk and Weinreb, 1993).

Homelessness as an Indicator of Nutrition and Health Risk

Although somewhat sparse, the empirical evidence, as identified below, documents poorer pregnancy outcomes, increased risk of malnutrition and health problems, low utilization of preventive health services, and a higher incidence of developmental delays and learning problems among homeless families with women and their children.

Women. In general, homeless women experience a variety of health disorders and problems. Higher than expected levels of iron deficiency anemia, overweight and obesity, and high serum cholesterol concentrations were found among single homeless women living in temporary housing shelters in Kansas City, Missouri (Drake, 1992), and among homeless men and women in New York City (Luder et al., 1990). Homeless women are also found to have higher prevalence of such chronic health problems as hypertension, diabetes mellitus, coronary heart disease, mental illness, alcoholism, and tuberculosis (Drake, 1992; Luder et al., 1990).

Pregnancy outcomes are worse for low-income homeless women than for other low-income women. A study of homeless pregnant women in New York City found significantly higher infant mortality rates and rates of low birth weight (LBW) among the homeless women than among women living in low-income public housing (Chavkin et al., 1987). Another study of birth outcomes in New York City found that pregnant WIC participants were three times more likely to have LBW newborns if they were homeless (Jaffee et al., 1992).

The explanation of the poorer pregnancy and health outcomes for homeless pregnant women is most likely a combination of inadequate prenatal care, poor nutrition, and other behavioral and health problems. In the 1982–1984 New York City study of homeless pregnant women and housed low-income pregnant women, 40 percent of the homeless women received no prenatal care, compared with less than 15 percent of the women living in public housing (Chavkin et al., 1987). In Jaffee's study of homeless pregnant women in New York City, pregnant homeless WIC program participants were four times more likely to lack prenatal care than similar WIC program participants with housing (Jaffee et al., 1992).

Studies of the diets and eating patterns of all homeless individuals suggest the following: increased risk of protein-energy malnutrition and chronic malnutrition; high intakes of sodium, saturated fat, and cholesterol; shortages of essential nutrients; low dietary adequacy scores; and primary sources of food that include fast-food restaurants, shelters, delicatessens, and garbage bins

(Luder et al., 1989, 1990; Wiecha et al., 1991; Wolgemuth et al., 1992). The few studies of dietary intakes by single homeless women living in shelters found (1) low mean intakes of iron, calcium, magnesium, zinc, and folate (< 50 percent of Recommended Dietary Allowances [RDAs]) (Drake, 1992); and (2) higher than recommended fat intake (Drake, 1992); and (3) low average intake of servings in each of four food groups and a high intake of foods of low nutrient density (28 percent of total food intake) (Bunston and Breton, 1990).

Children. The socioeconomic, health, and nutrition problems faced by homeless women are exacerbated for their homeless infants and children. Homeless children are at increased risks of infectious diseases, growth and developmental delays, behavioral and emotional problems, and a host of other biologic and developmental insults.

The frequency of health problems among homeless children exceeds that of housed comparison groups or standard reference populations with places to live. In particular, homeless children have very high rates of delayed immunizations (Acker et al., 1987; Alperstein et al., 1988; Miller and Lin, 1988). Other health problems experienced by homeless children include a high reported rate of child abuse and neglect; a higher incidence of asthma; and increased risks of infectious disease, especially conjunctivitis, ringworm, gastrointestinal disorders, upper respiratory infections, and scabies and lice infestations (Khan, 1991). High proportions of homeless children and their families have no regular source of medical care, and they over-rely on hospital emergency rooms for primary health care (Hu et al., 1989; Roth and Fox, 1990; Wood and Valdez, 1991). Homeless children also suffer disproportionately from significant behavioral and developmental problems that affect their cognitive growth and development (Bassuk and Rubin, 1987; Bassuk et al., 1986; Eddins, 1993; Parker et al., 1991).

Studies examining measures of physical growth of homeless children provide mixed evidence on the prevalence of acute and chronic malnutrition. Those studies differ considerably on the basis of the geographic areas studied and the age groups examined, but together, they present a broad-based overview of the physical growth status of homeless children. Some studies of homeless children reported weight-for-height and height-for-age measurements similar to those for other low-income children, suggesting that malnutrition is not disproportionately prevalent among homeless children (Lewis and Meyers 1989; Alperstein et al., 1988; Wood et al., 1990). In contrast, one study of homeless children in New York City reported a higher than expected prevalence of stunting (low height-for-age) but not wasting (low weight-for-height), suggesting moderate, chronic malnutrition (Fierman et al., 1991). Another study of homeless preschoolers in Baltimore found a higher than expected prevalence of wasting, suggesting that some homeless children may have experienced acute undernutrition (Taylor and Koblinsky, 1993).

The most typical growth problem found among homeless children is an increased risk of obesity. Estimates of the percentage of homeless children who are overweight range from 12 to 35 percent (Miller and Lin, 1988; Taylor and Koblinsky, 1993; Wood et al., 1990).

Estimates of the prevalence of anemia among homeless children vary widely across studies, ranging from 2 percent to nearly 50 percent (Acker et al., 1987; Arnstein and Alperstein, 1987; Wright and Weber-Burdin, 1987). Although limited in number, most studies find that the prevalence of anemia is significantly higher among homeless children than among other low-income children (Acker et al., 1987).

Higher than expected rates of obesity, anemia, and stunting among homeless children are consistent with poor dietary quality. One comprehensive study found a wide range of poor eating habits and inadequate diets among homeless children in two temporary housing shelters in Kansas City, Missouri, during 1989 (Drake, 1992). Although a sufficient quantity of food was available for these children, the foods offered were typically convenience and prepackaged foods that were high in fat and saturated fat and low in nutrient density. The most common method of food preparation was frying. Average intakes of iron, magnesium, zinc, and folate were about 50 percent of the RDA. Most mothers of infants did not use iron-fortified formulas, as recommended, but instead fed their infants homogenized whole milk from a bottle. Taylor and Koblinsky (1993) confirm the inadequate iron intakes of homeless children, and several studies find that diets of homeless children are lacking in fresh fruits and vegetables (Drake, 1992; Taylor and Koblinsky, 1993; Wood et al., 1990).

There are apparently no research studies that have investigated the dietary or health effects of WIC program participation on homeless women and their children.

Homelessness as an Indicator of Nutrition and Health Benefit

Despite the lack of empirical evidence, the nutrition and health problems experienced by homeless women and their children underscore their need for the nutrition education, nutritious foods, and referrals to health care provided through the WIC program. Low iron intakes and higher than expected prevalence of anemia could be addressed through the provision of supplemental food through the WIC program and education on food sources of iron, ways to increase iron absorption, and the appropriate use of iron supplements, especially iron-fortified formula for bottle-fed infants and iron-fortified infant cereal for all infants older than 3 to 4 months. Obesity and other growth problems could be diminished through the provision of supplemental nutritious foods through the WIC program and through education on food sources of nutrients and food preparation techniques. Finally, referrals to appropriate health care, and other services, such as the Food Stamp Program or prenatal care, would also hold potential for reducing nutrition risk.

Limited evidence suggests that WIC program participation by homeless families with women, infants, and children is less than that by similar low-income families with housing. In New York City in 1988, only 44 percent of homeless women who were pregnant or who had new infants were participating in the WIC program, compared with 60 percent of eligible housed women (Weitzman, 1989). In Boston, a study of homeless families with children reported a participation rate in the WIC program of 54 percent (Lewis and Meyers, 1989). The authors suggest that the lack of storage for perishable foods and the high mobility of homeless families contribute to low rates of WIC participation in the WIC program. Siegler and colleagues (1993) report on a WIC food package that was adapted for the living conditions of homeless families and nutrition education that focused on food safety, foods requiring little or no cooking, and healthful snacks for children.

Other factors that may contribute to low participation rates include the lack of adequate kitchen facilities in homeless shelters, lack of transportation, mistrust of health care providers, the lack of a safe and stable living environment, mental illness, domestic violence, alcoholism, and drug abuse.

Use of Homelessness as a Nutrition Risk Criterion in the WIC Setting

As discussed earlier, homelessness has only recently been allowed for use as a predisposing nutrition risk criterion by state WIC programs. Given the severe health and nutrition problems experienced by homeless women, infants, and children, it is highly likely that they are placed in a priority higher than VII by virtue of an anthropometric, medical, or dietary nutrition risk criterion or by virtue of the state's option to place homeless program applicants in Priorities IV through VI. This may be less likely for those who are newly homeless. In the face of the funding constraints encountered by the WIC program, concerns have been raised that homeless women, infants, and especially children may not be served because of the lower priority assigned to homelessness as a nutrition risk (Lenihan, 1994).

Recommendation for Homelessness

In summary, the scientific evidence unquestionably documents significant health and nutrition risks associated with *homelessness* and identification of homelessness is relatively straightforward. There is theoretical evidence of benefit from WIC program participation among homeless women, infants, and children. The committee recommends that *homelessness* be used as a nutrition risk criterion for women, infants, and children in the WIC program, at a priority level higher than VII, and emphasizes the value of specially tailored food packages for the homeless.

MIGRANCY

Testimony before the National Advisory Council on Migrant Health indicates that lack of permanent housing for the migrant population predisposes migrants to the same set of problems identified above for homeless individuals. As a result, the final WIC program regulations published in the April 19, 1995, *Federal Register* also included *migrancy* as a predisposing nutrition risk criterion certifying eligibility for participation in the WIC program. Migrant individuals who are eligible for participation in the WIC program on the basis of categorical criteria and income but who lack any other documented medical or nutrition risk criterion are placed in Priority VII, with the state having the option of placing individuals in Priorities IV through VI.

Prevalence of and Factors Associated with Migrancy

Lack of reliable data on the number of migrants makes it difficult to calculate rates of mortality and morbidity and the prevalence of health problems and disability. As with homelessness, estimates of the prevalence of migrancy reflect both variations in its definition and counting methods.

There is no standard definition of *migrant* among government agencies. WIC program regulations refer to the term *migrant* and *migrant farmworker* interchangeably and define a migrant farmworker as "an individual whose principal employment is in agriculture on a seasonal basis, who has been so employed within the last 24 months, and who establishes, for the purposes of such employment, a temporary abode" (*Federal Register*, 59(66):16,146–16,149).

Estimates from the USDA and the U.S. Department of Labor generally count only employed farmworkers over age 14 years, ignoring the dependents of migrant workers. Thus, those estimates are lower than estimates from the Department of Health and Human Services (DHHS). The DHHS Office of Migrant Health estimated that there were about 3 million migrant and seasonal farmworkers and their dependents in the mid-1980s (Rust, 1990), whereas more recent estimates range between 4 million and 5 million (DHHS, 1990; Mobed et al., 1992).

In general, migrant farmworkers have low incomes, live in crowded and unsanitary conditions, and perform strenuous physical labor for long hours. The migrant population comprises people of various racial and ethnic backgrounds, but the majority are Hispanic in origin. Although most migrant farmworkers are U.S. citizens, English is often not their primary language and many have low levels of education. Studies of migrant farmworkers in Wisconsin in 1978 reported that 35 percent of migrant women of childbearing age were functionally illiterate (4 or fewer years of schooling) (Slesinger et al., 1986). Literacy levels improved during the 1980s, but they are still below national levels (Slesinger and Ofstead, 1993). A very high proportion (63 percent) are children under the age of 16 years, a group that is particularly at risk of infectious diseases and other health problems from adverse and crowded living conditions (National Advisory Council on Migrant Health, 1992). The high rate of mobility of migrant farmworkers makes it difficult for these individuals to maintain continuous and comprehensive health care.

Migrancy as an Indicator of Nutrition and Health Risk

The array of health and nutrition problems experienced by migrant farmworkers and their dependents is different from that experienced by the general population. Common problems documented in the literature include increased risk of respiratory infections, gastroenteritis, intestinal parasites, skin infections, otitis media, scabies and head lice, pesticide exposure, tuberculosis, poor nutrition, anemia, short stature, obesity, hypertension, diabetes mellitus, congenital anomalies, delayed development, injuries, adolescent pregnancy, inadequate dental care, and delayed immunizations (AAP, CCHS, 1989; Dever, 1991). However, large gaps exist in the literature on the health status of migrant individuals, and on factors that contribute to their poor health and nutrition status (Rust, 1990).

Women. Most studies of the health and nutrition status of migrant farmworkers combine men and women in the analyses. Yet the data show convincingly that migrant farmworkers and their dependents experience poor health and both acute and chronic illnesses. Access to health care is limited, and most migrant and seasonal workers seek medical treatment for acute illnesses rather than for preventive services and the management of chronic conditions.

Recent data on pregnancy outcomes for migrant women are not available. The few older studies (Chase et al., 1971; Slesinger et al., 1986; de la Torre and Rush, 1989) demonstrated elevated infant mortality rates relative to the rate for the general U.S. population. Chase and co-workers (1971) reported an infant mortality rate that was nearly three times the U.S. infant mortality rate at that time. De la Torre and Rush (1989) found that 24 percent of the migrant women in their study had experienced one or more miscarriages or fetal death and that 8 percent had experienced at least one infant death.

Old data suggest that inadequate levels of prenatal care, lack of access to appropriate labor and delivery facilities, and poor nutrition contribute to these higher than average rates of infant mortality (Chase, 1971). Reasons cited for not receiving prenatal care included lack of money, lack of transportation, lack of child care, and lack of a perceived need for prenatal care (National Advisory Council on Migrant Health, 1992). One-fourth of farmworkers in Wayne County, New York, expressed a fear and distrust of the medical profession (Chi, 1985).

Data on the adequacies of the diets of migrant farmworkers are very limited (Cardenas et al., 1976). A study conducted by Public Voice in 1989 reported that one-half of migrant farmworkers had diets that did not meet the RDA for vitamin A, iron, or calcium; almost one-third reported running out of food sometime during the past year; and over one-fifth suffered from intestinal parasites. Finally, less than one-quarter of eligible migrant farmworkers participated in the Food Stamp Program—many migrants were not aware of their eligibility (Shotland et al., 1989).

Many aspects of the living conditions of migrant farmworkers and their families contribute to poor dietary patterns. Inadequate cooking and food storage facilities, lack of money for food purchases, limited access to supermarkets, long working hours, a lack of time to prepare nutritious meals, and overconsumption of prepackaged and convenience foods may all contribute to poor nutrition.

Children. Information on the health and nutrition status of migrant children is even more limited than that for migrant women and is similarly based on old survey data (Chase et al., 1971). In 1969, 55 percent of the preschool-age migrant children studied in Colorado had below-normal serum vitamin A concentrations. Other nutrition problems included anemia, stunting, low head circumference, and low alkaline phosphates concentrations, all suggestive of undernutrition among preschool-age migrant children.

Like Chase and colleagues, Slesinger provided further evidence of the high proportions of migrant children under 16 years of age who had not received basic health services. Chronic health conditions were more common among migrant children than among all U.S. children surveyed in the 1969 to 1970 National Health Interview Survey (11 percent of migrant children versus 3 percent of all U.S. children).

Migrancy as an Indicator of Nutrition and Health Benefit

There is no empirical evidence on migrancy as a predictor of nutrition and health benefit. However, the wide range of health and nutrition problems of migrant women and their children suggests that interventions like those provided through the WIC program have potentially large expected benefits. Poor dietary quality and the resulting high rates of vitamin deficiencies, stunting, obesity, and poor perinatal outcomes are evidence of the need for both nutrition education and WIC program foods that are high in key nutrients. Health care and social service referrals and education on the importance of health care could address perceptions among migrants that preventive health care and prenatal care are not needed, ways to get appropriate health care, and the importance of timely immunizations.

Many local agencies have developed programs to overcome language barriers and cultural differences, transportation problems, lack of child care, and long working hours of their clientele. Sometimes working in combination with the Expanded Food and Nutrition Education Program, they adapt their educational programs to the needs of migrants. Through referral systems, they strive to achieve a comprehensive approach to meeting their clients' health needs.

Very little information is available on the WIC program participation rate by migrant women and their children, and no published studies have investigated the effects of the WIC program on the health of migrant participants. However, a joint project in North Carolina that includes a WIC program (Watkins et al., 1990) provides some useful data: (1) more than 90 percent of migrant farmworker women and children were enrolled in the center's WIC program; (2) by the third year, there were increases in the average number of prenatal visits (7 to 10), and in the proportion of women entering prenatal care in the first trimester (from 41 percent to 51 percent); (3) there was a decrease in the percentage of women with low-birth-weight newborns in the 1986 and 1987 cohorts; (4) the proportion of children receiving development screens increased (34 percent to more than 75 percent), and the proportion of children with complete immunization rose (40 percent to more than 60 percent); and (5) although anemia remained a common problem throughout the study period, a higher proportion of returning children than children coming to the center for only one season had a normal hematocrit level.

In that health center, some nutrition problems have persisted. Although the women's diets did not include excessive amounts of high-calorie, nutrient-poor foods, and pica was not a common problem, both women and children reported low intakes of foods in the dairy and the fruit and vegetable groups. Moreover, 18 percent of infants and children were classified as obese, defined as weight-for-height at or above the 90th percentile, and the prevalence of stunting was more than twice the expected rate (Watkins et al., 1990).

This project and its evaluation demonstrate the kind of data collection and analysis that are needed both to assess the nutrition and health risks of migrant women and children and to determine the effectiveness of the WIC program in addressing these risks.

Use of Migrancy as a Nutrition Risk Criterion in the WIC Setting

FCS has long recognized the special needs of migrant populations and has incorporated special regulations addressing the unique circumstances of migrant farmworkers. The Child Nutrition Act of 1966, as amended, stipulates that not less than 0.9 percent of the sums appropriated for the WIC program must be made available to eligible members of migrant populations. In addition, state WIC program plans are required to include information on how program benefits will be provided to migrant farmworkers and their families, nutrition education plans must address the special needs of migrant families, and states must provide expedited processing services for migrant applicants. Migrant participants in the WIC program are not required to be recertified if they move to a different state during the middle of an eligibility period.

The recent addition of migrancy as an explicit predisposing nutrition risk criterion allows migrant women, infants, and children eligible for participation in the WIC program on the basis of categorical criteria and income to be certified under Priority VII. However, in the face of funding constraints, migrants eligible only under Priority VII may not be served. However, states have the option of placing migrants in Priorities IV through VI.

Data from the 1992 Study of WIC Participant and Program Characteristics (PC92) provide limited information on the extent to which using Priority VII for migrancy actually results in unserved migrant individuals. PC92 data were derived directly from certification records of individuals certified for participation in the WIC program in April 1992, before migrancy was allowed as a predisposing nutrition risk criterion. Data on the nutrition risks show that biochemical risks (hematocrit or hemoglobin level) were reported more frequently for migrant WIC program participants than for the overall caseload in the WIC program (USDA, 1994), suggesting that migrant workers are likely to have some other documented medical or nutrition risks that would place them in a higher priority. On the other hand, the proportion of migrant WIC participants without a reported categorization of risk priority is higher than for the WIC program overall, suggesting that migrancy itself might serve as the predisposing nutrition risk criterion.

Recommendations for Migrancy

The nutrition and health risks associated with *migrancy* are well documented in women, infants, and children and it is easy to identify migrancy. There is a theoretical basis for benefit from participation in the WIC program. Therefore, the committee recommends use of *migrancy* as a nutrition risk criterion for women, infants, and children by the WIC program.

However, because evidence on the nutrition risk of migrancy was obtained 15 to 20 years ago and is based on either small clinic-based samples or a few regional or statewide surveys of the health status of migrant individuals, research is needed—including a focus on other nutritional status measures such as obesity, iron deficiency anemia, and poor eating habits.

PASSIVE SMOKING

Exposure to tobacco smoke includes exposure during pregnancy and after birth to tobacco-smoke-contaminated air either at home or in other environmental contexts (Samet et al., 1994). Generally, the sources of air contamination are side-stream smoke from the cigarette's burning end and the smoke exhaled by the smokers. *Passive smoking* and *involuntary smoking* are terms frequently used to refer to exposure to tobacco-contaminated air, which is the topic in this section. Maternal smoking, which causes even higher fetal exposure to substances in smoke, is addressed in Chapter 5.

Prevalence of and Factors Associated with Passive Smoking

Since 1964, the prevalence of tobacco use has decreased dramatically as a result of educational efforts to discourage tobacco use among adults (DHHS, 1994a). However, smoking continues to be a major public health threat in the United States among families who meet the criteria for eligibility for participation in the WIC program.

Of interest to the WIC program is that young females with low levels of education have shown the least reduction in their smoking habits (U.S. Bureau of the Census, 1993) (see Chapter 5). Young pregnant women may discontinue smoking during pregnancy, but smokers are likely to resume smoking after giving birth and thus expose their young children to tobacco-contaminated air.

Concern over the exposure to tobacco smoke among young children is rising, as observed in the results of a 1988 nationwide survey (Overpeck and Moss, 1991). Almost one-half of all U.S. children (42 percent) under age 5 years were exposed to tobacco smoke. As income and maternal education levels decreased, the probability of children's exposure to tobacco smoke increased. In addition, a recent survey in California found that 25 percent of female nonsmokers 18 to 44 years of age were exposed to passive smoking at work and 34 percent were exposed at work and at home (Burns and Pierce, 1992). Exposure rates were higher in Hispanics, Asians, and women with less than 12 years of education.

Passive Smoking as an Indicator of Nutrition and Health Risk

The level of contamination of indoor air secondary to tobacco use depends on the number of smokers, the intensity of smoking, the size of the indoor space, the rate of exchange of indoor and outdoor air, and the use of air cleaning devices (Samet et al., 1994). Empirical evidence shows increased levels of nicotine and cotinine (a metabolic by-product of nicotine and a very good indicator of nicotine exposure) in the serum, urine, and umbilical cord blood of women exposed to passive smoking (Jordanov, 1990; and Ueda et al., 1989).

Studies of the association between passive smoking during pregnancy and birth outcomes provide mixed findings. Some studies reported a reduction in mean birth weight of infants whose mothers were exposed to passive smoking during pregnancy (Martin and Bracken, 1986; Rubin et al., 1986), whereas other studies found either no relationship between mean birth weight and passive smoking (Chen et al., 1989) or an increase in mean birth weight of infants born to mothers exposed to passive smokers (MacArthur and Knox, 1987). Studies that examined the relative risk of low birth weight of infants born at term generally find that maternal exposure to passive smoking during pregnancy is not associated with an increased risk of term infants being born small-for-gestational-age (Chen and Petitti, 1995).

A study of day care centers showed that the nicotine exposure for children from homes where at least one person smoked was ten times higher than that for children from homes where no one smoked (cited in Samet et al., 1994). More recently, a study on exposure to tobacco smoke among 6- to 8-week-old infants living in homes where one member of the family (other than the mother) smoked showed that their level of urine cotinine was five to six times higher than the level in infants not exposed to smoking. The infants of mothers and fathers who both smoked had cotinine concentrations 12 times greater than the concentrations in infants whose parents that did not smoke (Chilmonczyk et al., 1990).

Recent reviews have extensively documented the effects of involuntary smoking on children (DHHS, 1989; Poswillo and Alberman, 1992; Samet et al., 1994). The data consistently show that children of smokers experience an increased risk of lower respiratory infections, respiratory symptoms, reduced lung growth, exacerbation of asthma, and irritation of eyes, nose, throat, and lower respiratory tract (Samet et al., 1994).

Recent evidence from the National Longitudinal Survey of Youth (1992), based on a nationally representative sample, indicates that involuntary smoking may lead to behavioral problems in children (Weitzman et al., 1992). Independently of duration, 4- to 11-year-olds exposed to maternal cigarette smoking showed increased occurrences of behavioral problems (as indicated by a behavior problem index). In this sample, which included 2,252 children, 54 percent of the mothers reported smoking during and/or after pregnancy.

There was a dose-response relationship for children whose mothers smoked either after pregnancy or both before and after pregnancy. In the group whose mothers smoked only after pregnancy, children had an average of 0.7 additional behavior problems ($p = .10$) if their mothers smoked less than a pack per day and 2.1 additional behavior problems ($p = .0004$) if their mothers smoked a pack or more per day, compared to those who did not smoke.

Despite the apparent health risks, however, there is little evidence of specific risk to the nutrition status of women infants and children exposed to tobacco-smoke-contaminated air.

Passive Smoking as an Indicator of Nutrition and Health Benefit

While the health benefits of smoking cessation by parents to the overall health of women, infants, and children in the household are clear, there is no indication that supplemental food, nutrition education, or participation in the WIC program can abate the risk posed by passive smoking.

Passive Smoking as a Nutrition Risk Criterion in the WIC Setting

Three state WIC agencies used passive smoking as a nutrition risk criterion for women in 1992 (see Table 7-1).

Recommendation for Passive Smoking

Biologic markers indicate that infants and children exposed to particles from secondhand smoke are at risk for impaired health, growth, and development. Similarly, exposure to tobacco smoke is associated with upper and lower respiratory problems, asthma, and irritation of sensory channels. The health risk from *passive smoking* is documented, but nutrition risk and evidence of benefit from WIC participation are not. Therefore, the committee recommends discontinuation of use of *passive smoking* as a risk criterion for women, infants, and children in the WIC program.

LOW LEVEL OF MATERNAL EDUCATION AND ILLITERACY

In public health programmatic and research activities, *education* is generally defined by the number of years of formal schooling. Years of education are often classified into such broad categories as less than 12 years, 12 years, and greater than 12 years (Kramer et al., 1995). A *low level* of parental education is also defined as less than a 9th-grade education. In some instances, *illiteracy* is the indicator of choice.

Immigrants and Puerto Ricans represent a substantial portion of the U.S. population and some of them may be unable to speak, read, or write in English. WIC offices may require appropriate bilingual personnel and offer materials written in their native language.

Prevalence of and Factors Associated with Low Level of Maternal Education and Illiteracy

Participants in the WIC program have, on average, comparatively low levels of education. In the National WIC Evaluation, 55 percent of the pregnant women enrolled had less than 12 years of education (Rush et al., 1988). In the general population of women (18 years of age and over) in the 1990 census, 21 percent had less than 12 years of education (U.S. Bureau of the Census, 1993).

Low Level of Maternal Education and Illiteracy as Indicators of Nutrition and Health Risk

Maternal education is negatively associated with infant and childhood mortality, low birth weight, and mild mental retardation. It is positively associated with the health (including cognitive development) and nutrition of the offspring. Children of illiterate women are especially at risk for poor health and nutrition. In some international studies, maternal literacy was the most powerful of numerous social and economic predictors for positive child health outcomes (Hobcraft et al., 1984).

Because maternal education is associated with family income, wealth, parental occupation, and quality of housing, there is concern whether maternal education and literacy are the explanatory variables. Preliminary data suggest that these two variables are causally related to the health and nutrition of the offspring. Following tight control of potential confounders, numerous studies have shown that maternal education accounts for significant percentages of differences in health and nutrition outcomes (Cleland and Van Ginneken 1988; Victora et al., 1992). Cleland and Van Ginneken (1988) attribute about 50 percent of the variability of childhood mortality to low levels of maternal education, but this research was conducted in developing countries and may have limited applicability to the WIC program setting.

Data from the 1980 National Natality Survey show that mothers with less than 12 years of education were at a higher risk of having an LBW baby than those with 12 or more years of education. After controlling for maternal smoking, height, and weight, women with less than 12 years of education had an LBW odds ratio of 1.6. However if women with less than 12 years of education stopped smoking during pregnancy, the incidence of LBW would decline by

35 percent (Kleinman and Madans, 1985), bringing the odds ratio much closer to 1.0. In a study of newborns served by Medicaid in five states, low maternal education was associated with significant decreases in newborn birth weight and an increase in the incidence of LBW (Devaney et al., 1990).

Dietary information gathered in the Hispanic Health and Nutrition Examination Survey and the second National Health and Nutrition Examination Survey (NHANES II) shows that the educational level of Hispanic women and of white, non-Hispanic women predicts the quality of their diet (Guendelman and Abrams, 1995). In particular, the lower their education level, the higher the risk of poor dietary intake as defined by an average consumption of less than 50 percent of the RDA for eight nutrients (protein, calcium, iron, zinc, folate, and vitamins A, C, and E).

As the level of maternal education (and literacy) increases, the mother's use of health services increases, and women assume a greater role in making child care decisions (Weiss et al., 1991).

Low Level of Maternal Education and Illiteracy as Indicators of Nutrition and Health Benefit

Increasingly, WIC programs are designing their educational programs to be useful to a clientele with low literacy. For example, Navaje and co-workers (1994) found that WIC clients processed and retained nutrition education messages better if they were simple and few in number. Videos and food demonstrations in the WIC program provide a very useful method for increasing the nutrition knowledge and skills of women with low literacy even for those who do not speak English. This suggests good potential for women with low literacy to benefit from the WIC program. A few WIC programs have joined forces with adult education and offer GED courses that center on food and nutrition. Women with low literacy would have few other opportunities to gain this information.

Although formal schooling and literacy are not prerequisites for the good health of the offspring, it is likely that the identification of illiterate women or women with low levels of education within the WIC program will also identify children at some degree of risk for poor health and nutrition status.

Use of Low Level of Maternal Education and Illiteracy as a Nutrition Risk Criterion in the WIC Setting

The two states that used low maternal education as a nutrition risk criterion (see Table 7-1) used cutoff values of 8th grade or 9th grade. The use of less than 9 years of formal schooling as a cutoff point for low level of maternal education is supported by evidence that a 10th grade reading level is required to comprehend reading materials from the American Academy of Pediatrics, the Centers for Disease Control and Prevention, and the March of Dimes (Davis et al., 1994). However, up to 11 to 14 years of education is required to comprehend hospital forms and many patient education materials (Davis et al., 1990).

Self-reported education is often not a reliable marker for determining the reading ability required to understand and use written health and nutrition materials. Many individuals with reading problems are unwilling to acknowledge them to care providers. To the extent possible, validated instruments such as the Rapid Estimate of Adult Literacy in Medicine (Davis et al., 1993) are recommended for evaluating reading comprehension.

Recommendation for Low Level of Maternal Education and Illiteracy

A *low level of maternal education* and a *low literacy level* appear to be linked to measures of poor health outcomes and inadequate dietary patterns. There is a theoretical basis for benefit from participation in the WIC program. Therefore, the committee recommends use of *low level of maternal education* and *illiteracy* as a nutrition risk criterion for women, infants, and children in the WIC program. At this time, scientific evidence is inadequate to recommend a definitive cutoff value for low level of maternal education and literacy.

MATERNAL DEPRESSION

Maternal depression was reviewed by the committee in lieu of mental illness since the relevant information in the scientific literature addresses only maternal depression. *Depression* is a term used to characterize either depressive symptoms or a clinical diagnosis of depression. Depressive symptoms include a variety of emotions and feelings—sadness, helplessness, gloom, loss of interest, emotional emptiness, and feeling of flatness. A clinical diagnosis of depression includes both depressive and somatic symptoms that last for an extended period (Zuckerman and Beardslee, 1987). Depression can vary in severity, from mild swings in moods to extreme psychosis.

Prevalence of and Factors Associated with Depression

Estimates of the prevalence of depression vary widely by the population group studied, the assessment tools used, and the definitions of depression used. In general, however, the prevalence of depressive symptoms is higher than that of diagnosed depression (Zuckerman and Beardslee, 1987). Based on the fourth edition of the *Diagnostic and Statistical Manual of Mental Disorders,* roughly 2 to 3 percent of men and between 5 and 9 percent of women can be diagnosed as depressed (APA, 1994). In contrast, depression measures from population-based, self-reported data from the first National Health and Nutrition Examination Survey (NHANES I) show that roughly 10 percent of men and 20 percent of women report depressive symptoms (Eaton and Kessler, 1981).

Several factors are associated with depressive symptoms. Prevalence of depression is significantly higher among low-income individuals. In particular, low-income blacks have extremely high rates of depression, with nearly 50 percent reporting depressive symptoms (Eaton and Kessler, 1981; Orr and James, 1984). Mothers of young children, especially those without a strongly supportive social network, report high rates of depression. Estimates of these rates range from 12 percent, by using strict diagnostic criteria, to 52 percent, by using self-reports of depressive symptoms (Parker et al., 1988). Other factors that have been associated with maternal depression include immigrant status, housing dissatisfaction, low education, poor marital relationship, and stressful life events (Williams and Carmichael, 1985; Zuckerman and Beardslee, 1987).

Depression during the postpartum period is common among women. Postpartum depression ranges from "postpartum blues," which is a transient change in mood affecting 50 to 60 percent of all women, through postpartum depression, which lasts 5 to 6 weeks and affects roughly 20 percent of all women, to postpartum psychosis, which is very rare (Zuckerman and Beardslee, 1987).

Maternal Depression as an Indicator of Nutrition and Health Risk

Appetite changes are a distinguishing feature of depression; 77 to 90 percent of all depressed individuals show appetite changes (Casper et al., 1985; Leckman et al., 1984; Maes et al., 1991). The most common change is a reduction in appetite, although sometimes the opposite occurs. In one study of appetite and weight change in 193 patients with depressive symptoms who were ages 20 to 65 years, 54 percent of patients had a decreased appetite, 27 percent had an increased appetite, and the remainder had no change in appetite (Harris et al., 1984). Other studies confirm this pattern (Casper et al., 1985; Paykel, 1977). In addition, greater appetite change in both directions is related to increased severity of depression (Harris et al., 1984; Paykel, 1977). Severe depression is often associated with anorexia, bulimia, and weight loss (Hudson and Pope, 1990; Maes et al., 1991).

The relationship between maternal psychological status and pregnancy outcomes has long been of interest, although little systematic research has been conducted (Wolkind, 1981). A recent review of prior studies presented evidence that maternal depressive symptoms are associated with preterm birth among low-income urban African-American women (Orr and Miller, 1995). Other studies have found that depressed pregnant women are more likely to smoke during pregnancy, attend prenatal care less frequently, have a higher incidence of LBW infants, and experience higher perinatal mortality rates than non-depressed pregnant controls (Wolkind, 1981; Zax et al., 1977). A study of depressed parents and their children found: (1) increased use of mid or high forceps at delivery, (2) a weak or abnormal cry at birth, and (3) a higher incidence of not breathing for one or more minutes after birth (Weissman et al., 1986). Maternal depression was also associated with recurrent stomachaches and headaches in a community study of preschool-age children (Zuckerman et al., 1987).

Maternal depression is strongly associated with children's emotional well-being and development. Specifically, maternal depression is linked with delayed achievement of developmental milestones (Weissman et al., 1986), long-term child behavior problems (Ghodsian et al., 1984), and a host of negative behavioral and developmental outcomes, including sleep problems, feeding problems, attention deficit disorders, child depression, socially isolating behavior, and withdrawn and defiant behaviors (Parker et al., 1988).

Maternal Depression as an Indicator of Nutrition and Health Benefit

There is little evidence that maternal depression can serve as an indicator of potential benefit from WIC participation, either for women or for their children. However, given the empirical evidence showing appetite changes among depressed patients, it is likely that depressed women and their families would benefit from participation in the WIC program. The nutrition education and supplemental foods provided through the WIC program could help mitigate the relationship between depression and eating habits, and the social service and medical referrals and support could potentially address the social and emotional isolation typically experienced by low-income depressed mothers.

Use of Depression as a Nutrition Risk Criterion in the WIC Setting

Depression is not currently used as a nutrition risk criterion in the WIC program. Diagnosis of depression could be reported to WIC personnel by a health care professional or self-reported measures of depression could be collected during nutrition assessments at WIC program clinics.

Several measures of depression are available that could be used in the WIC setting. One widely used depression measure is the Center for Epidemiologic Studies Depression Scale (CES-D), which is designed to measure the symptoms of clinical depression (Radloff, 1977; Weissman et al., 1977). This scale includes 20 items that ask for the frequency with which a given symptom was experienced during the previous week. The standard cutoff of 16 or more depressive symptoms is used to identify depression; this cutoff includes a high proportion of individuals with a major depressive disorder and dysthymia (less severe clinical depression), as well as some individuals who suffer from depressive symptoms but who do not satisfy the diagnostic criteria (Eaton and Kessler, 1981). The CES-D has been extensively validated and correlates well with other self-reported depression measures and with clinical ratings of depression. It has been used in many previous studies of low-income populations and evaluations of demonstration programs including the JOBS evaluation, the evaluation of the Teenage Parent Demonstration (in progress), and the evaluation of the Comprehensive Child Development Program (DHHS, 1994b).

Recommendation for Maternal Depression

Depression presents health and nutrition risks to the mother and her children, and a suitable method for identifying the risk is available. There is a theoretical basis for benefit from participation in the WIC program. Therefore, the committee recommends use of *maternal depression* as a nutrition risk criterion for women in all state WIC programs. This is a recommendation for a new nutrition risk criterion.

BATTERING

Battering refers to violent assaults on women by their husbands, ex-husbands, boyfriends, or lovers (Rudolf, 1990).

Prevalence of and Factors Associated with Battering

The prevalence of physical assault of pregnant women has been estimated to be around 8 percent among a random sample drawn from public and private clinics and between 7 and 11 percent among nonrandom samples drawn from university obstetrics clinics (Newberger et al., 1992). In a prospective study of 1,203 pregnant women, 24 percent reported experiencing physical or sexual abuse during the previous year (Parker et al., 1994). In another prospective study of 275 women, 19 percent reported experiencing moderate or severe violence during pregnancy; this increased to 25 percent during the postpartum period (Gielen et al., 1994). Data from the 1990 and 1991 Pregnancy Risk Assessment Monitoring System (PRAMS) suggested that the prevalences of battering (self-reports of being physically hurt by a husband or partner during the 12 months prior to delivery) were 6.1, 3.8, 6.9, and 5.1 percent for Alaska, Maine, Oklahoma, and West Virginia, respectively (CDC, 1994).

Two studies identified young maternal age, late prenatal care, substance abuse, poverty, a low level of education, a history of emotional problems, and previous history of abuse as more prevalent among battered pregnant women than among nonabused pregnant women (Parker et al., 1994; Stewart and Cecutti, 1993). In the PRAMS study, nonwhite race, unplanned pregnancies, and WIC program participation were associated with higher rates of physical abuse. The proportion of women reporting physical abuse was two to three times higher among WIC program participants than among nonparticipants (CDC, 1994).

Battering as an Indicator of Nutrition and Health Risk

Several mechanisms have been proposed to explain a link between battering and pregnancy outcome (Newberger et al., 1992). Maternal trauma resulting from battering could cause preterm labor, bleeding, infection, or other conditions that threaten maternal or fetal health and survival. Even when maternal trauma is not serious enough to directly cause poor health consequences, battering may produce intermediate risks for poor pregnancy outcome. For example, the social isolation often experienced by battered women could limit their access to health care; the stress of battering might encourage substance abuse; or inadequate income or denial of food as part of the pattern of victimization could lead to poor nutrition (Newberger et al., 1992).

Relatively few studies have examined pregnancy outcomes in battered women. Some evidence indicates that battering during pregnancy is associated with increased risks of low birth weight (Parker et al., 1994), preterm delivery, and chorioamnionitis (Berenson et al., 1994). Other studies have found no increased risk of poor pregnancy outcome (O'Campo et al., 1994). The lack of consistency in the results may reflect methodologic constraints in carrying out this research.

Battering is associated with poor nutrition and health behaviors. Compared with women not exposed to domestic violence, battered women are more likely to have a low maternal weight gain (< 7 kg), to be anemic, to consume an unhealthy diet, and to abuse drugs, alcohol, and cigarettes (Parker et al., 1994; Stewart and Cecutti, 1993).

Battering as an Indicator of Nutrition and Health Benefit

The committee identified no reports of trials of the effects of provision of WIC nutrition services to abused or battered pregnant women that measured improvement of pregnancy outcome and no studies providing indirect evidence of benefit. There is good potential for battered women to benefit from the supplemental food provided by the WIC program. Moreover, battered women require immediate access to protection, crisis intervention, and support services (Newberger et al., 1992), which WIC referrals could facilitate.

Use of Battering as a Nutrition Risk Criterion in the WIC Setting

In 1992, seven state WIC agencies used battering during pregnancy as a nutrition risk criterion (see Table 7-1).

Recommendation for Battering

The nutrition risk of *battering* is documented for women. There is a theoretical basis but no documentation of benefit via improved outcome of pregnancy as a result of WIC participation. The committee recommends use of *battering* as a nutrition risk criterion for women by the WIC program, unless contradictory information becomes available, and that it remain in the predisposing risks category.

CHILD ABUSE OR NEGLECT

Child neglect is defined as an omission of care by a child's primary caregiver that produces harm, such as inadequate nutrition, clothing, or medical attention (Children's Bureau, DHEW, 1978; Gaudin, 1993). Child maltreatment includes physical abuse, sexual abuse, neglect and emotional maltreatment (NRC, 1993).

Prevalence of and Factors Associated with Child Abuse or Neglect

Reports of child abuse or neglect have increased dramatically, perhaps because of increased reporting, but the actual prevalence of this condition is not known (Johnson, 1995; Wilcox and Marks, 1995). Surveillance of child abuse is limited by a lack of consistent definitions, differences in legal requirements, and the lack of standardization of recordkeeping (Wilcox and Marks, 1995). It has been estimated that each year approximately 2 million children in the United States are seriously abused by their caregivers, and this leads to death in about 1,000 of these cases (AMA, 1992).

Child abuse or neglect can occur in any family. Abuse or neglect is more likely to occur when parents or other caregivers who live under difficult social conditions have little knowledge of child development and unrealistic expectations of child behavior (Johnson, 1995). Child abuse or neglect is reported more frequently among poor families, perhaps in part because of increased attention to the health and social issues among the poor. Psychosocial stress, unplanned pregnancy, teenage parents, low levels of education, and substance abuse are all associated with child abuse and neglect. Child abuse and spousal abuse are related, and parents who were themselves abused as children are more likely to be abusive. The risk of physical abuse is higher for infants and children with chronic medical conditions or physical or mental disabilities.

Child Abuse or Neglect as an Indicator of Nutrition and Health Risk

Serious neglect and physical, emotional, or sexual abuse have short- and long-term physical, emotional, and functional consequences. Nutrition neglect, which is a form of child abuse, is the most common cause of poor growth in infancy and may account for as much as half of all cases of nonorganic failure to thrive (Johnson, 1995) (see also Chapter 5). It has been reported that preschool-age children who were abused were more than 16 times more likely to be malnourished than nonabused children from the same neighborhood (Karp et al., 1989). Other data suggest that among abused children with poor growth, those who were placed in long-term foster care demonstrated catch-up growth that was not observed in children who remained in their original families (King and Taitz, 1985).

It may be possible to identify infants at risk of child abuse early in the postpartum period (Leventhal et al., 1989). The ability to target high-risk families may allow the application of educational and social interventions to prevent child abuse and neglect.

Child Abuse or Neglect as an Indicator of Nutrition and Health Benefit

Through intensive and comprehensive treatment, 80 to 90 percent of families involved in child neglect or abuse can become able to provide adequate care to the children, but this is more difficult when substance abuse is involved (Johnson, 1995). In examining mechanisms to prevent child abuse and neglect, the National Research Council Panel on Child Abuse and Neglect recognized the potential benefit of participation in the WIC program (NRC, 1993). The provision of nutritionally dense foods and education about appropriate feeding practices is especially important for those children with nonorganic failure to thrive, but these interventions, as well as linkages to the medical and social systems, are also likely to benefit children who have been traumatized by physical, emotional, or sexual abuse.

Use of Child Abuse or Neglect as a Risk Criterion in the WIC Program

In 1992, seven state WIC agencies considered abuse or neglect to be a nutrition risk criterion for children, and nine considered physical abuse to be a nutrition risk criterion for infants (see Table 7-1).

Recommendation for Child Abuse or Neglect

There is empirical and theoretical evidence that *child abuse* or *neglect* pose nutrition risks. There is a theoretical basis for benefit from participation in the WIC program. Therefore, the committee recommends use of reported or diagnosed *child abuse* or *neglect* as a nutrition risk criterion for infants and children in the WIC program.

CHILD OF A YOUNG CAREGIVER

There is little disagreement that adolescent women generally are less prepared economically, emotionally, socially, and physically for motherhood than their somewhat older counterparts (Hofferth, 1987; Phipps-Yonas, 1980; Trussel, 1988). By and large, the scientific community has focused on the physical risk that early pregnancy imposes on young women and on its potential for poor pregnancy outcomes and health problems (see Chapter 5). Adolescent pregnancies and motherhood, however, impose risks that go well beyond the medical consequences of teenage pregnancies.

Prevalence of and Factors Associated with Child of a Young Caregiver

Currently, about 1 million adolescent women (12 percent of women 15 to 19 years of age) become pregnant, and about half give birth (Guttmacher Institute, 1994). More than 80 percent of young women who give birth are poor.

Although older teenagers (ages 18 to 19 years) account for most teenage pregnancies and births, 9,000 women under age 15 gave birth and 161,000 women ages 15 to 17 years gave birth in 1988. Virtually all of these births were outside of marriage (Trussel, 1988).

According to USDA (1994), just under 1.3 million women participated in the WIC program in 1992. Of the women whose age was reported in that study, 11 percent (over 136,000) were age 17 years and under. At the time of the study, 68 percent of these young mothers were pregnant, 6 percent were breastfeeding mothers, and 26 percent were postpartum, nonnursing mothers.

Child of a Young Caregiver as an Indicator of Nutrition and Health Risk

Despite the wide array of literature on teenage motherhood and its health consequences for children, young age is seldom isolated from other contributing factors, such as economic and social status, family support, motivation, educational performance, and achievement (Phipps-Yonas, 1980; Trussel, 1988). Thus, there is little research directly linking nutrition status among infants and children to young age of their mother. Since parental diet and eating habits influence the diet and eating habits of children, this could be a fruitful line of research.

Children born to teenage mothers are at higher risk of abuse, neglect, maltreatment, poor growth, and problems in mother-child interaction than other children (Earp and Ory, 1980; Egeland and Brunnquell, 1979; Herrenkohl and Herrenkohl, 1979; Steir et al., 1993). The study by Steir and colleagues (1993), a longitudinal, cohort study of 219 children born to women 18 years of age or younger and of 219 children born to women 19 years of age or older, is notable for its careful design. These investigators reviewed birth records to match children by date of birth, ethnicity, gender, birth order, and method of payment for the hospitalization (Medicaid, private insurance, or self-payment) as a marker for socioeconomic status. Analysis of the records revealed that maltreatment (abuse, neglect, or sexual abuse) occurred twice as frequently among the children of the younger mothers, and that poor growth occurred in 6.9 percent of the children of the young mothers compared with 4.1 percent of the children of the older mothers.

Child of a Young Caregiver as an Indicator of Nutrition and Health Benefit

The committee found no direct or indirect empirical evidence evaluating the benefit of participation in the WIC program on the children of young caregivers. Although adult age of the caregiver is not a prerequisite for infants' and children's good health, it is likely that identifying young caregivers will identify infants and children who can benefit from WIC participation. There is potential for the children to benefit from the provision of nutritious food and nutrition education of their caregivers, as well as from referrals.

Use of Child of a Young Caregiver as a Risk Criterion in the WIC Program

Of the five states that included young age of the mother as a nutrition risk criterion for infants (see Table 7-1), two broadened the definition to include a nonmaternal caregiver. The specific age of a young mother or caregiver ranged from less than 18 to less than 19 years of age.

Recommendations for Child of a Young Caregiver

Child of a young mother or *caregiver* thus far has been found to be a weak indicator of nutrition risk among infants and children. Even though there is a theoretical basis for benefit from participation in the WIC program, the benefit is expected to be minor. However, the lack of empirical evidence for young caregiver is a result of lack of studies of this risk criterion, rather than studies showing no risk or benefit. Therefore, the committee recommends using *child of a young caregiver* as a risk criterion for infants and children in the WIC program pending further scientific evidence. The committee recommends research on young age of caregivers and the health and nutrition status of the children in their care.

CHILD OF A MENTALLY RETARDED PARENT

Prevalence of and Factors Associated with a Child of a Mentally Retarded Parent

The committee found no data on the prevalence of children with a mentally retarded parent in the U.S. population or in the WIC program population. However, on the basis of a study of parents considered to have intellectual impairment in the state of Oregon, the Association for Retarded Citizens estimates that approximately 32,500 U.S. parents are mentally retarded (Ingram, 1993).

Mentally Retarded Parent as an Indicator of Nutrition and Health Risk

Although it is likely that many mentally retarded parents are adequate care providers, parents with intellectual disabilities frequently have problems in ensuring that a child's physical, nutrition, health, and safety needs are met (Feldman, 1994). If abuse and neglect occur, children of parents with mental retardation are at risk of poor outcomes (medical, cognitive, and emotional problems) (Accardo and Whitman, 1990; Whitman et al., 1990). The occurrence of neglect appears to be secondary to a lack of parental education in combination with the unavailability of supportive services (Schilling et al., 1982; Seagull and Scheurer, 1986). In fact, the best predictor of neglect appears to be the lack of familial or societal supports that can help prevent the circumstances leading to neglect (Tymchuk, 1992). Without information about such supports, an intelligence (IQ) quotient score below a certain level, usually taken to be 60, may be useful as a predictor of neglect. Many parents with a low IQ have other risk factors that are associated with child maltreatment such as poverty, personality disorders, low self-esteem, history of abuse, unemployment, and transient living arrangements (Belsky, 1984; Tymchuk and Feldman, 1991).

In 13 of the 14 studies reviewed by Schilling and colleagues (1982), mentally retarded parents were overrepresented in samples of parents who abused or neglected their children. They concluded that research suggests there is an increased risk of maltreatment of children raised by mentally retarded parents.

The infants of mentally retarded mothers can be at risk of poor health from circumstances existing prior to their birth. Mentally retarded mothers may not receive optimal prenatal care if they are unaware of the need for prenatal care or they lack access to it. Their infants are at higher than normal risk of malnutrition, alcohol or lead exposure, infection, and other prenatal complications (Rolfe, 1990).

Assessment of growth and development in the infant or child may reveal much about the adequacy of the child's environment. Nonorganic failure to thrive in the infant or child of a mentally retarded parent is a reliable indicator of neglect (Rolfe, 1990).

Mentally Retarded Parent as an Indicator of Nutrition and Health Benefit

The children of mentally retarded parents can benefit from educational interventions for their parents. Educational programs for mentally retarded adults with preschool-age children have been shown to improve their parenting skills (Whitman et al., 1990). A parent training program conducted in St. Louis combined basic teaching at their center with one or two observational home visits weekly. Child care and parent-child relationships were the major areas covered, with food preparation being an important component. All families made progress in selected parenting skills.

In earlier research, teaching mentally retarded adults grocery shopping and menu planning skills assisted them in serving more nutritious meals (Feldman, 1994; Sarber et al., 1983). Feldman and colleagues (1992a, b) studied mothers with developmental disabilities who lacked child care skills. Instruction in proper feeding techniques, correct formula preparation, bottle cleaning techniques, and meal planning and preparation improved the mothers' skills and was associated with such benefits as increased weight gain and fewer illnesses in their children. Research indicates that the most effective training for parents with intellectual disabilities should be performance based and should use modeling, practice, feedback, and praise (Feldman, 1994).

The WIC program's supplemental food package and nutrition education could help mentally retarded parents provide nutritionally balanced diets to infants and children. Although some WIC programs teach participants grocery shopping skills and menu planning, the specialized training required by an intellectually disabled parent to acquire child care skills is most likely beyond the scope of the WIC program. Nonetheless, WIC program referrals can direct the mentally retarded parent to other social and health services that can improve parenting skills.

Use of Mentally Retarded Parent as a Risk Criterion in the WIC Program

Documentation or a diagnosis of mental retardation in a parent is generally done outside of the WIC program setting by a medical or mental health professional. If an initial certification for participation in the WIC program identifies gross indicators of abuse or neglect this could lead to a finding of mental retardation in a parent.

Recommendation for Child of a Mentally Retarded Parent

The risk for a *child of a mentally retarded parent* is well documented. Many families with a mentally retarded parent experience poverty and have difficulty maintaining their family because of a lack of support systems. On a theoretical basis, WIC program services and referrals may help to prevent or treat problems resulting from the parenting inadequacies of a mentally retarded parent. Therefore, the committee recommends use of *child of a mentally retarded parent* as a nutrition risk criterion for infants and children by the WIC program at a higher priority.

SUMMARY

The assessment of conditions that may predispose low-income individuals to health or nutrition risks has become an important part of the WIC program. Some predisposing risk criteria have been used by state WIC agencies for many years, and some have been adopted recently. A summary of the risk and potential to benefit with predisposing risks covered in this chapter appears above in Table 7-2.

Based on available evidence concerning nutrition and health risks and potential to benefit, the committee recommends use of nutrition risk criteria as shown previously in Table 7-3.

REFERENCES

AAP, CCHS (American Academy of Pediatrics, Committee on Community Health Services). 1989. Health care for children of migrant families. Pediatrics 84:739–740.

Accardo, P.J., and B.Y. Whitman. 1990. Children of parents with mental retardation: Problems and diagnoses. Pp. 123–131 in When a Parent is Mentally Retarded, B.Y. Whitman and P.J. Accardo, eds. Baltimore, Md.: Paul H. Brookes Pub. Co.

Acker, P.J., A.H. Fierman, and B.P. Dreyer. 1987. An assessment of parameters of health care and nutrition in homeless children. Am. J. Dis. Child. 141:388.

Alperstein, G., C. Rappaport, and J.M. Flanigan. 1988. Health problems of homeless children in New York City. Am. J. Public Health 78:1232–1233.

AMA (American Medical Association). 1992. Diagnostic treatment guidelines on child physical abuse and neglect. Arch. Fam. Med. 1:187–197.

APA (American Psychiatric Association). 1994. Diagnostic and Statistical Manual of Mental Disorders, 4th ed. Washington, D.C.: APA.

Arnstein, E., and G. Alperstein. 1987. Health care for the homeless. Public Health Currents 27:29–34.

Bassuk, E., and L. Rubin. 1987. Homeless children: A neglected population. Am. J. Orthopsychiatry 57:279–286.

Bassuk, E.L., and L. Weinreb. 1993. Homeless pregnant women: Two generations at risk. Am. J. Orthopsychiatry 63:348–355.

Bassuk, E.L., L. Rubin, and A.S. Lauriat. 1986. Characteristics of sheltered homeless families. Am. J. Public Health 76:1097–1101.

Becker, J., A. Robinson, S. Gortmaker, L. Weinreb, and E. Bassuk. 1992. Reproductive health Status of Homeless Pregnant Women. Paper presented at the National Conference of American Public Health Association, Washington, D.C.: American Public Health Association.

Belsky, J. 1984. The determinants of parenting: A process model. Child Dev. 55:83–96.

Berenson, A.B., C.M. Wiemann, G.S. Wilkinson, W.A. Jones, and W.G. Anderson. 1994. Perinatal morbidity associated with violence experienced by pregnant women. Am. J. Obstet. Gynecol. 170:1760–1769.

Bunston, T., and M. Breton. 1990. The eating patterns and problems of homeless women. Women Health 16:43–62.

Burns, D., and J.P. Pierce. 1992. Tobacco use in California, 1990–1991. Sacramento, Calif.: California Department of Health Services.

Cardenas, J., C.E. Gibbs, and E.A. Young. 1976. Nutritional beliefs and practices in primagravid Mexican-American women. J. Am. Diet. Assoc. 69:262–265.

Casper, R.C., D.E. Redmond, Jr., M.M. Katz, C.B. Schaffer, J.M. Davis, and S.H. Koslow. 1985. Somatic symptoms in primary affective disorder. Presence and relationship to the classification of depression. Arch. Gen. Psychiatry 42:1098–1104.

CDC (Centers for Disease Control and Prevention). 1994. Physical violence during the 12 months preceding childbirth—Alaska, Maine, Oklahoma and West Virginia, 1990–1991. Morbid. Mortal. Weekly Rep. 43(8):132–137.

Chase, H.P., V. Kumar, J.M. Dodds, H.E. Sauberlich, R.M. Hunter, R.S. Burton, and V. Spalding. 1971. Nutritional status of preschool Mexican-American migrant farm children. Am. J. Dis. Child. 122:316–324.

Chavkin, W., A. Kristal, C. Seabron, and P.E. Guigli. 1987. The reproductive experience of women living in hotels for the homeless in New York City. N.Y. State J. Med. 87:10–13.

Chen, L.H., and D.B. Petitti. 1995. Case-control study of passive smoking and the risk of small-for-gestational-age at term. Am. J. Epidemiol. 142:158–165.

Chen, Y., L.L. Pederson, and N.M. Lefcoe. 1989. Passive smoking and low birth weight. Lancet 2:54–55.

Chi, P.S. 1985. Medical utilization patterns of migrant farm workers in Wayne County, New York. Public Health Rep. 100:480–490.

Children's Bureau, DHEW (U.S. Department of Health, Education, and Welfare). 1978. Interdisciplinary Glossary on Child Abuse and Neglect: Legal, Medical, Social Work Terms. Washington, D.C.: Government Printing Office.

Chilmonczyk, B.A., G.J. Knight, G.E. Palomaki, A.J. Pulkkinen, J. Williams, and J.E. Haddow. 1990. Environmental tobacco smoke exposure during infancy. Am. J. Public Health. 80:1205–1208.

Cleland, J.G., and J.K. Van Ginneken. 1988. Maternal education and child survival in developing countries: The search for pathways of influence. Soc. Sci. Med. 27:1357–1368.

Davis, T.C, M.A. Crouch, G. Wills, S. Miller, and D.M. Abdehou. 1990. The gap between patient reading comprehension and the readability of patient education materials. J. Fam. Pract. 31:533–538.

Davis, T.C., S.W. Long, R.H. Jackson, E.J. Mayeaux, R.B. George, P.W. Murphy, and M.A. Crouch. 1993. Rapid estimate of adult literacy in medicine: A shortened screening instrument. Fam. Med. 25:391–395.

Davis, T.C., E.J. Mayeaux, D. Fredrickson, J.A. Bocchini, Jr., R.H. Jackson, and P.W. Murphy. 1994. Reading ability of parents compared with reading level of pediatric patient educational materials. Pediatrics 93:460–468.

de la Torre, A., and L.M. Rush. 1989. The effects of health care access on maternal and infant health among migrant and seasonal farmworker women in California. Migrant Health Newsline Clin. 6 (suppl.):1–2.

Devaney, B., L. Bilheimer, and J. Schore. 1990. The Savings in Medicaid Costs for Newborns and Their Mothers from Prenatal Participation in the WIC Program, Vol. I. Food and Nutrition Service, Office of Analysis and Evaluation, U.S. Department of Agriculture. Washington, D.C.: U.S. Government Printing Office.

Dever, G.E.A. 1991. Migrant Health Status: Profile of a Population with Complex Health Problems. Austin, Tex.: Migrant Clinicians Network.

DHHS (U.S. Department of Health and Human Services). 1989. Reducing the Health Consequences of Smoking: 25 Years of Progress. A Report of the Surgeon General DHHS Publication No. (CDC) 89–8411. Washington D.C.: U.S. Government Printing Office.

DHHS (U.S. Department of Health and Human Services). 1990. An Atlas of State Profiles Which Estimate Number of Migrant and Seasonal Farmworkers and Members of Their Families. Public Health Service, Health Resources and Services Administration, Bureau of Health Care Delivery and Assistance, Division of Primary Care Services, Migrant Health Branch. Washington, D.C.: USDHHS.

DHHS (U.S. Department of Health and Human Services). 1994a. Preventing Tobacco Use Among Young People. A Report of the Surgeon General. Washington, D.C.: U.S. Government Printing Office.

DHHS (U.S. Department of Health and Human Services). 1994b. Comprehensive Child Development Program: A National Family Support Demonstration. Interim Report to Congress, May 6, 1994. Washington, D.C.: U.S. DHHS.

Drake, M.A. 1992. The nutritional status and dietary adequacy of single homeless women and their children in shelters. Public Health Rep. 107:312–319.

Earp, J.A., and M.G. Ory. 1980. The influence of early parenting on child maltreatment. Child Abuse and Neglect 4:237–245.

Eaton, W.W., and L.G. Kessler. 1981. Rates of symptoms of depression in a national sample. Am. J. Epidemiol. 14:528–538.

Eddins, E. 1993. Characteristics, health status, and service needs of sheltered homeless families. Assoc. Black Nursing Faculty J. 4:40–44.

Egeland, B., and D. Brunnquell. 1979. An at-risk approach to the study of child abuse: Some preliminary findings. J. Am. Acad. Child Psychiatry 18:219–235.

Feldman, M.A. 1994. Parenting education for parents with intellectual disabilities: A review of outcome studies. Res. Dev. Disabil. 15:299–332.

Feldman, M.A., L. Case, M. Garrick, W. MacIntyre-Grande, J. Carnwell, and B. Sparks. 1992a. Teaching child-care skills to mothers with developmental disabilities. J. Appl. Behav. Anal. 25:205–215.

Feldman, M.A., L. Case, and B. Sparks. 1992b. Effectiveness of a child-care training program for parents at-risk for child neglect. Can. J. Behav. Sci. 24:14–28.

Fierman, A.H., B.P. Dreyer, L. Quinn, S. Shulman, C.D. Courtlandt, and R. Guzzo. 1991. Growth delay in homeless children. Pediatrics 88:918–925.

Fischer, P.J. 1991. Alcohol, Drug Abuse, and Mental Health Problems Among Homeless Persons: A Review of the Literature, 1980–1990. Executive Summary. DHHS Pub. No. (ADM) 91-1763(B). Rockville, Md.: U.S. Dept. of Health and Human Services, Public Health Service, Alcohol, Drug Abuse, and Mental Health Administration.

Gaudin, J.M., Jr. 1993. Child Neglect: A Guide for Intervention. U.S. Department of Health and Human Services, National Center on Child Abuse and Neglect. Washington, D.C.: U.S. Department of Health and Human Services.

Ghodsian, M., E. Zajicek and S. Wolkind. 1984. A longitudinal study of maternal depression and child behaviour problems. J. Child Psychol. Psychiatry 25:91–109.

Gielen, A.C., P.J. O'Campo, R.R. Faden, N. Kass, and X. Xue. 1994. Interpersonal conflict and physical violence during the childbearing year. Soc. Sci. Med. 39:781–787.

Guendelman, S., and B. Abrams. 1995. Dietary intake among Mexican-American women: Generational differences and a comparison with white non-Hispanic women. Am. J. Public Health 85:20–25.

Guttmacher Institute. 1994. Sex and America's Teenagers. New York: The Alan Guttmacher Institute.

Harris, B., J. Young, and B. Hughes. 1984. Appetite and weight change in patients presenting with depressive illness. J. Affect. Disord. 6:331–339.

Herrenkohl, E.C., and R.C. Herrenkohl. 1979. A comparison of abused children and their nonabused siblings. J. Am. Acad. Child Psychiatry 18:260–269.

Hobcraft, J.N., J.W. McDonald, and S.O. Rutstein. 1984. Socioeconomic factors in infant and child mortality: A cross-national comparison. Population Studies 38:189–223.

Hofferth, S.L. 1987. The children of teen childbearers. Chapter 8 in Risking the Future: Adolescent Sexuality, Pregnancy, and Childbearing. Volume II: Working Papers and Statistical Appendixes. Report of the Panel on Adolescent Pregnancy and Childbearing, Committee on Child Development Research and Public Policy, Commission on Behavioral and Social Sciences and Education. Washington, D.C.: National Academy Press.

Hu, D.J., R.M. Covell, J. Morgan, and J. Arcia. 1989. Health care needs for children of the recently homeless. J. Community Health 14:1–8.

Hudson, J.I., and H.G. Pope. 1990. Depression and Eating Disorders. In Eating Disorders, L.K. Hsu, ed. New York: Guilford Press.

Ingram, D. 1993. Parents Who Have Mental Retardation. The Association for Retarded Citizens (ARC) Q & A. Arlington, Tex.: Association for Retarded Citizens.

Jaffee, K., T. Melnick, and M. Sawyer. 1992. A Comparison of Birth Outcomes and Risk Factors for Homeless and Domiciled African-American Women Enrolled in WIC: New York City, 1989–1990. Washington, D.C.: American Public Health Association.

Johnson, C. 1995. Abuse and neglect of children. Pp. 112–120 in Nelson Textbook of Pediatrics, 15th ed., R.E. Behrman, R.M. Kliegman, and A. Arvin, eds. Philadelphia: W.B. Saunders.

Jordanov, J.S. 1990. Cotinine concentrations in amniotic fluid and urine of smoking, passive smoking and non-smoking pregnant women at term and in the urine of their neonates on the 1st day of life. Eur J. Pediatr. 149:734–737.

Karp, R.J., T.O. Scholl, E. Decker, and E. Ebert. 1989. Growth of abused children contrasted with non-abused in an urban poor community. Clin. Pediatr. Phila. 28:317–320.

King, J.M., and L. Taitz. 1985. Catch up growth following abuse. Arch. Dis. Child. 60:1152–1154.

Kleinman, J.C., and J.H. Madans. 1985. The effects of maternal smoking, physical stature, and educational attainment on the incidence of low birth weight. Am. J. Epidemiol. 121:843–855.

Kramer, R.A., L. Allen, and P.J. Gergen. 1995. Health and social characteristics and children's cognitive functioning: Results from a national cohort. Am. J. Public Health 85:312–318.

Leckman, J.F., K.A. Caruso, B.A. Prusoff, M.M. Weissman, K.R. Merikangas, and D.L. Pauls. 1984. Appetite disturbance and excessive guilt in major depression. Arch. Gen. Psychiatry 41:839–844.

Lenihan, A. 1994. Scientific Base for the Nutrition Risk Criteria Used in the Special Supplemental Food Program for Women, Infants, and Children. Statement at the First Public Meeting, May 19, of the Committee on Scientific Evaluation of WIC Nutrition Risk Criteria, Food and Nutrition Board, Institute of Medicine, Washington, D.C.

Leventhal, J.M., R.B. Garber, and C.A. Brady. 1989. Identification during the postpartum period of infants who are at high risk of child maltreatment. J. Pediatr. 114:481–487.

Lewis, M.R., and A.F. Meyers. 1989. The growth and development status of homeless children entering shelters in Boston. Public Health Rep. 104:247–250.

Link, B.G., E. Susser, A. Stueve, J. Phelan, R.E. Moore, and E. Struening. 1994. Lifetime and five-year prevalence of homelessness in the United States. Am. J. Public Health 84:1907–1912.

Luder, E., E. Boey, B. Buchalter, and C. Martinez-Weber. 1989. Assessment of the nutritional status of urban homeless adults. Public Health Rep. 104:451–457.

Luder, E., E. Ceysens-Okada, A. Koren-Roth, and C. Martinez-Weber. 1990. Health and nutrition survey in a group of urban homeless adults. J. Am. Diet. Assoc. 90:1387–1392.

MacArthur, C., and E.G. Knox. 1987. Passive smoking and birth weight. Lancet 1:37–38.

Maes, M., M. Vandewoude., S. Scharpe, L. De Clarcq, W. Stevens, L. Lepoutre, and C. Schotte. 1991. Anthropometric and biochemical assessment of the nutritional state in depression: Evidence for lower visceral protein plasma levels in depression. J. Affect. Disord. 23:25–33.

Martin, T.R., and M.B. Bracken. 1986. Association of low birth weight with passive smoking exposure in pregnancy. Am. J. Epidemiol. 124:633–642.

Miller, D.S., and E.H.B. Lin. 1988. Children in sheltered homeless families: Reported health status and use of health services. Pediatrics 81:668–673.

Mobed, K., E.B. Gold, and M.B. Schenker. 1992. Occupational health problems among migrant and seasonal farm workers. West. J. Med. 157:367–373.

National Advisory Council on Migrant Health. 1992. Farmworker Health for the Year 2000: 1992 Recommendations of the National Advisory Council on Migrant Health. Austin, Tex.: National Migrant Resource Program, Inc.

Navaje, M., D. Glik, and K. Saluja. 1994. Communication effectiveness of postnatal nutrition education in a WIC program. J. Nutr. Educ. 26:211–217.

Newberger, E.H., S.E. Barkan, E.S. Lieberman, M.C. McCormick, K. Yllo, L.T. Gary, and S. Schechter. 1992. Abuse of pregnant women and adverse birth outcome: Current knowledge and implications for practice. J. Am. Med. Assoc. 267:2370–2372.

New York Coalition for the Homeless. 1986. Hungry Children and Mr. Cuomo: Time for Action. New York: New York Coalition for the Homeless.

NRC (National Research Council). 1993. Understanding Child Abuse and Neglect. Report of the Panel on Research on Child Abuse and Neglect, Commission on Behavioral and Social Sciences and Education. Washington, D.C.: National Academy Press.

O'Campo, P., A.C. Gielen, R.R. Faden, and N. Kass. 1994. Verbal abuse and physical violence among a cohort of low-income pregnant women. Womens Health Issues 4:29–37.

Orr, S.T., and C.A. Miller. 1995. Maternal depressive symptoms and the risk of poor pregnancy outcome. Epidemiol. Rev. 17(1):165–171.

Orr, S.T., and S. James. 1984. Maternal depression in an urban pediatric practice: Implications for health care delivery. Am. J. Public Health 74:363–365.

Overpeck, M.D., and Moss, A.J. 1991. Children's exposure to environmental cigarette smoke before and after birth. Hyattsville, Md.: U.S. Department of Health and Human Services.

Parker, B., J. McFarlane, and K. Soeken. 1994. Abuse during pregnancy: Effects on maternal complications and birth weight in adult and teenage women. Obstet. Gynecol. 84:323–328.

Parker, R.M., L.A. Rescorla, J.A. Finkelstein, N. Barnes, J.H. Holmes, and P.D. Stolley. 1991. A survey of the health of homeless children in Philadelphia shelters. Am. J. Dis. Child. 145:520–526.

Parker, S., S. Greer, and B. Zuckerman. 1988. Double jeopardy: The impact of poverty on early child development. Pediatr. Clin. North Am. 35:1227–1239.

Paykel, E.S. 1977. Depression and appetite. J. Psychosom. Res. 21:401–407.

Phipps-Yonas, S. 1980. Teenage pregnancy and motherhood. A review of the literature. Am. J. Orthopsychiatry 50:403–431.

Poswillo, D., and E. Alberman. 1992. Effects of Smoking on the Fetus, Neonate and Child. New York: Oxford Medical Publishers.

Radloff, L.S. 1977. The CES-D Scale: A self-report depression scale for research in the general population. J. Appl. Psychol. Meas. 1:385–401.

Rolfe, U.T. 1990. Children of parents with mental retardation: The pediatrician's role. Pp. 133–146 in When a Parent is Mentally Retarded, B.Y. Whitman and P.J. Accardo, eds. Baltimore, Md.: Paul H. Brookes Pub. Co.

Rossi, P.H., J.D. Wright, G.A. Fisher, and G. Willis. 1987. The urban homeless: Estimating composition and size. Science 235:1336–1341.

Roth, L., and E.R. Fox. 1990. Children of homeless families: Health status and access to care. J. Community Health 15:275–284.

Rubin, D.H., P.A. Krasilnikoff, J.M. Leventhal, B. Weile, and A. Berget. 1986. Effect of passive smoking on birth-weight. Lancet 2:415–417.

Rudolf, C. 1990. Prenatal Care to Reduce Family Violence. In New Perspectives on Prenatal Care, I.R. Merkatz and J.E. Thompson, eds. New York: Elsevier Science Pub. Co.

Rush, D., D.G. Horvitz, W. Burleigh Seaver, J. Leighton, N.L. Sloan, S.S. Johnson, R.A. Kulka, J.W. Devore, M. Holt, J.T. Lynch, T.G. Virag, M. Beebe Woodside, and D.S. Shanklin. 1988. The National WIC Evaluation: Evaluation of the Special Supplemental Food Program for Women, Infants, and Children. IV. Study methodology and sample characteristics in the longitudinal study of pregnant women, the study of children, and the food expenditures study. Am. J. Clin. Nutr. 48:429–438.

Rust, G.S. 1990. Health status of migrant farmworkers: A literature review and commentary. Am. J. Public Health 80:1213–1217.

Samet, J.M., E.M. Lewit, and K.E. Warner. 1994. Involuntary smoking and children's health. Future Child. 4(3):94–114.

Sarber, R.E., M.M. Halasz, M.C. Messmer, A.D. Bickett, and J.R. Lutzker. 1983. Teaching menu planning and grocery shopping skills to a mentally retarded mother. Ment. Retard. 21:101–106.

Schilling, R.F., S.P. Schinke, B.J. Blythe, and R.P. Barth. 1982. Child maltreatment and mentally retarded parents: Is there a relationship? Ment. Retard. 20:201–209.

Seagull, E.A.W., and S.L. Scheurer. 1986. Neglected and abused children of mentally retarded parents. Child Abuse Negl. 10:493–500.

Shotland, J., D. Loonin, and E. Haas. 1989. Full Fields, Empty Cupboards: The Nutritional Status of Migrant Farmworkers in America. Washington, D.C.: Public Voice for Food and Health Policy.

Siegler, M.B., G.K. Franklin, and M.A. Lynch. 1993. Lesson plans for WIC homeless. J. Nutr. Educ. 25:294A.

Slesinger, D.P., and C. Ofstead. 1993. Economic and health needs of Wisconsin migrant farm workers. J. Rural Health 9(2):138–148.

Slesinger, D.P., B.A. Christenson, and E. Cautley. 1986. Health and mortality of migrant farm children. Soc. Sci. Med. 23:65–74.

Steir, D.M., J.M. Leventhal, A.T. Berg, L. Johnson, and J. Mezger. 1993. Are children born to young mothers at increased risk of maltreatment? Pediatrics 91:642–648.

Stewart, D.E., and A. Cecutti. 1993. Physical abuse during pregnancy. Can. Med. Assoc. J. 149:1257–1263.

Taylor, M.L., and S.A. Koblinsky. 1993. Dietary intake and growth status of young homeless children. J. Am. Diet. Assoc. 93:464–466.

Trussell, J. 1988. Teenage pregnancy in the United States. Fam. Plann. Perspect. 20:262–272.

Tymchuk, A.J. 1992. Predicting adequacy of parenting by people with mental retardation. Child Abuse Negl. 16:165–178.

Tymchuk, A.J., and M.A. Feldman. 1991. Parents with mental retardation and their children: Review of research relevant to professional practice. Can. Psychol. 32:486–494.

Ueda, Y., H. Morikawa, T. Punakoshi et al. 1989. Estimation of passive smoking during pregnancy by cotinine measurement and its effect on fetal growth. Acta Obstet. Gynaecol. Jpn 41:454–460.

U.S. Bureau of the Census. 1993. Statistical Abstract of the United States: 1993, 113th ed. Washington, D.C.: U.S. Government Printing Office.

U.S. Conference of Mayors. 1984. Homeless in America. Washington, D.C.: U.S. Government Printing Office.

U.S. Conference of Mayors. 1986. The Continued Growth of Hunger, Homelessness, and Poverty in America's Cities: A 25-City Survey. Washington, D.C.: U.S. Government Printing Office.

U.S. Conference of Mayors. 1987. A Status Report on the Homeless Families in American's Cities: A 29-City Survey. Washington, D.C.: U.S. Government Printing Office.

USDA (U.S. Department of Agriculture). 1991. Homeless Mothers and Children: What is the Evidence of Nutritional Risk? Report no. 12 in Technical Papers: Review of WIC Nutritional Risk Criteria. Prepared for the Food and Nutrition Service by the Department of Family and Community Medicine, College of Medicine, University of Arizona, Tucson. Washington, D.C.: USDA.

USDA (U.S. Department of Agriculture). 1992. 1992 Biennial Report on the Special Supplemental Food Program for Women, Infants and Children and on the Commodity Supplemental Food Program. National Advisory Council on Maternal, Infant, and Fetal Nutrition. Food and Nutrition Service. Washington, D.C.: USDA.

USDA (U.S. Department of Agriculture). 1994. Study of WIC Participant and Program Characteristics, 1992. Final Report. Office of Analysis and Evaluation, Food and Nutrition Service. Washington, D.C.: USDA.

Victora, C.G., S.R. Huttly, F.C. Barros, C. Lombardi, and J.P. Vaughan. 1992. Maternal education in relation to early and late child health outcomes: Findings from a Brazilian cohort study. Soc. Sci. Med. 34:899–905.

Watkins, E.L., K. Larson, C. Harlan, and S. Young. 1990. A model program for providing health services for migrant farmworker mothers and children. Public Health Rep. 105:567–575.

Weiss, B.D., G. Hart, and R.E. Pust. 1991. The relationship between literacy and health. 1:351–363.

Weissman, M.M., D. Sholomskas, M. Pottenger, B.A. Prusoff, and B.Z. Locke. 1977. Assessing depressive symptoms in five psychiatric populations: A validation study. Am. J. Epidemiol. 106:203–214.

Weissman, M.M., K. John, K.R. Merikangas, B.A. Prusoff, P. Wickramaratne, D. Gammon, A. Angold, and V. Warner. 1986. Depressed parents and their children: General health, social, and psychiatric problems. Am. J. Dis. Child. 140:801–805.

Weitzman, B.C. 1989. Pregnancy and childbirth: Risk factors for homelessness? Fam. Plann. Perspect. 21:175–178.

Weitzman, M., S. Gortmaker, and A. Sobol. 1992. Maternal smoking and behavior problems of children. Pediatrics 90:342–349.

Whitman, B.Y., B. Graves, and P.J. Accardo. 1990. Parents learning together I: Parenting skills training for adults with mental retardation. Pp. 51–65 in When a Parent is Mentally Retarded, B.Y. Whitman and P.J. Accardo, eds. Baltimore, Md.: Paul H. Brookes Pub. Co.

Wiecha, J.L., J.T. Dwyer, and M. Dunn-Strohecker. 1991. Nutrition and health services needs among the homeless. Public Health Rep. 106:364–374.

Wilcox, L.S., and J.S. Marks, eds. 1995. From Data to Action: CDC's Public Health Surveillance for Women, Infants and Children. Atlanta: Centers for Disease Control.

Williams, H., and A. Carmichael. 1985. Depression in mothers in a multi-ethnic urban industrial municipality in Melbourne. Aetiological factors and effects on infants and preschool children. J. Child Psychol. Psychiatry 26:277–288.

Wolgemuth, J.C., C. Myers-Williams, P. Johnson, and C. Henseler. 1992. Wasting, malnutrition, and inadequate nutrient intakes identified in a multiethnic homeless population. J. Am. Diet. Assoc. 92:834–839.

Wolkind, S. 1981. Prenatal emotional stress: Effects on the fetus. Pp. 177–193 in Pregnancy: A Psychological and Social Study, S. Wolkind and E. Zajicek, ed. New York: Grune & Stratton.

Wood, D., and R.B. Valdez. 1991. Barriers to medical care for homeless families compared with housed poor families. Am. J. Dis. Child. 145:1109–1115.

Wood, D.L., R.B. Valdez, T. Hayashi, and A. Shen. 1990. Health of homeless children and housed, poor children. Pediatrics 86:858–866.

Wright, J.D., and L.E. Weber-Burdin. 1987. Homelessness and Health. Washington, D.C.: McGraw Hill.

Zax, M., A.J. Sameroff, and H.M. Babigian. 1977. Birth outcomes in the offspring of mentally disordered women. Am. J. Orthopsychiatry 47:218–230.

Zuckerman, B.S., and W.R. Beardslee. 1987. Maternal depression: A concern for pediatricians. Pediatrics 79:110–117.

Zuckerman, B., J. Stevenson, and V. Bailey. 1987. Stomachaches and headaches in a community sample of preschool children. Pediatrics 79:677–682.

8

Conclusions and Recommendations

The concept of nutrition risk assessment is integral to the design and operation of the WIC program. Nutrition risk is a criterion for program eligibility, and nutrition risk criteria are used to assign a priority level to women, infants, and children. By serving those at the highest priority levels first, the WIC priority system is used to allocate limited program resources among eligible individuals. In addition, the nutrition risk assessments are used to tailor the WIC intervention and, in some cases, to monitor the health and nutrition status of program participants.

This report is a scientific assessment of the WIC nutrition risk criteria as they are currently used to establish WIC eligibility and the priority of the WIC eligible individuals. Based on this scientific assessment, this final chapter provides general conclusions, recommendations for specific nutrition risk criteria, and recommendations for future research and action.

The framework that was used in the scientific assessment conducted for this report has two key features. The first is the exposition and utilization of the concept of potential to benefit from the delivery of interventions and services provided by the WIC program. This concept differs from the approach that has guided the development of risk criteria used by the WIC program, namely, assessment of the individual's risk of a poor outcome. This application of the concept of potential to benefit moves the program focus from curative (tertiary prevention) to risk reduction (secondary prevention). Utilizing such an approach can provide for more efficient targeting of the scarce resources available to the WIC program and also improve outcomes.

A second important feature of the analytical framework is the explicit consideration of the concepts of yield of risk, yield of benefit, and sensitivity of the nutrition risk criteria used by the WIC program. These concepts, in conjunction with the concepts of indicators of risk and indicators of benefit, have implications that underlie both the assessments of the nutrition risk criteria used by the WIC program and the development of the report's conclusions and recommendations. In particular, risk indicators and cutoff points should be chosen such that the highest proportion of those who are truly at risk can be identified and the highest proportion of those identified can benefit from WIC program participation. With limited program resources, cutoff points should be set with less than perfect sensitivity to increase yield, recognizing that as cutoff points become more restrictive, some individuals who could benefit from WIC services will not be served. The decision process presented in Chapter 3 can be used to review other risk criteria that the WIC program may be asked to approve in the future.

GENERAL CONCLUSIONS

The committee reached seven general conclusions about the WIC nutrition risk criteria and priority system:

• *A body of scientific evidence supports a majority of the nutrition risk criteria used by the WIC program.* For some of the risk criteria, however, there are serious gaps in the evidence.

• *Nutrition risk criteria used by many states have a high sensitivity and low yield of benefit.* This is because the prevalence of many of the risk conditions is low and the cutoffs used are generous, resulting in both the selection of many of those who have the risk condition (high sensitivity) and the selection of many individuals who do not have the risk condition (low yield of risk, which results in low yield of benefit).

• *Use of generous cutoff points or loosely defined conditions in categories designated by federal regulation to receive high priority for eligibility may result in denial of services to individuals who are actually at higher nutrition risk.* When resources are limited, individuals in lower priority categories may not be served even if their true risk is very high, while those in high priority categories must be served. Very generous cutoff points produce a low yield of benefit without any increase in sensitivity (serving more of those truly at risk). Loosely defined risk conditions are those that encompass a broad range of medical problems with varying degrees of nutrition risk or potential to benefit from WIC participation. Such loosely defined nutrition risk criteria include endocrine disorders, renal disease, chronic and recurrent infections, food allergies, and genetic and congenital disorders.

• *There is some inconsistency between the WIC program's goals, design, and implementation.* The goal of the WIC program is one of primary prevention—to prevent the occurrence of health problems. Through the use of nutrition risk criteria, the WIC priority system is designed in principle to be a secondary/tertiary prevention program to reduce or cure identified risk. However, through the use of generous cutoff points, loosely defined risk conditions, and a priority system that places pregnant women and infants at the highest priorities, in general, the WIC program operates as a primary prevention program for pregnant women and infants and a secondary and tertiary prevention program for children and postpartum women.

- *The WIC priority system should be reexamined.* Many individuals now classified in low priority categories have more potential to benefit from WIC services than some individuals placed in higher priority categories. For example, a child of a mentally retarded parent (currently priority VII) or an anemic child age 3 years with a very low hemoglobin (currently priority III) may have a greater potential to benefit than an infant classified as anemic (currently priority I) by a criterion with a too generous cutoff point.

- *It is important that the WIC program reevaluate the criteria in use every 5 to 10 years and change cutoffs and incorporate new criteria as necessary.* This is because the yield of risk of a criterion increases as the prevalence of the risk in the population increases, and it decreases as the prevalence of the risk in the population decreases. For example, the yield of risk of the nutrition risk criterion for poor growth has decreased over time as the prevalences of wasting and stunting have declined. The addition of homelessness as a nutrition risk criterion by the WIC program reflects, in part, increases in the prevalence of homelessness.

- *There is a need to identify or develop additional nutrition risk criteria that select those individuals who are at risk of developing specific health and nutrition problems if they do not receive WIC benefits.* Since the WIC program is believed to be a major contributor to the decline in the prevalence of health and nutrition problems (for example, iron deficiency anemia), it is important to identify practical indicators of the risk of developing the problem so that the WIC program can maintain its preventive function. Dietary risk criteria or predisposing risk criteria may do this, but data are limited. Setting high cutoff points for anemia or poor growth does not effectively identify those at risk of developing the problem.

In addition, the committee emphasizes the importance of the systematic collection of data about the prevalence of individuals meeting specific WIC nutrition risk criteria.

RECOMMENDATIONS FOR SPECIFIC NUTRITION RISK CRITERIA

Table 8-1 summarizes the committee's recommendations for use of nutrition risk criteria, cutoff values, and the segments of the population to which they apply. For greater specificity, the name of the criterion used occasionally

TABLE 8-1 Nutrition Risk Criteria and Committee Recommendations for the Specific WIC Population, by Category of Nutrition Risk

Risk Criterion	Committee Recommendation	Pregnant Women	Postpartum Women Lactating	Postpartum Women Nonlactating	Infants	Children
Anthropometric Risk Criteria						
Women						
Prepregnancy underweight	Use with cutoff value of IBW <90% or BMI <19.8	✓				
Low maternal weight gain	Use with cutoff value of <0.9 kg/mo for nonobese and <0.45 kg/mo for obese	✓				
Maternal weight loss during pregnancy	Use with cutoff value of >2 kg first trimester, >1 kg 2nd or 3rd trimesters	✓				
Prepregnancy overweight	Use with cutoff value of IBW >120% or BMI >26	✓	✓	✓		
High gestational weight gain	Use with cutoff value of >3 kg/mo	✓	✓	✓		
Maternal short stature	Do not use					
Postpartum underweight	Use with cutoff value of IBW <90% or BMI <19		✓	✓		
Postpartum overweight	Use with cutoff value of IBW >120% or BMI >26 after 6 weeks postpartum		✓	✓		
Abnormal postpartum weight change	Do not use					

Infants and Children

Low birth weight	Use with cutoff value of <2,500 g				✓
Small for gestational age	Use with cutoff value of <10th percentile			✓	✓
Short stature	Use with cutoff value of <5th percentile			✓	✓
Underweight	Use with cutoff of 5th percentile			✓	✓
Low head circumference	Use with cutoff value of <5th percentile			✓	✓
Large for gestational age	Do not use				
Overweight	Use with cutoff value of >95th percentile			✓	✓
Slow growth	Use with cutoff value of <3rd percentile			✓	✓

Biochemical and Other Medical Risk Criteria

Criteria Related to Nutrient Deficiencies

Anemia	Use with CDC or IOM cutoffs	✓	✓	✓	✓
Failure to thrive	Use[a]	✓	✓	✓	✓
Nutrient deficiency diseases	Use[a]	✓	✓	✓	✓

Medical Conditions Applicable to the Entire WIC Population[b]

Gastrointestinal disorders	Use	✓	✓	✓	✓
Nausea and vomiting during pregnancy	Use only if serious and prolonged	✓	✓	✓	✓
Diabetes mellitus	Use	✓	✓	✓	✓
Gestational diabetes	Use	✓		✓	✓

Continued

TABLE 8-1 Continued

Risk Criterion	Committee Recommendation	Pregnant Women	Postpartum Women Lactating	Postpartum Women Nonlactating	Infants	Children
Biochemical and Other Medical Risk Criteria *(Continued)*						
Medical Conditions Applicable to the Entire WIC Population[b] (Continued)						
Thyroid disorders	Use	✓	✓	✓	✓	✓
Chronic hypertension	Use	✓	✓	✓	✓	✓
Renal disease	Use, but not for chronic urinary tract infections	✓	✓	✓	✓	
Cancer	Use	✓	✓	✓	✓	✓
Central nervous system disorders	Use	✓	✓	✓	✓	✓
Genetic and congenital disorders	Use	✓	✓	✓	✓	✓
Pyloric stenosis	Do not use					
Inborn errors of metabolism	Use[a]	✓	✓	✓	✓	✓
Chronic or recurrent infections	Use, with exceptions	✓	✓	✓	✓	✓
Upper respiratory infections	Do not use					
Bronchitis	Do not use					
Otitis media	Do not use					
Urinary tract infections	Do not use					
HIV infections and AIDS	Use	✓	✓	✓	✓	✓
Recent major surgery, trauma, burns, or severe acute infections	Use	✓	✓	✓	✓	✓

Other medical conditions (juvenile rheumatoid arthritis, lupus erythematosus, and cardiorespiratory disorders)	Use	✓		✓	✓	

Conditions Related to the Intake of Specific Foods

Food allergies	Use	✓	✓	✓	✓	✓
Celiac disease	Use	✓	✓	✓	✓	✓
Lactose intolerance	Use	✓	✓	✓	✓	✓
Other food intolerance	Do not use					
Asthma	Do not use					

Conditions Specific to Pregnancy

Pregnancy at a young age	Use with cutoff value of 2 years postmenarche	✓
Pregnancy age older than 35 years	Do not use	
Closely spaced pregnancies	Use with an interconceptional interval of 6 months (9 months if concurrently lactating)	✓
High parity	Do not use	
History of preterm delivery	Use	✓
History of postterm delivery	Do not use	
History of low birth weight	Use	✓
History of neonatal loss	Do not use	
History of birth with congenital or birth defect	Use	✓

Continued

341

TABLE 8-1 *Continued*

Risk Criterion	Committee Recommendation	Pregnant Women	Postpartum Women Lactating	Postpartum Women Nonlactating	Infants	Children
Biochemical and Other Medical Risk Criteria *(Continued)*						
Conditions Specific to Pregnancy (Continued)						
Lack of prenatal care	Use with cutoff value of care beginning after 1st trimester or long intervals between visits[c]	✓				
Multifetal gestation	Use	✓	✓			
Fetal growth restriction	Use	✓		✓		
Preeclampsia and eclampsia	Do not use					
Placental abnormalities	Do not use					
Conditions Specific to Infants and/or Children						
Prematurity	Use with cutoff value of ≤37 weeks' gestation; do not use for children				✓	✓
Hypoglycemia	Use				✓	✓
Potentially Toxic Substances						
Long-term drug-nutrient interactions	Use for selected drugs	✓	✓			
Maternal smoking	Use, with cutoff of any smoking[c,d]	✓	✓			
Alcohol and illegal drug use	Use with cutoff of any use[c,e]	✓	✓	✓	✓	
Lead poisoning	Use with cutoff value of >10 μg/dl	✓	✓	✓	✓	✓

Dietary Risk Criteria

Failure to meet Dietary Guidelines	Use; develop valid assessment tools		✓	✓	
Vegan diets	Use		✓	✓	✓
Other vegetarian diets	Do not use		✓	✓	
Highly restrictive diets	Use	✓	✓		✓
Inappropriate infant feeding	Use	✓		✓	
Early introduction of solid foods	Use	✓		✓	
Feeding cow milk during 1st 12 months	Use			✓	
No dependable source of iron after 4–6 months	Use			✓	
Improper dilution of formula	Use			✓	
Feeding other foods low in essential nutrients	Use			✓	
Lack of sanitation in preparation of nursing bottles	Use			✓	
Infrequent breastfeeding as sole source of nutrients	Use			✓	
Inappropriate use of nursing bottle	Use			✓	
Excessive caffeine intake	Do not use		✓		
Pica	Use				✓

Continued

TABLE 8-1 Continued

Risk Criterion	Committee Recommendation	Pregnant Women	Postpartum Women Lactating	Postpartum Women Nonlactating	Infants	Children
Dietary Risk Criteria *(Continued)*						
Inadequate diet	Do not use; use diet recall or FFQ to tailor nutrition education; develop valid assessment tools	✓				
Food insecurity	Use; develop valid assessment tools		✓	✓	✓	
Predisposing Risk Criteria						
Homelessness	Use	✓	✓	✓	✓	✓
Migrancy	Use	✓	✓	✓	✓	✓
Passive smoking	Do not use					
Low level of maternal education or illiteracy	Use	✓	✓	✓	✓	✓
Maternal depression	Add	✓	✓	✓	✓	✓
Battering	Use	✓	✓	✓		
Child abuse or neglect	Use				✓	✓
Child of a young caregiver	Use				✓	✓
Child of a mentally retarded parent	Use				✓	✓

345

NOTE: ✓ = subgroup to which the recommendation applies; IBW = ideal body weight; BMI = body mass index; CDC = Centers for Disease Control; IOM = Institute of Medicine; FFQ = food frequency questionnaire.

[a] This criterion merits higher priority among children.
[b] Diagnosis of the condition is the cutoff point used.
[c] This criterion merits lower priority.
[d] Two committee members (Barbara Abrams and Barbara Devaney) preferred to (1) set a higher cutoff point that would more clearly identify women whose cigarette use places them at higher risk of poor outcomes and (2) maintain this criterion at high priority.
[e] Three committee members (Barbara Abrams, Barbara Devaney, and Roy Pitkin) preferred to (1) set a higher cutoff point that would more clearly identify women whose alcohol use places them at higher risk of poor outcomes and (2) maintain these criteria at high priority.

differs from that used by the WIC program. The recommendations are intended to apply to all states unless otherwise indicated. Exceptions may be made if the meaning of the criterion in a particular context is different or the condition (e.g., pica) is common in one state and uncommon in another. Brief supplementary information about these recommendations follows for each of the categories of nutrition risk criteria. The full report provides the basis for each recommendation. For convenience, Table 8-2 lists those nutrition risk criteria that the committee recommends adding and those that it recommends discontinuing.

Anthropometric Risk Criteria

Anthropometric risk criteria are used in the WIC program to assess individuals for nutrition risk and to monitor their nutrition status or their response to WIC program interventions over time. The committee's review indicated that the WIC anthropometric risk indicators are predictors both of nutrition and health risks and of benefit from participation in the WIC program. The cutoff points used for anthropometric risk indicators among WIC programs vary substantially, however, with resulting effects on yield. Therefore, the committee recommends that cutoff points for anthropometric measures be limited to those that are scientifically justified. It further points out that there is no obvious justification for the use of symmetric cutoff points (for example, at the 5th and 95th percentiles).

Risk criteria for which there was very little evidence of nutrition risk or benefit from WIC participation include maternal short stature, abnormal postpartum weight change, and infants large for gestational age. Therefore, the committee recommends discontinuing use of these nutrition risk criteria.

Biochemical and Other Medical Risk Criteria

In general, the biochemical and other medical risk criteria predict nutrition and health risk, with varying degrees of benefit. The most common concern of the committee was the lack of scientific justification for the generous cutoff points for biochemical and certain other medical risk criteria currently used by many state WIC agencies.

Of the biochemical and other medical risk criteria, anemia is used most frequently in the WIC program to establish the eligibility of women, infants, and children to participate in the program. Cutoff values for anemia vary substantially among state WIC agency programs, with little or no scientific justification for variation from standard definitions. The committee recommends

TABLE 8-2 Committee Recommendations for Changes in Risk Criteria

Nutrition Risk Criteria That Should Be Added:
Dietary
    Food insecurity
Predisposing
    Maternal depression

Nutrition Risk Criteria That Should Not Be Used:
Anthropometric
    Maternal short stature
    Large for gestational age
    Abnormal postpartum weight change
Medical
    Arthritis, general
    Asthma
    Bronchitis
    Food intolerance, except lactose intolerance
    High parity
    History of neonatal loss
    History of postterm delivery
    Nausea and vomiting, mild
    Otitis media
    Placental abnormalities
    Preeclampsia and eclampsia
    Pregnancy age older than 35 years
    Prematurity for children
    Pyloric stenosis
    Upper respiratory infection
    Urinary tract infection except chronic pyelonephritis with persistent proteinuria
Dietary
    Inadequate diet
    Excessive caloric intake
    Excessive caffeine intake
    Vegetarian diets except vegan
Predisposing
    Passive smoking

that anemia continue to be used as a risk criterion in the WIC program but discourages the use of high cutoff points because of the resulting low yield from increasing their iron intake. That is, the high cutoff values for anemia used by many state WIC programs result in the inclusion of many who do not have and are not at risk of anemia and, thus, are unlikely to benefit from provision of WIC's supplemental food.

Many biochemical and other medical nutrition risks are documented as the result of diagnosis by a medical care provider of an existing medical condition that affects nutritional needs or may be improved by dietary management. These diagnosed conditions are reported to WIC program staff. The committee recommends that most of these nutrition risk criteria continue to be used in the WIC program, using cutoff points that generally are documentation or diagnosis of the disease or disorder.

Maternal cigarette, alcohol, and drug use among pregnant and lactating women pose significant health risks but uncertain benefit from participation in the WIC program. On an interim basis, the committee recommends that these nutrition risk indicators be used in the WIC program, with a cutoff of "any use."[1]

Risk criteria for which there was risk and benefit only under specific conditions included long-term drug-nutrient interactions and chronic and recurrent infections. The committee feels that these criteria were too vague to be useful in their current form. It recommends that a listing of drugs for which there are clear drug-nutrient interactions or potential for misuse be developed. The use of other medications would not be associated with nutrition risk or benefit, and thus their use would not provide a basis for eligibility. For chronic and recurrent infections, evidence of risk and benefit was available only for certain chronic infections for which there were documented nutrition deficits, and the committee recommends that states should clearly define "chronic" or "recurrent" in determining cutoff points for these indicators.

Risk criteria for which there was very limited evidence of nutrition risk or benefit from participation in the WIC program included food intolerance other than lactose intolerance, high age at conception, previous placental abnormalities, history of postterm delivery, high parity, preeclampsia and eclampsia, and prematurity as a risk criterion for children ages 1 to 5 years. The committee recommends that these nutrition risk criteria no longer be used in the WIC program.

Dietary Risk Criteria

Three major categories of dietary risk criteria are reviewed: inappropriate dietary patterns, inadequate diets, and food insecurity. Risk criteria classified as inappropriate dietary patterns are listed in Table 8-1. The committee found that there are clear health and nutrition risks associated with selected inappropriate dietary patterns and that the potential to benefit from participation in the WIC program is high. For women and for children at least 2 years of age, failure to

---

[1] Three committee members preferred to set higher cutoff points that would more clearly delineate women whose substance use places them at higher risk for poor outcomes. Barbara Abrams and Barbara Devaney preferred to set higher cutoff points for cigarette and alcohol use; Roy Pitkin preferred a higher cutoff point only for alcohol use.

meet Dietary Guidelines for Americans is a dietary risk criterion that receives increased attention in this report.

As long as the food provided by the supplemental food package is eaten, the WIC program is likely to improve the diets of those WIC participants with inadequate diets. In the WIC setting, however, diet recalls and food frequency questionnaires that compare estimated nutrient intake with Recommended Dietary Allowances have poor ability to ascertain who actually has inadequate diets. Thus, even though the WIC program is likely to improve dietary intake, the committee recommends discontinuing use of *inadequate diets* as a nutrition risk criterion because it has a very low yield. Nonetheless, diet recalls or food frequency questionnaires are useful in the WIC program for identifying foods commonly consumed and providing a starting point for nutrition education.

Food insecurity is defined as the lack of predictable, sustainable access in socially acceptable ways to enough food of adequate quality to sustain health. Although this risk criterion is just beginning to be used by state WIC agencies, and there is limited evidence to evaluate causal links to nutrition and health risk, the committee believes that there is a fundamental value to addressing the risk to health and nutrition related to a lack of access to food. The benefit of participation in the WIC program for those at risk of food insecurity is high. Therefore, the committee recommends use of food insecurity as a nutrition risk criterion in the WIC program. At present, however, there is insufficient scientific evidence on which to select a cutoff point that would identify those most likely to benefit from the WIC program.

Predisposing Nutrition Risk Criteria

Currently, predisposing nutrition risk criteria receive a low priority within the WIC program. The use of predisposing nutrition risk criteria warrants additional attention. If an individual has a predisposing risk but no other risk, he or she will be placed in a priority category that is usually unserved by the WIC program. This may limit the WIC program's ability to serve as a preventive program. Additional attention to the predisposing nutrition risk criteria is warranted because (1) they have a high yield for risk and a high, but as yet unknown, potential for benefit from WIC services, and (2) the prevalence of some of these factors (e.g., homelessness) is increasing, thus increasing the overall yield of these criteria.

The committee supports the use of most of the predisposing risk criteria that have been used in the WIC program for women, infants, and children (see Table 8-1).

The committee recommends that a diagnosis of depression be added as a predisposing risk criterion for women, and that diagnosed maternal depression be added as a predisposing risk criterion for infants and children. Because of the lack of evidence that nutrition will benefit those exposed to passive smoking, the committee recommends that this risk criterion no longer be used in the WIC program.

RECOMMENDATIONS FOR FUTURE RESEARCH AND ACTION

Research Recommendations

Regarding the nutrition risk criteria reviewed in the report, the committee recommends the following areas for future research:

- Develop anthropometric standards (including weight change velocity) for pregnant and lactating women, including adolescents. These standards should be suitable to assess the likelihood that these women would benefit from nutrition intervention and to achieve improved reproductive outcomes.
- Evaluate whether the use of a combination of criteria (e.g., an anthropometric risk criterion plus a dietary risk criterion) may be more effective than the use of a single risk criterion in predicting a benefit from participation in the WIC program.
- Evaluate whether overweight or obese mothers and their infants and children benefit from current WIC program interventions. The prevalence of overweight and obesity among low-income women, infants, and children is increasing over time, and the health and nutrition risks of obesity are well-documented.
- Evaluate the yields of benefit for the various cutoff points used for anthropometric risk criteria—recognizing that there is no obvious justification for symmetric high and low cutoff points. It is possible that current cutoff points are so generous that the yield of benefit from WIC program interventions is low.
- Examine how the WIC program affects nutrition outcomes for individuals with selected medical risk factors.
- Determine the extent to which women who use cigarettes, alcohol, and/or illegal drugs benefit from the WIC program and the level of use of these substances that should be set as the cutoff point, if applicable.
- Invest in the development and validation of practical dietary assessment instruments that can be used across WIC programs for the identification of inappropriate dietary patterns, inadequate dietary intake, and food insecurity, recognizing that adaptations may be needed for culturally diverse populations.
- Examine the utility of predisposing factors (such as homelessness, migrancy, low level of maternal education, child abuse and neglect, and maternal depression) as predictors of benefit from WIC program services.

Action Recommendations

In addition to these research recommendations, the committee recommends the following actions be taken by the Food and Consumer Service, U.S. Department of Agriculture, to provide guidance to state WIC agencies in the development of nutrition risk criteria:

- Adopt scientifically justified cutoff values for anemia and for anthropometric criteria among women, infants, and children, realizing that they may be different across populations as prevalences change.
- Define *preterm* consistently as delivery before the end of the 37th postmenstrual week for both mothers and their infants.
- Adopt scientifically justified cutoff points for *young maternal age* (chronological or gynecological, or both), because increased risks associated with births to these women cannot be entirely explained by poverty.
- Distinguish among some of the broadly defined medical and dietary conditions used by the WIC program in order to identify eligible WIC participants truly at high nutrition risk. These broad nutrition risk categories include *endocrine disorders*, renal disease, *chronic and recurrent infections, food allergies,* and *genetic and congenital disorders*. They include a broad range of medical problems with varying degrees of nutrition risk or potential to benefit from participation in the WIC program. Similarly, the category *inappropriate diet* includes some behaviors for which little nutrition risk is evident. The list in Table 8-1 distinguishes among criteria in the broad nutrition risk categories.
- Appoint an expert committee to provide guidance on cutoff points for cigarette, alcohol, and illegal drug use that will identify pregnant and lactating women who are most likely to benefit from the WIC program. Members of the expert committee should have expertise in substance abuse during pregnancy and lactation, assessment and treatment of substance abuse, public policy, nutrition, and epidemiology.
- Identify the specific drugs that place individuals at nutrition risk with prolonged use and for which WIC program interventions could provide some benefit. The current nutrition risk criteria *drug-nutrient interactions* and *inappropriate use of medications* are too broadly defined and likely to produce very low yield of benefit.
- Disseminate information about risk criteria widely.
- Consider changing the current WIC priority system to give higher priority to those nutrition risk criteria identified in this report as having strong relationships to risk and potential to benefit and lower priority to nutrition risk criteria with weaker relationships to risk and potential to benefit.

1. *Risk criteria that merit higher priority*: vegan diets, highly restrictive diets, selected aspects of inappropriate infant feeding, food insecurity, homelessness, child of a mentally retarded parent.

2. *Risk criteria that merit higher priority among children*: nutrient deficiency diseases, failure to thrive, gastrointestinal disorders, inborn errors of metabolism.

3. *Risk criteria that merit lower priority*: mild nausea and vomiting during pregnancy; lack of prenatal care; cigarette, alcohol, and illegal drug use.[2]

Such a change in the priority system would require disaggregating the current categories (anthropometric, medical, dietary, and predisposing) that are used for ranking each risk criterion into one of seven priorities. It would also mean that in some cases children could be given priority over pregnant women. Such a change should improve the targeting of the program in terms of both risk and benefit.

---

[2] Three committee members (Barbara Abrams, Barbara Devaney, and Roy Pitkin) prefer retaining high priority for the criteria *alcohol use* and *illegal drug use*. Barbara Abrams and Barbara Devaney prefer retaining the high-priority level for the criterion *cigarette use* as well. See footnote 1 concerning cutoff points for these criteria.

Appendix A

Participants at the First Public Meeting May 19, 1994

ORGANIZATIONS AND INDIVIDUALS MAKING ORAL PRESENTATIONS OR SUBMITTING WRITTEN COMMENTS

AMERICAN SOCIETY FOR CLINICAL NUTRITION, Bethesda, MD
PHYLLIS A. BRAMSON, WIC Supplemental Food Branch, California Department of Health Services, Sacramento, CA
FRANCES H. COOK, Office of Nutrition, Georgia Department of Human Resources, Atlanta, GA
PAULA EUREK, Nebraska WIC Program, Department of Health, Lincoln, NE
CATHY FRANKLIN, Department of Health, Community and Family Health, Washington State WIC Program, Olympia, WA
STEFAN HARVEY, Center on Budget and Policy, Washington, DC
JULIE KRESGE, Food and Consumer Services, U.S. Department of Agriculture, Alexandria, VA
ALICE J. LENIHAN, National Association of WIC Directors, Washington, DC
NATIONAL ASSOCIATION OF WIC DIRECTORS, Washington, DC
LARRY R. PROHS, Bureau of Women, Infants, and Children, Ohio Department of Health, Columbus, OH
JUDITH SOLBERG, Public Policy and Legislation, Association of State and Territorial Public Health Nutrition Directors, Washington, DC
CAROL WEST SUITOR, Bethesda, MD

OBSERVERS

TODD ASKEW, American Academy of Pediatrics, Washington, DC
CHRISTINA BLUE, Olsson, Frank and Weeda, Washington, DC
DOUG GREENAWAY, National Association of WIC Directors, Washington, DC
JAY HIRSCHMAN, Food and Consumer Services, U.S. Department Agriculture, Alexandria, VA
DAVID HOYT, Budget Office, U.S. Department of Agriculture, Washington, DC
LINDA JUPIN, Food and Consumer Service, U.S. Department of Agriculture, Alexandria, VA
ELLEN LAZZARO, National Association of WIC Directors, Washington, DC
HELEN MARTIN, Food and Consumer Services, U.S. Department of Agriculture, Alexandria, VA
CATHERINE PAPPAS, March of Dimes, White Plains, NY
JANET TOGNETTI SCHILLER, Food and Consumer Service, U.S. Department of Agriculture, Alexandria, VA
CYNTHIA SCOTT, March of Dimes, White Plains, NY
JANICE STEINSCHNEIDER, Center on Budget and Policy Priorities, Washington, DC

Appendix B

Participants at the Second Public Meeting September 19–20, 1994

ORGANIZATIONS AND INDIVIDUALS MAKING ORAL PRESENTATIONS OR SUBMITTING WRITTEN COMMENTS

J. A. ANDERSON, Los Angeles County Department of Public Health. Los Angeles, CA
ROSA AVELAR, REI WIC Program, Inglewood, CA
MARION TAYLOR BAER, University of Southern California Affiliated Program, Children's Hospital of Los Angeles, Los Angeles, CA
CARLA BOUCHARD, Children's Medical Service, California Department of Health Services, Sacramento, CA
TINA CIFUENTES, Public Health Foundation WIC Program, Los Angeles, CA
CASWELL A. EVANS, Jr., Los Angeles County Department of Health, Los Angeles, CA
PAULA GREGG, Maricopa County Department of Public Health Services, Phoenix, AZ
ELOISE JENKS, Public Health Foundation WIC Program, Irwindale, CA
SHARON JONES, REI WIC Program, Inglewood, CA
LOIS JOVANOVIC-PETERSON, Sansum Medical Research Foundation, Santa Barbara, CA
MARY KELLIGREW KASSLER, The Commonwealth of Massachusetts Department of Public Health; Boston, MA
LYNN KERSEY, Children's Advocacy Institute, Los Angeles, CA
WILLIAM J. KLISH, American Academy of Pediatrics, Houston, TX
ROBERT and STACY PALACIO, Public Health Foundation, Los Angeles, CA
DEBORAH PELLEGRINI, WIC Supplemental Food Branch, California Department of Health Services, Sacramento, CA

CHARLES M. PETERSON, Sansum Medical Research Foundation, Santa Barbara, CA
MARGARITA POSADAS, Clinica Sierra Vista WIC Program, Bakersfield, CA
BRUCE E. SMITH, San Bernadino County Department of Public Health, San Bernadino, CA
LAURIE TRUE, California Food Policy Advocates, San Francisco. CA
GERALD WAGNER, Adult and Child Health Services, County of Orange Health Care Agency, Santa Ana, CA
KIMBERLEY K. YEAGER, California Department of Health Services, Sacramento, CA
DOROTHY M. YONEMITSU, San Diego WIC Program, San Diego, CA

OBSERVERS

BETSY CLINE, San Bernadino County, Department of Public Health, San Bernadino, CA
LYNN FRAZIN, Public Health Foundation–WIC, Irwindale, CA
JENNIFER JEFFRIES, Public Health Foundation, Irwindale, CA
SARAH KELLOGG, Food and Consumer Service, U.S. Department of Agriculture, San Francisco, CA
GAIL KIBBY, Public Health Foundation, Inglewood, CA
HEIDI KUO, Public Health Foundation, REI WIC Program, Inglewood, CA
SALLY M. LIVINGSTON, Clinica Sierra Vista WIC, Bakersfield, CA
SAMAR McGREGOR, Public Health Foundation, Irwindale, CA
LAURENCE J. OBAID, County of Orange Health Care–WIC, Santa Ana, CA
DURREEN QURESHI, County of Orange Health Care–WIC, Santa Ana, CA
MANDET UBANEZ, County of Orange Health Care–WIC, Santa Ana, CA
MICHELE Y. VAN EYKEN, County of Orange Health Care–WIC, Santa Ana, CA
KNAN YALEYA, Public Health Foundation, REI WIC Program, Inglewood, CA

Appendix C

WIC Program: Common Nutritional Risk Criteria

GROUP A

Closely Spaced Pregnancies
Hematocrit
Hemoglobin
High Parity
High Weight Gain
Low Age at Conception
Low Birthweight
Low Weight Gain
Obesity Percentile
Overweight
Short Percentile
Underweight
Underweight Percentile
Weight Loss During Pregnancy

GROUP B

Abnormal Weight Gain/Loss
Alcohol or Other Substance Abuse or Addicted Infant
Chronic Disorders
Excessive Dietary Intake

Food Allergies/Intolerance
History of Infectious Conditions
HIV Positive
Inadequate Dietary Intake
Inappropriate Dietary Intake
Long-term Intake of Medication with Known Drug-Nutrient Interaction
Major Infections Conditions
Metabolic Disorders
Pica
Preeclampsia/Eclampsia or History of Eclampsia
Small for Gestational Age
Year Post-Menarche

GROUP C

Caretaker Currently Drug/Alcohol Abuser, or Physically or Mentally Disabled
Excessive Caffeine
Inappropriate Feeding Behavior or Techniques
Inadequate Facilities for Food Preparation or Storage
Passive Smoking
Young Caretaker (< 18 Years of Age)

SOURCE: J. Hirschman, Food and Consumer Service, U.S. Department of Agriculture, personal communication, 1993.

Appendix D

Definitions of Yield and Sensitivity of Cutoff Points for Nutrition Risk

Efficacy of WIC interventions: the proportion of individuals selected for WIC whose bad outcomes will be prevented or reduced =

$$Y/(Y + w), \qquad (D-1)$$

where

   Y = those identified who have the risk and will benefit
   w = those identified who have the risk and will not benefit

	Overall benefit from WIC	
Identified by criterion	Yes	No
Yes	Y	w

Yield of risk[1]: the proportion of those identified at risk who are at risk =

$$B/(B + o), \qquad (D-2)$$

where

   B = those identified at risk who are at risk
   o = those identified at risk who are not at risk

---

[1] Yield of risk is called *positive predictive value* in epidemiology (Last, 1988).

| | At risk of bad outcome ||
Identified by criterion	Yes	No
Yes	B	o
No	b	O

Not all those who have the risk and are identified at risk (B) will benefit, thus:

$$B = Y + w \qquad (D\text{-}3)$$

Combining equations D-2 and D-3:

Yield of risk = $B/(B + o) = (Y + w)/(Y + w + o)$

Yield of benefit: proportion of those identified at risk who will benefit =

$$Y/(B+o) = [B/(B + o)] \times [(Y/B)] \quad = [B/(B + o)] \times [Y/(Y + w)] \qquad (D\text{-}4)$$
$$= [\text{yield of risk}] \times [\text{efficacy of WIC}]$$

Sensitivity for risk[2] =

$$B/(B + b) \qquad (D\text{-}5)$$

Sensitivity for benefit:

$$Y/(Y+w+b) \qquad (D\text{-}6)$$

REFERENCES

Habicht, J-P. 1980. Some characteristics of indicators of nutritional status for use in screening and surveillance. Am. J. Clin. Nutr. 33:531–535.

Habicht, J-P., L.D. Meyers, and C. Brownie. 1982. Indicators for identifying and counting the improperly nourished. Am. J. Clin. Nutr. 35:1241–1254.

Last, J.M. 1988. A Dictionary of Epidemiology. London: Oxford University Press.

---

[2] Nutritional examples of tradeoffs between specificity and sensitivity are discussed in Habicht (1982), and the relationship of specificity-sensitivity tradeoffs to the positive predictive value are discussed in Habicht (1980).

Appendix E

Biographical Sketches

COMMITTEE

RICHARD E. BEHRMAN (*Chair*) currently serves as the Managing Director of the David and Lucile Packard Foundation Center for the Future of Children in Los Altos, California. Previously, he was at the Case Western Reserve University School of Medicine, where he was vice president of medical affairs and dean. Dr. Behrman graduated from Amherst College and received his J.D. degree from Harvard University and M.D. degree from the University of Rochester. Former positions include professor and department chair of pediatrics at the College of Physicians and Surgeons at Columbia University and at Case Western Reserve University, chairman of the Department of Perinatal Physiology at the Oregon Regional Primate Research Center, and section chief for physiology and biochemistry at the National Institute for Neurological Diseases and Blindness. As a member of the Institute of Medicine, Dr. Behrman served as vice chair for the Committee on Department of Energy Radiation Epidemiological Research Programs for the Board on Radiation Effects Research. He holds memberships in the American Academy of Pediatrics, the American Pediatrics Society, the Perinatal Research Society, Sigma Xi, and the Society for Pediatric Research, for which he served a term as vice president. At the National Research Council he served on the Board of Maternal, Child, and Family Health Research.

BARBARA ABRAMS is an Associate Professor of Public Health, Nutrition, and Epidemiology, School of Public Health at the University of California, Berkeley. She has a cross appointment in maternal and child health while holding membership in the Graduate Group in Nutrition. Concurrently, she is an assistant professor in the Department of Obstetrics, Gynecology, and Reproductive Sciences at the University of California, San Francisco, where she had been a lecturer and clinical nutritionist. Previously, she was a lecturer at Stanford University and a research nutritionist at the University of California, Berkeley and the Kaiser Foundation Research Institute. Dr. Abrams received her B.S. in nutrition and dietetics from Simmons College in Boston. She continued her education at the University of California, Berkeley, where she earned her M.P.H. in nutrition, M.S. in epidemiology, and Dr.P.H. in nutrition. For the National Academy of Sciences, Dr. Abrams served on the Food and Nutrition Board's Committee on Nutritional Status During Pregnancy and Lactation and its Subcommittee for a Clinical Application Guide. She currently is a panel member for the WIC Eligibility Study II and the Low Birthweight in Minority and High-Risk Women PORT Project. Dr. Abrams is a member of the American Dietetic Association, American Institute of Nutrition, American Public Health Association, American Society for Clinical Nutrition, Jacobs Institute of Women's Health, Society for Epidemiologic Research, and Society for Nutrition Education.

MARY ELLEN COLLINS is the Director of the Department of Nutrition at Brigham and Women's Hospital in Boston. She formerly held the directorships of dietetics and nutrition and of the dietetic internship at the hospital. Her responsibilities include managing the development, coordination, implementation, and evaluation of nutrition services and programs in tertiary, ambulatory, clinical research, and community settings. As such, she manages the Neighborhood Health Center's Women, Infants, and Children Nutrition Programs. Ms. Collins earned her B.S. in nutrition from Framingham State College in Massachusetts and her M.Ed. in nutrition education from Tufts University Graduate School. She was awarded the Medallion Award from the American Dietetic Association, a World Health Organization Fellowship to University of London, New Zealand, and a Churchill Fellowship to the University of London—the first given to an American dietitian. Additional special assignments include the National Nutrition Policy Study, nutrition consultant to the Office of Economic Opportunity-Apache Tribal Council, and Scientific Liaison Staff, White House Conference on Food, Nutrition, and Health. Ms. Collins is a member of the American Dietetic Association, the American Diabetes Association, and the American Heart Association.

CATHERINE COWELL is a Clinical Professor of Public Health at the Center for Population and Family Health, Columbia University, School of Public Health. She also held positions at New York University, City University of New York, University of Iowa, and Albert Einstein School of Medicine. Dr. Cowell is a former director of the Bureau of Nutrition in the New York City Department of Health, where staff provided public health nutrition services for at risk subpopulation groups including a large WIC program serving infants and young children enrolled in well-baby clinics. She serves as both a federal and regional nutrition consultant to the Head Start program. Dr. Cowell is a member of several committees and governing boards regarding children and nutrition in New York and held the top leadership positions in several of these over the years. She is an American Public Health Association fellow and an associate fellow for the New York Academy of Medicine. Likewise, she is a member of the American Association of Family and Consumer Sciences, Omicron Nu, and Pi Delta Kappa. After receiving her B.S. in nutrition and home economics from the Hampton University in Hampton, Virginia, she earned her M.S. in nutrition from the University of Connecticut and Ph.D. in nutrition from the New York University.

BARBARA L. DEVANEY is a Senior Fellow at Mathematica Policy Research, Inc., Princeton, New Jersey. Dr. Devaney has 18 years of experience in designing and conducting program evaluations, and has conducted numerous studies of the WIC program. She was the principal investigator of the WIC-Medicaid study that estimated the effects of prenatal WIC participation and prenatal care adequacy on birth outcomes and Medicaid costs during the first 60 days after birth. In addition, she conducted analyses of the effects of WIC participation on infant mortality and very low birthweight among Medicaid newborns, and has investigated the infant feeding practices, health care utilization, and immunization status of infant WIC participants. Her other work at MPR focuses on maternal and child health policy. Dr. Devaney previously taught courses in economics and statistics at Duke University and The Johns Hopkins University. Dr. Devaney received her B.A. in economics from Mount Holyoke College and her Ph.D. in economics from the University of Michigan.

LEON GORDIS is a Professor in the Department of Pediatrics in The Johns Hopkins School of Hygiene and Public Health and in the Department of Pediatrics at The Johns Hopkins School of Medicine, where he also is Associate Dean for Admissions and Academic Affairs. He earned a B.A. from Columbia University, B.H.L. from the Jewish Theological Seminary in New York, M.D. from the State University of New York's Downstate Medical Center, and M.P.H. and Dr.P.H. at The Johns Hopkins University School of Hygiene and Public Health. He is a member of the Board of Scientific Counselors of the National Institute of Child Health and Human Development, and chairman of the Fox Chase Cancer Center's External Advisory Committee to the Population Science Program. He chaired the Society for Epidemiologic Research's Committee on Access to Research Data; NIH-NIA's ad-hoc Scientific Advisory Committee for the Epidemiology, Demography, and Biometry Program; and Institute of Medicine's Section IX Membership Committee. Dr. Gordis' professional memberships include the American Epidemiological Society, Society for

Epidemiologic Research, American Pediatric Society, Society for Pediatric Research, Ambulatory Pediatric Society, and American Public Health Association. He has served as president of the Society for Epidemiologic Research and of the American Epidemiological Society. He has served as an editor of *Epidemiologic Reviews* and edited a monograph on *Epidemiology and Health Risk Assessment.*

JEAN-PIERRE HABICHT is a Professor of Nutritional Epidemiology in the Division of Nutrition Sciences at Cornell University. His other professional experience includes special assistant to the director of Division of Health Examination Statistics at the National Center for Health Statistics, WHO medical officer at the Instituto de Nutricion de Centro America y Panama, and professor of maternal and child health at the University of San Carlos in Guatemala. Currently, Dr. Habicht serves as an advisor to United Nations and government health and nutrition agencies. He is a member of the Expert Advisory Panel on Nutrition, World Health Organization, and has been a member of the Food and Nutrition Board and the UN Advisory Group on Nutrition. He has served as a consultant to the Ford Foundation's Urban Poverty Program for design of a technical review of the follow-up study of children for the National WIC program. He is a fellow of the American College of Epidemiology. Dr. Habicht received his M.D. from the Universities of Geneva and Zurich, his M.P.H. from the Harvard School of Public Health, and the Ph.D. from the Massachusetts Institute of Technology.

K. MICHAEL HAMBIDGE is a Professor of Pediatrics at the University of Colorado Health Science Center. Concurrently, he is the director of the Children's Clinical Research Center and the Center for Human Nutrition. He has received both the Borden Award from the American Institute of Nutrition and the Nutrition Award form the American Academy of Pediatrics. He is a member of the Food and Nutrition Board (FNB) and serves as the FNB liaison to this committee. From Cambridge University, he received his B.A. and an honorary Sc.D. Dr. Hambidge also earned his M.B. and B.Chir. from the Westminster Medical School.

GAIL G. HARRISON is a Professor in the Department of Community Health Sciences at the UCLA School of Public Health. Prior to this, she was professor in the Department of Family and Community Medicine at the University of Arizona. Dr. Harrison is a former member of the Food and Nutrition Board and has served on several of its committees, including the Committee on International Nutrition Program. She chaired the Panel on Factors Affecting Food Selection for the Committee on Food Consumption Patterns and the National Research Council's U.S. National Committee to the International Union of Nutritional Sciences. She has served in various capacities for NIH, USDA, WHO, and UNICEF. She directed a technical review of several issues relative to the nutritional risk criteria for the WIC program in 1990–1991, and has served as a technical consultant to the WIC program of the Public Health Foundation of Los Angeles. Dr. Harrison belongs to the American Anthropological Association, the American Institute of Nutrition, the Society for International Nutrition, the Western Society for Pediatric Research, and the Society for Pediatric Research. Dr. Harrison earned a B.S. degree in foods and nutrition from the University of California, Santa Barbara, a M.N.S. from Cornell University, and a Ph.D. in physical anthropology at the University of Arizona.

JEAN YAVIS JONES is a Legislative Specialist and Head of the Food and Agriculture Section of the Environment and Natural Resources Division for the Library of Congress' Congressional Research Service. Her responsibilities cover research, policy analysis and counsel on legislation and public policy issues. Her areas of specialty include domestic hunger and food programs such as WIC, school food programs, and food stamps. Ms. Jones has developed a close working relationship with various congressional committees and Department of Agriculture agencies. She has served on various USDA panels, including the National Hunger Forum, is a member of the Institute for Educational Leadership, and is on the faculty of the CRS Legislative Institute. Ms. Jones is a member of the Library of Congress Professional Association, American Historical Association, Organization of American Historians, and Congressional Research Employees Association, for which she served on the Board of Governors and as vice president and president. Ms. Jones completed a B.A. in history at Rutgers University and an M.A. in History at the University of Maryland.

ROY PITKIN is the Chair of and a Professor in the Department of Obstetrics and Gynecology at the UCLA School of Medicine. Formerly, he served as department chair and was a professor of obstetrics and gynecology at the University of Iowa College of Medicine; prior to that, he was an assistant professor at the University of Illinois. Dr. Pitkin received both his B.A. and M.D. from the University of Iowa and has been certified in maternal-fetal medicine for 20 years. As a member of the Institute of Medicine, he recently chaired the activities of the Food and Nutrition Board's Committee on Nutrition During Pregnancy and Lactation. Additionally, Dr. Pitkin is a member of the American College of Obstetrics and Gynecology and chaired its Committee on Nutrition. Other memberships include Society for Gynecological Investment, for which he served as president; Perinatal Research Society; Society for Experimental Biology and Medicine; American Gynecology and Obstetrics Society; AMA, from which he received the Joseph B. Goldberger Award; Society for Perinatal Obstetricians, for which he served as president; and American Federation for Clinical Research.

ERNESTO POLLITT is a Professor of Human Development in the Department of Pediatrics at the University of California, Davis School of Medicine. Additionally, he is a professor of graduate group of nutrition and of human development and a child psychologist in the agricultural experiment station. He received his B.A. at the Catholic University of Lima, Peru, where he also become a psychologist at the Institute of Psychology; he earned his Ph.D. in the Department of Child Development and Family Relationships at Cornell University. Dr. Pollitt's prior teaching experience includes professorships at the University of California, Davis, and the University of Texas Health Science Center in Houston. He is a Human Biology Council fellow and member of American Society of Clinical Nutrition, Society for Research in Child Development, and American Public Health Association. On numerous occasions, Dr. Pollitt provided technical assistance as a consultant to the World Bank, UNESCO, WHO, and UNICEF. Currently, he is chair of the Nutrition and Behavioral Development Committee of the International Union of Nutrition Scientists, member of the Long Range Planning Committee and Advisory Committee of IDECG, and senior advisor to the Food Biotechnology and Poverty Program of the United Nations University in Tokyo.

KATHLEEN M. RASMUSSEN is Professor in the Division on Nutritional Sciences at Cornell University, where her research focuses on maternal and child nutrition, particularly pregnancy and lactation. She is program director of an NIH-sponsored training program in maternal and child nutrition. Dr. Rasmussen previously served on two Food and Nutrition Board committees, the Committee on Nutrition During Pregnancy and Lactation as well as its Subcommittee on Nutrition During Lactation. Dr. Rasmussen was a Pew Faculty Scholar in Nutrition; she earned her A.B. degree at Brown University and her Sc.M. and Sc.D. degrees from Harvard University, and is a registered dietitian.

EARNESTINE WILLIS is Director, Center for the Advancement of Urban Children, and Associate Professor, Department of Pediatrics at the Medical College of Wisconsin, MACC Fund Research Center. Formerly, Dr. Willis was associate section chief of general pediatrics at the University of Chicago, associate professor of clinical pediatrics, and medical director of the Woodlawn Maternal and Child Health Center. Dr. Willis was a recent Robert Wood Johnson Health Policy Fellow, working as a health aide to Senator Robert Dole. Among her many professional activities, she actively serves on the Illinois Governor's Task Force on Health Care Reform; past activities include serving as vice president of Leadership Greater Chicago and as a board of directors member of Chicago Children's Museum. Dr. Willis was the recipient of the 1992 Colgate-Palmolive "Model of Excellence Award." She earned her B.S. in mathematics from Tougaloo College in Mississippi, her M.D. from Harvard Medical School, and her M.P.H. from Harvard School of Public Health.

STAFF

ROBERT EARL, Study Director until November 1995, Committee on Scientific Evaluation of WIC Nutrition Risk Criteria, has been a Program Officer with the Food and Nutrition Board (FNB) since 1990. In addition to his most recent service as Program Officer for the Committee on the Prevention, Detection, and Management of Iron Deficiency Anemia Among U.S. Children and Women of Childbearing Age, he was Director of the FNB's Food Forum and was Program Officer of studies by the Committee on Opportunities in the Nutrition and Food Sciences, the Committee on the Nutrition Components of Food Labeling, and the Committee on State Food Labeling. Prior to joining the Institute of Medicine, Mr. Earl was Administrator of Government Affairs for the American Dietetic Association, Washington, D.C. Previously, he was statewide nutrition consultant with the Texas Department of Health, Austin. Mr. Earl is a member of Delta Omega National Public Health Honorary Society. He is a member of the American Dietetic Association and the Institute for Food Technologists and serves on the Governing Council the American Public Health Association. Mr. Earl holds a B.S. in human nutrition from the University of Michigan, Ann Arbor, an M.P.H. from the University of North Carolina at Chapel Hill, and is working on a doctorate in public policy at the Center for Public Administration and Policy at Virginia Polytechnic Institute and State University, Falls Church.

CAROL WEST SUITOR, Study Director beginning November 1995, served as a Program Officer for the Food and Nutrition Board from 1988 to 1992 and returned to serve as Senior Program Officer in 1994. She served as Study Director for the Committee on Nutritional Status During Pregnancy and Lactation and its four subcommittees and for the Committee on Defense Women's Health Research. She is currently Study Director for the Committee on Military Nursing Research. At Harvard School of Public Health, Dr. Suitor worked on the development and testing of instruments for collecting dietary information from low-income women. At the National Center for Education in Maternal and Child Health, Georgetown University, Dr. Suitor managed projects on maternal and child nutrition, breastfeeding, cultural diversity, and children with special health care needs. Dr. Suitor earned a B.S. degree from Cornell University, an M.S. from the University of California at Berkeley, and an Sc.M. and Sc.D. from Harvard School of Public Health.

ALLISON A. YATES is the Director of the Food and Nutrition Board. She is a registered dietitian, having completed a master of science in public health at U.C.L.A. and a dietetic internship at the Los Angeles Veteran's Administration Hospital, prior to working for the Los Angeles County Department of Health as a public health nutritionist. She earned a doctorate in human nutrition from the

University of California at Berkeley, did postdoctoral work there, and has since served as a faculty member in nutrition and dietetics at the University of Texas Health Science Center in Houston and at Emory University School of Medicine in Atlanta. She currently is on leave from the University of Southern Mississippi in Hattiesburg, where she has served as Dean of the College of Health and Human Sciences for the past 7 years and as Professor of Foods and Nutrition. Dr. Yates is a member of the American Institute of Nutrition, the American Dietetic Association, the Institute of Food Technologists, and the American Public Health Association, and served on the Committee on Military Nutrition Research of the FNB from 1981–1985 and 1991–1994. She has conducted research on essential fatty acid and vitamin E deficiencies in animals, soy protein utilization and methionine requirements in men, and protein and energy requirements in older men and women.

SANDRA A. SCHLICKER is a senior program officer with the Food and Nutrition Board and serves as Study Director for the Food Forum. Prior to joining the Food and Nutrition Board, Dr. Schlicker was Vice-President of a consulting/research firm that focused on public policy issues in the fields of nutrition, health, and agriculture. She came to Washington, D.C. in 1982 as the Nutrition Advisor to the Administrator of USDA's Food and Consumer Service after several years as a nutritionist with the food industry. After earning a B.S. in Science and M.S. and Ph.D. degrees in Foods and Nutrition from The Pennsylvania State University, she became a faculty member at Purdue University.

SHEILA MOATS has been a Research Associate with the Food and Nutrition Board (FNB) since 1990. She has worked on a number of studies, including those of the Committee to Develop Criteria for Evaluating the Outcomes of Approaches to Prevent and Treat Obesity, the Committee on Opportunities in the Nutrition and Food Sciences, the Committee on Nutrition During Pregnancy and Lactation and the Subcommittee for a Clinical Application Guide, the Committee on the Food Chemicals Codex, and the Food Additives Survey Committee. Ms. Moats received the Institute of Medicine Staff Achievement Award in 1993. Prior to joining the Institute of Medicine, she was coordinator of patient information for the national office of the American Diabetes Association, worked in the department of dietetics at the Alexandria Hospital in Alexandria, Virginia, and assisted in nutrition research at the University of Colorado Health Sciences Center. Ms. Moats received her B.S. degree in Nutrition Science from The Pennsylvania State University.

KIMBERLY A. BREWER is a Research Assistant in the Institute of Medicine's Food and Nutrition Board and Board on International Health. Ms. Brewer's focus has been on environmental health, epidemiology, international health policy and programs, and maternal and child health promotion. Ms.

APPENDIX E 369

Brewer received a B.A. from Colby College in government and her M.P.H. in international health policy and programs from the George Washington University. Prior to her work with the Committee on Scientific Evaluation of WIC Nutrition Risk Criteria, Ms. Brewer worked with the Committee to Reduce Lead Exposure in the Americas and with the Steering Committee on the Implications of Trade Liberalization for the Health Sector with the Board on International Health.

Acronyms

ACOG	American College of Obstetrics and Gynecologists
AFDC	Aid to Families with Dependent Children
AIDS	acquired immunodeficiency syndrome
BMI	body mass index
CDC	U.S. Centers for Disease Control and Prevention
CES-D	Center for Epidemiologic Studies Depression Scale
CN-AAP	Committee on Nutrition of the American Academy of Pediatrics
CNS	central nervous system
CP	cerebral palsy
CPI	Consumer Price Index
CSFII	Continuing Survey of Food Intakes of Individuals
FAS	fetal alcohol syndrome
FCS	Food Consumer Service
FFQ	food frequency questionnaire
FNS	Food and Nutrition Service
FTT	failure to thrive
FY	fiscal year
GAO	U.S. Government Accounting Office
HIV	human immunodeficiency virus
IBW	ideal body weight
IgE	immunoglobulin E
IOM	Institute of Medicine
IQ	intelligent quotient
JRA	juvenile rheumatoid arthritis

LBW	low birth weight
LHC	low head circumference
LGA	large for gestational age
NCHS	National Center for Health Statistics
NHANES I–III	National Health and Nutrition Examination Surveys
NLSY	National Longitudinal Survey of Youth
NMIHS	National Maternal and Infant Health Survey
NTD	neural tube defects
OBRA	Omnibus Budget Reconciliation Act
PC92	1992 WIC Participant and Program Characteristics
PedNSS	Pediatric Nutrition Surveillance System
PEM	protein energy malnutrition
PKU	phenylketonuria
PNSS	Pregnancy Nutrition Surveillance System
PRAMS	Pregnancy Risk Assessment Monitoring System
RDA	Recommended Dietary Allowance
SGA	small for gestational age
USDA	U.S. Department of Agriculture
WIC	Special Supplemental Nutrition Program for Women, Infants, and Children

Index of Risk Criteria

This index identifies the first page of text for each risk criterion reviewed by the committee. For the table that summarizes all the committee's recommendations for the use of risk criteria, see Chapter 8, page 338.

A

Abnormal postpartum weight change, 96
Abuse or neglect, child, 319
Age older than 35 years, pregnancy, 197
Age, pregnancy at young, 195
AIDS and HIV infections, 185
Alcohol and illegal drug use, 226
Allergies, food, 192
Anemia, 154
Anthropometric Risk Criteria, 67
Asthma, 192

B

Battering, 317
Biochemical and Other Medical Risk Criteria, 149
Birth or congenital defect, history of birth with, 207
Birth weight, history of low, 206
Birth weight, low, 97
Birth with congenital or birth defect, history of, 207
Bottle, inappropriate use of, 265
Bottles, lack of sanitation in preparation of nursing, 261
Breastfeeding as sole source of nutrients, infrequent, 261
Bronchitis, 183
Burns, major surgery or trauma, and severe acute infections, 188

C

Caffeine intake, excessive, 269
Cancer, 175
Cardiorespiratory disorders, 190
Celiac disease, 192
Central nervous system disorders, 177
Child abuse or neglect, 319
Child of a mentally retarded parent, 323
Child of a young caregiver, 321
Children and/or infants, conditions specific to, 215
Chronic hypertension, 172
Chronic or recurrent infections, 183
Closely spaced pregnancies, 197
Conditions related to the intake of specific foods, 192
Conditions specific to infants and/or children, 215
Conditions specific to pregnancy, 195
Congenital and genetic disorders, 179
Congenital or birth defect, history of birth with, 207
Cow milk feeding during 1st 12 months, 261
Criteria related to nutrient deficiencies, 154

D

Deficiency diseases, nutrient, 159
Delivery, history of postterm, 206
Delivery, history of preterm, 204
Depression, maternal, 314
Diabetes mellitus, 169
Diabetes, gestational, 169

Diet, inadequate, 272
Dietary Guidelines, failure to meet, 253
Dietary Risk Criteria, 251
Diets, highly restrictive, 260
Diets, vegan, 259
Diets, vegetarian, 259
Disease, renal, 174
Diseases, nutrient deficiency, 159
Disorders, gastrointestinal, 166
Disorders, genetic and congenital, 179
Disorders, thyroid, 170
Drug and alcohol use, 226
Drug-nutrient interactions, 218

E

Early introduction of solid foods, 261
Eclampsia and preeclampsia, 213
Education or illiteracy, low level of maternal, 311
Essential nutrients, feeding other foods low in, 261
Excessive caffeine intake, 269

F

Failure to meet Dietary Guidelines, 253
Failure to thrive, 159
Feeding cow milk during 1st 12 months, 261
Feeding other foods low in essential nutrients, 261
Feeding, inappropriate infant, 261
Fetal growth restriction, 211
Food allergies, 192
Food insecurity, 279

Food intolerances, other, 194
Foods, conditions related to the intake of specific, 192
Foods, early introduction of solid, 261
Formula, improper dilution of, 261

G

Gastrointestinal disorders, 166
Genetic and congenital disorders, 179
Gestation, multifetal, 210
Gestational age, large for, 117
Gestational age, small for, 100
Gestational diabetes, 169
Gestational weight gain, high, 84
Growth restriction, fetal, 211
Growth, slow, 123

H

Head circumference, low, 114
High gestational weight gain, 84
High parity, 200
Highly restrictive diets, 260
History of birth with congenital or birth defect, 207
History of low birth weight, 206
History of neonatal loss, 207
History of postterm delivery, 206
History of preterm delivery, 204
HIV infection and AIDS, 185
Homelessness, 297
Hypertension, chronic, 172
Hypoglycemia, 217

I

Illegal drug and alcohol use, 226
Illiteracy or education, low level of maternal, 311
Improper dilution of formula, 261
Inadequate diet, 272
Inappropriate infant feeding, 261
Inappropriate use of nursing bottle, 265
Inborn errors of metabolism, 181
Infant feeding, inappropriate, 261
Infants and/or children, conditions specific to, 215
Infections, chronic or recurrent, 183
Infections, HIV and AIDS, 185
Infections, severe acute; major surgery or trauma; and burns, 188
Infections, upper respiratory, 183
Infections, urinary tract, 183
Infrequent breastfeeding as sole source of nutrients, 261
Insecurity, food, 279
Intake of specific foods, conditions related to, 192
Intolerance, lactose, 194
Intolerances, other food, 194
Iron after 4–6 months, no dependable source, 261

L

Lack of prenatal care, 208
Lack of sanitation in preparation of nursing bottles, 261
Lactose intolerance, 194
Large for gestational age, 117
Lead poisoning, 229
Low birth weight, 97

Low birth weight, history of, 206
Low head circumference, 114
Low level of maternal education or illiteracy, 311
Low maternal weight gain, 73
Lupus erythematosus, 190

M

Major surgery, trauma, burns, or severe acute infections, 188
Maternal depression, 314
Maternal education or illiteracy, low level of, 311
Maternal short stature, 87
Maternal smoking, 220
Maternal weight loss during pregnancy, 79
Medical conditions (Juvenile rheumatoid arthritis, lupus erythematosus, and cardiorespiratory disorders), 190
Mentally retarded parent, child of, 323
Metabolism, inborn errors of, 181
Migrancy, 304
Multifetal gestation, 210

N

Nausea and vomiting during pregnancy, 166
Neglect or abuse, child, 319
Neonatal loss, history of, 207
Nervous system disorders, central, 177
No dependable source of iron after 4–6 months, 261
Nursing bottle, inappropriate use of, 265
Nursing bottles, lack of sanitation in preparation, 261
Nutrient deficiencies, criteria related to, 154
Nutrient deficiency diseases, 159
Nutrient-drug interactions, 218
Nutrients, feeding other foods low in essential, 261
Nutrition Risk Criteria, Predisposing, 295

O

Other food intolerance, 194
Other medical conditions (juvenile rheumatoid arthritis, lupus erythematosus, and cardiorespiratory disorders), 190
Otitis media, 183
Overweight, 118
Overweight, postpartum, 92
Overweight, prepregnancy, 80

P

Parity, high, 200
Passive smoking, 309
Pica, 270
Placental abnormalities, 214
Poisoning, lead, 229
Postterm delivery, history of, 206
Postpartum overweight, 92
Postpartum underweight, 89
Postpartum weight change, abnormal, 96
Potentially toxic substances, 218
Predisposing Nutrition Risk Criteria, 295
Preeclampsia and eclampsia, 213
Pregnancies, closely spaced, 197

INDEX OF RISK CRITERIA

Pregnancy age older than 35 years, 197
Pregnancy at a young age, 195
Pregnancy, conditions specific to, 195
Pregnancy, maternal weight loss during, 79
Pregnancy, nausea and vomiting during, 166
Prematurity, 215
Prenatal care, lack of, 208
Prepregnancy overweight, 80
Prepregnancy underweight, 70
Preterm delivery, history of, 204
Pyloric stenosis, 179

R

Renal disease, 174
Restrictive diets, 260
Rheumatoid arthritis, juvenile, 190
Risk Criteria, Anthropometric, 67
Risk Criteria, Biochemical and Other Medical, 149
Risk Criteria, Dietary, 251
Risk Criteria, Predisposing Nutrition, 295

S

Short stature, 104
Slow growth, 123
Small for gestational age, 100
Smoking, maternal, 220
Smoking, passive, 309
Solid foods, early introduction of, 261
Stature, maternal short, 87
Stature, short, 104
Surgery, trauma, burns, or severe acute infections, 188

T

Thrive, failure to, 159
Thyroid disorders, 170
Toxic substances, 218
Trauma, major surgery, burns, or severe acute infections, 188

U

Underweight, 110
Underweight, postpartum, 89
Underweight, prepregnancy, 70
Upper respiratory infections, 183
Urinary tract infections, 183

V

Vegan diets, 259
Vegetarian diets, 259
Vomiting and nausea during pregnancy, 166

W

Weight change, abnormal postpartum, 96
Weight gain, high gestational, 84
Weight gain, low maternal, 73
Weight loss during pregnancy, maternal, 79
Weight, low birth, 97

Y

Young caregiver, child of, 321

*U.S. GOVERNMENT PRINTING OFFICE:1997-519-132/83745